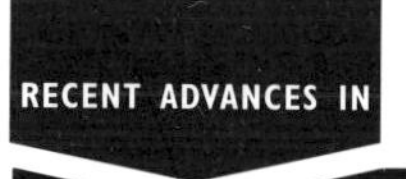

Surgery

RECENT ADVANCES IN SURGERY

Contents of Number 18
Edited by I. Taylor C. D. Johnson

Pathogenesis of pancreatitis
C. D. Johnson
Non-biliary laparoscopic surgery
J. J. T. Tate
Non-surgical treatment of oesophageal cancer
C. S. Robertson
Screening for colorectal cancer
D. H. Bennett, J. D. Hardcastle
Penetrating chest injury
S. S Ashraf, G. Grötte
Management of advanced breast cancer
I. S. Fentiman
Parathyroid surgery
A. W. Goode
The critically ischaemic limb
W. G. Tennant, C. V. Ruckley
Surgical aspects of urinary incontinence
A. R. Mundy
Modern hernia management
A. N. Kingsnorth
Oncology for surgeons: monoclonal antibodies
C. Y. Yiu
Surgical lasers and photodynamic technology
S. Evrard, J. Marescaux
Innovations in paediatric surgery
R. Wheeler
Recent advances in general surgery
I. Taylor

ISBN 0443 051321

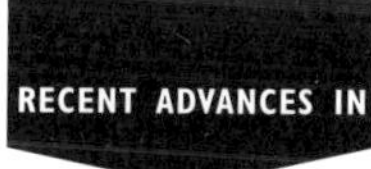

Surgery

Edited by

C. D. Johnson MChir FRCS
Senior Lecturer in Surgery,
University of Southampton,
Southampton, UK

I. Taylor MD ChM FRCS
Professor and Head, Department of Surgery,
University College London,
London, UK

NUMBER NINETEEN

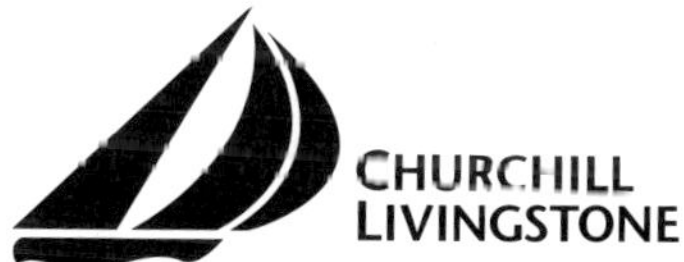

NEW YORK EDINBURGH LONDON MADRID MELBOURNE SAN FRANCISCO AND TOKYO 1996

CHURCHILL LIVINGSTONE
Medical Division of Pearson Professional Limited

Distributed in the United States of America by
Churchill Livingstone Inc., 650 Avenue of the Americas,
New York, N.Y. 10011, and by associated companies,
branches and representatives throughout the world.

First published 1996

ISBN 0443 053170
ISSN 0143-697X

British Library Cataloguing in Publication Data
A catalogue record for this book is available from the
British Library.

Library of Congress Cataloging in Publication Data
is available

Note
Medical knowledge is constantly changing. As new information becomes available, changes in treatment, procedures, equipment and the use of drugs become necessary. The editors/authors/contributors and the publishers have, as far as it is possible, taken care to ensure that the information given in this text is accurate and up to date. However, readers are strongly advised to confirm that the information, especially with regard to drug usage, complies with latest legislation and standards of practice.

Page layout: Gerard Heyburn, Janet Smith

Printed in Singapore

The publisher's policy is to use **paper manufactured from sustainable forests**

Contents

1. The management of malignant large bowel obstruction 1
N. J. Carty, D. Ravichandran

2. Aortic aneurysm update 19
M. M. Thompson, P. R. F. Bell

3. Recent advances in cardiopulmonary support 43
A. A. Majid

4. *Helicobacter pylori:* an update for surgeons 61
M. M. Ozmen, R. Patankar, C. D. Johnson

5. The management of superficial bladder cancer 77
T. R. L. Griffiths, D. E. Neal

6. Trauma centres 93
R. M. Kirby, J. B. Elder, J. Templeton

7. Bone metastases 109
S. E. Downey, N. J. Bundred

8. CT and MRI in general surgery 129
R. M. Blaquière

9. Recent advances in nutritional support of surgical patients 149
B. J. Moran

10. Wound healing and the plastic surgeon 169
A. D. Wilmshurst

11. Peptide receptors and gastrointestinal cancers 183
S. A. M. Laws, H. S. Chave

12. Surgical treatment of obesity 199
J-C. Gazet

13. The surgical management of cutaneous malignant melanoma 215
D. S. Soutar

14. What's new in general surgery – a review of the journals 235
I. Taylor

Index 261

Preface

This issue of *Recent Advances in Surgery* once again addresses the topical subjects of general surgery and allied disciplines. We hope that our readers will find this volume of interest. It has been designed with the needs of two particular groups in mind: the busy general surgeon who wishes to have an easy source of reference for recent developments in the surgical world which might be difficult to obtain from other sources, and trainees who are preparing for specialist examinations in surgery, who will find this book a useful collection of up-to-date reviews.

We are grateful to our contributors who have willingly put enormous effort into ensuring a uniform high quality. As usual we have spread the net wide, and we are pleased to be able to include contributions dealing with aortic aneurysm surgery, large bowel obstruction, various aspects of malignant disease, nutritional support along with a definitive review of surgery for obesity, and a contribution which reviews the administrative aspects of setting up a trauma centre. There is also a well illustrated description of the value of new cross-sectional imaging techniques in general surgery. We conclude with a review of the journals for 1994, a feature which continues to be popular with our readers.

We hope that those who have enjoyed previous volumes in this series will find this volume a useful addition to their library, and that new readers will be tempted to explore the fascinating variety of subjects covered by our contributors.

Southampton
London
1996

C.D.J.
I.T.

Contributors

Peter R.F. Bell MD, FRCS
Professor of Surgery, Department of Surgery, University of Leicester, Leicester Royal Infirmary, Leicester, UK

Richard M. Blaquière
Consultant Surgeon, Department of Radiology, Southampton General Hospital, Southampton, UK

Nigel J. Bundred MD, FRCS
Senior Lecturer and Consultant Surgeon, Department of Surgery, University Hospital of South Manchester, Manchester, UK

Nicholas James Carty MD, FRCS
Consultant Surgeon, Salisbury District Hospital, Odstock, Salisbury, Wiltshire, UK

Helen Sally Chave MBBS, FRCS
Surgical Research Registrar, University Department of Surgery, Southampton General Hospital, Southampton, UK

Sarah E. Downey FRCS
Research Registrar, Breast Unit, Department of Surgery, University Hospital of South Manchester, Manchester, UK

James B. Elder MD, FRCS
Professor of Surgery, School of Postgraduate Medicine, University of Keele, Stoke on Trent, UK

Jean-Claude Gazet
Consulting Surgeon to St George's and the Royal Marsden Hospitals, London, UK

T. R. Leyshon Griffiths BSc FRCS (Ed)
Clinical Research Associate, Department of Surgery, University of Newcastle upon Tyne, Newcastle upon Tyne, UK

Colin D. Johnson MChir, FRCS
Senior Lecturer and Honorary Consultant, University Surgical Unit, Southampton General Hospital, Southampton, UK

Robert M. Kirby MD, FRCS
Consultant Surgeon and Senior Clinical Lecturer, Department of Surgery, North Staffordshire Hospital and School of Postgraduate Medicine, University of Keele, Stoke-on-Trent, UK

Siobhan A.M. Laws MBBS, FRCS
Guernsey Research Fellow, University Department of Surgery, Southampton General Hospital, Southampton, UK

Aljafri Abdul Majid MBBS, BMedSci, FRCS(Ed)
Professor and Head, Department of Surgery, Faculty of Medicine, University of Malaya, Kuala Lumpur, Malaysia

Brendan J. Moran
Consultant Surgeon, Colorectal Research Unit, North Hampshire Hospital, Basingstoke, UK

David E. Neal MS, FRCS
Professor of Surgery, University of Newcastle Upon Tyne; Honorary Consultant Urological Surgeon, Freeman Hospital, Newcastle Upon Tyne, Newcastle upon Tyne, UK

M. Mahir Ozmen MD
Visiting Senior Registrar in Surgery and Research Fellow, University Surgical Unit, Southampton General Hospital, Southampton, UK

R. Patankar MS, FRCS(Ed), FRCS(Glas)
Research Registrar, University Surgical Unit, Southampton General Hospital, Southampton, UK

Duraisamy Ravichandran FRCS
Research Registrar, Southampton General Hospital, Southampton, UK

David S. Soutar ChM, FRCS(Ed), FRCS(Glas), MB ChB
Consultant Plastic Surgeon, West of Scotland Regional Plastic & Maxillofacial Surgery Unit, Canniesburn Hospital, and Honorary Clinical Senior Lecturer, University of Glasgow, Glasgow, UK

Irving Taylor MD, ChM, FRCS
David Patey Professor of Surgery and Head of Department of Surgery, University College London Medical School, London UK

John Templeton FRCS
Professor of Orthopaedic Surgery, School of Postgraduate Medicine, University of Keele, Stoke-on-Trent, UK

Matthew M. Thompson MD, FRCS
Lecturer in Surgery, Department of Surgery, University of Leicester, Leicester Royal Infirmary, Leicester, UK

Andrew D. Wilmshurst MB, FRCS
Consultant Reconstructive Plastic Surgeon, Department of Plastic Surgery, Dundee Royal Infirmary, Dundee, UK

1

The management of malignant large bowel obstruction

N. J. Carty D. Ravichandran

The optimal management of large bowel obstruction remains controversial despite an extensive literature on the subject. Interpretation of this literature is complicated by the fact that the individual reports include heterogeneous groups of patients, who have been treated in a variety of ways with little to indicate the rationale underlying the management decisions. Prospectively gathered data are rare (Fielding et al 1979) and there has been only one, incomplete, randomized trial (Kronborg 1986).

Large bowel obstruction is caused by a variety of conditions. Obstruction is most commonly the result of carcinoma, which accounts for about 90% of patients (Koruth et al 1985a, Stewart et al 1993). Less common causes include diverticular disease, ischaemic strictures and inflammatory bowel disease (Koruth et al 1985a). While volvulus is common in underdeveloped countries, this is the mechanism of obstruction in less than 5% of patients in Western series (Koruth et al 1985b). A substantial minority of patients thought clinically to have mechanical obstruction will be found to have a functional (pseudo-) obstruction.

The proportion of large bowel carcinomas that present with obstruction is, in the largest studies, about 15% (Phillips et al 1985, Kyllonen 1987). The risk that a colorectal cancer will cause obstruction varies with its site along the colon. The risk is highest for lesions at the splenic flexure, nearly half of which present with obstruction, while less than one tenth of all rectal carcinomas present in this manner (Phillips et al 1985, Waldron & Donovan 1986, Kyllonen 1987). At other sites in the colon, the risk of a lesion causing obstruction is similar at about 20% (Phillips et al 1985). However, given the unequal distribution of colorectal carcinoma, which is most common in the distal colon, approximately three-quarters of all malignant large bowel obstructions are situated in the left colon, i.e. at or distal to the splenic flexure (Serpell et al 1989, Sjodahl et al 1992).

DIAGNOSIS

The diagnosis of large bowel obstruction is based on the clinical features, radiological appearance and operative findings (Phillips et al 1985). Large bowel obstruction classically presents with abdominal pain, distension, absolute constipation and vomiting. Although abdominal pain is a feature in about 90% of patients (Umpelby & Williamson 1984, Serpell et al 1988), it is often less well defined in nature and less prominent a symptom compared to the pain of small bowel obstruction (Matheson 1989). A plain abdominal radiograph usually confirms the diagnosis with gaseous dilatation of the large bowel proximal to the site of obstruction and a distal cut-off (Fig. 1.1). Finally, at operation the proximal large bowel is dilated and oedematous.

The clinical features and plain radiographic findings can be misleading and the diagnosis should be confirmed by an urgent single contrast enema (Fig. 1.2). Of those patients thought clinically to have mechanical obstruction, over 10% in fact have pseudo-obstruction (Stewart et al 1984, Matheson 1989). These patients can usually be managed non-operatively and the routine use of a contrast enema in the assessment of patients with clinical large bowel obstruction reduces the rate of unnecessary operations (Koruth et al 1985a). Of patients who have clinical pseudo-obstruction a similar proportion (10%)

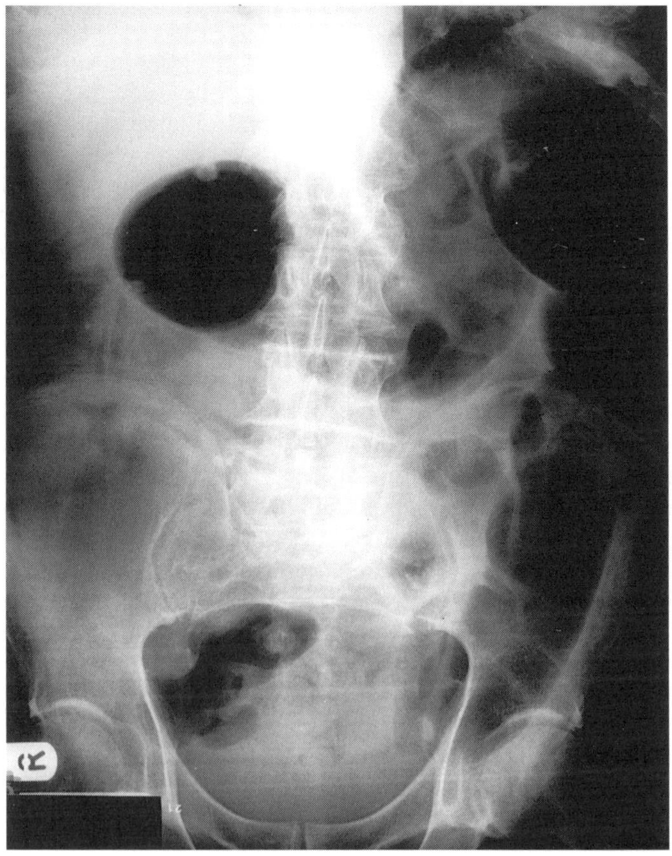

Fig. 1.1 Plain abdominal X-ray showing dilated proximal colon with cut-off in pelvis.

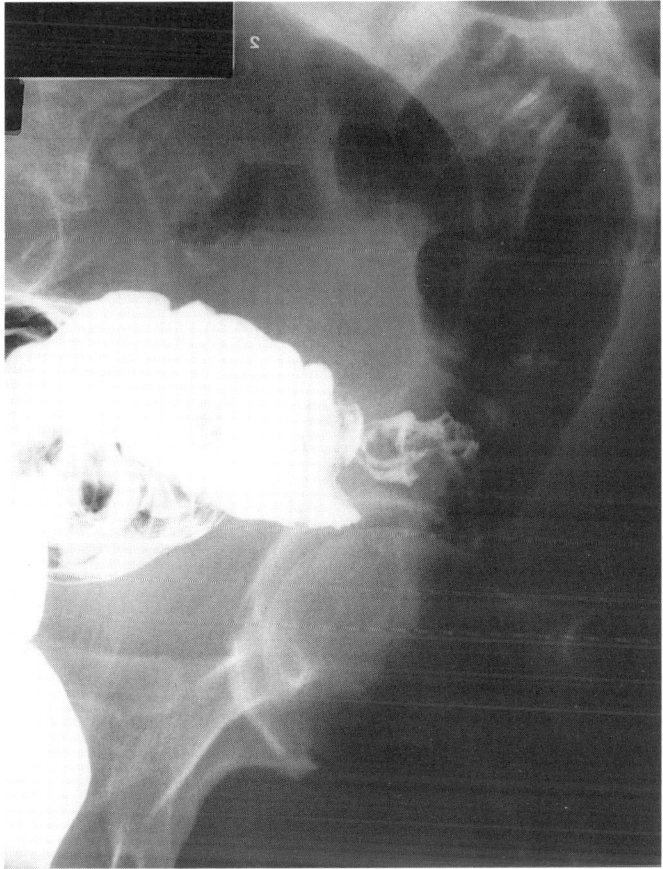

Fig. 1.2 Single contrast enema (same patient as in Fig. 1), showing typical apple-core stricture of an obstructing sigmoid carcinoma.

are found on imaging to have an obstructing carcinoma (Stewart et al 1984, Matheson 1989). An additional benefit of a contrast enema is the demonstration of the site of the obstruction, which allows planning of the operative strategy.

MANAGEMENT

Large bowel obstruction does not require emergency surgery unless the degree of abdominal tenderness suggests perforation or the caecum is larger than 9 cm in diameter on an abdominal radiograph signalling impending perforation (Matheson 1989). There is time for resuscitation with correction of fluid and electrolyte deficiencies. It is of value to pass a urinary catheter, and it may be prudent to insert a central venous line, to help to monitor fluid balance and guide intravenous fluid requirements. In elderly patients, over-enthusiastic fluid replacement can be at least as hazardous as under-replacement. During this period of resuscitation, the opportunity should be taken to assess and treat any pre-existing medical conditions. In those patients with an incompetent ileo-caecal valve, a nasogastric tube will be of value to decompress the small bowel. Antibiotic prophylaxis effective against both aerobic and anaerobic bacteria should be initiated. Finally, it is imperative that effective thromboembolism prophylaxis be given to these high risk patients (Campling et al 1993). Once the patient has been resuscitated and prophylactic therapies have been instituted, the ideal is for a planned operation to be performed during daylight hours by senior surgical and anaesthetic staff (Campling et al 1993).

SURGICAL OPTIONS

The aim in the management of these patients is to relieve the obstruction with low mortality and morbidity, to ensure long-term survival in a minority, but also to provide good palliation for the remainder. This last factor includes minimizing hospital stay and the number of patients with a colostomy.

It is now generally accepted that for obstruction proximal to the splenic flexure, resection and primary anastomosis is optimal therapy. This form of treatment was used in 96% of obstructed patients included in the Large Bowel Cancer Project (Phillips et al 1985). However, care is still required since right-sided anastomoses may leak in up to 10% of cases (Gandrup et al 1992) and the overall mortality in these patients can be as high as 20–35% (Clark et al 1975, Irvin & Greaney 1977, Runkel et al 1991). An internal bypass will be more appropriate in patients with an irresectable tumour and in high risk patients with extensive distant spread of disease.

The management of the more distal lesions is controversial. Traditional therapy has been to initially decompress the bowel by transverse colostomy or by caecostomy. At a second operation the obstruction is resected with anastomosis and finally the colostomy closed (this can be combined with the second phase). Recently, small numbers of patients have been treated by a variant of this technique; a lumen is re-established through the tumour using laser ablation or a stent to allow decompression of the bowel, routine bowel preparation and subsequent resection with immediate anastomosis.

Concerns that staged tumour resection may result in a worsening of long-term prognosis led to the increased performance of primary tumour resection. Most surgeons have been reluctant to ignore the traditional wisdom that it is unwise to anastomose dilated, oedematous, unprepared bowel and still elect for delayed anastomosis (Pain & Cahill 1991). However, recent years have seen the popularisation of techniques that allow safer primary bowel anastomosis.

These options for the treatment of left-sided large bowel obstruction will now be discussed.

Decompression and delayed resection

Bowel decompression can be accomplished by a transverse colostomy or, more controversially, by caecostomy. The decompression phase of a staged resection is not without complications. Decompression is contraindicated in patients with an associated perforation and this may be missed especially if a limited laparotomy is performed (Clark et al 1975). Decompression is inadequate in up to 5% of patients (Clark et al 1975). This figure may be higher if a caecostomy is favoured (Hoffmann & Jensen 1984). Finally, the stoma itself is liable to the complications of prolapse, retraction or necrosis in 5–10% of patients (Clark et al 1975, Waldron & Donovan 1986, Runkel et al 1991).

Although there are reports of good results using caecostomy (Brewer & Brewer 1993), in general, despite the minimal intervention this involves, the results of decompression by caecostomy have been disappointing. The relief of obstruction is incomplete in over 5% of patients and the quality of bowel preparation for the second operation is good in only half of the patients (Hoffmann & Jensen 1984). Consequently there are high mortality rates for resection and few patients complete the planned operations with restoration of bowel continuity (Hoffmann & Jensen 1984, Kristiansen et al 1990). A single report illustrates the use of percutaneous decompression of the caecum and transverse colon using suprapubic catheters (Salim 1991). The bowel was decompressed and washed out prior to elective resection. There was only one death in the treatment of 28 consecutive patients and all survivors were apparently discharged by 5 days postoperatively. This is certainly a novel and ingenious approach, but seems unlikely to gain widespread application.

The results of staged resection in a selection of series is shown in Table 1.1. When used as the usual treatment staged resection has been completed with low mortality, ranging from 4–12% (Hughes 1966, Fielding & Wells 1974, Ohman 1982, Gandrup et al 1992). However, these seemingly impressive figures need to be interpreted with caution. These series exclude a number of patients who had decompression only (Fielding & Wells 1974, Sjodahl et al 1992), while prospective data indicate that some of these patients will have initially been intended to complete staged excision (Phillips et al 1985). Inclusion of these patients raised the mortality of staged excision from 6% to 22% in this study. Higher mortality rates of over 20% are reported in series where, as is usually the case, this technique has been reserved for the less well patients (Umpelby & Williamson 1984, Vidger et al 1985, Waldron & Donovan 1986). Indeed, the overall mortality rate for the 16 series included in Table 1.1 is 21%; 16% for the decompression phase and an additional 5% for those who underwent resection.

There are major disadvantages to staged resection. Of those patients who embark on a programme of staged tumour excision, less than half emerge with bowel continuity restored (Clark et al 1975, Irvin & Greaney 1977, Waldron & Donovan 1986). This is because of disease progression, poor general health, and the cumulative operative mortality. Since these patients will die with their colostomy *in situ* they would appear to have been given poor palliation.

Table 1.1 The results of staged resection for obstructing colorectal cancer: values in parentheses are percentages

Reference	Number of patients	Number of deaths		Number who completed all stages
		First stage	Subsequent stages	
Hughes 1966	81	10 (12)	5 (6)	63 (78)
Clark et al 1975	42	10 (24)	3 (7)	29 (69)
Fielding & Wells 1974	28	1 (4)	0 (0)	27 (96)
Irvin & Greaney 1977	34	10 (29)	5 (15)	13 (38)
Fielding et al 1979	47	11 (23)	2 (4)	29 (62)
Hoffmann & Jensen 1984	57	8 (14)	11 (19)	30 (53)
Phillips et al 1985	157	28 (18)	7 (4)	114 (73)
Vidger et al 1985	24	4 (17)	2 (8)	18 (75)
Kronborg 1986	28	2 (7)	1 (4)	16 (57)
Huddy et al 1988	12	0 (0)	0(0)	10 (83)
Kristiansen et al 1990	135	32 (24)	0 (0)	84 (62)
Runkel et al 1991	29	7 (24)	1 (3)	12 (41)
Salim 1991	28	1 (4)	0 (0)	27 (96)
Gandrup et al 1992	53	1 (2)	1 (2)	45 (85)
Sjodahl et al 1992	48	3 (6)	4 (8)	36 (75)
Allen-Mersh 1993	10	1 (10)	0 (0)	9 (90)
Total	813	129 (16)	42 (5)	562 (69)

Secondly, the overall hospital stay at 40–60 days is at least twice as long as in those patients treated by one of the alternative options (Phillips et al 1985, Huddy et al 1988, Allen-Mersh 1993).

Recently, reports have been published in which bowel decompression has been performed using either a trans-tumoral stent or laser recanalization of the tumour. Following relief of obstruction by either of these techniques, the bowel is prepared and definitive surgery is performed. Stents have been used in a small number of patients with lesions in the rectum or sigmoid (Keen & Orsay 1992, Tejero et al 1995) and in these instances have given excellent results. Laser can be used to treat lesions at all sites in the colon with a high rate of recanalization and low risk of perforation (Kiefhaber et al 1987, Eckhauser & Mansour 1992). Further operative therapy may not be appropriate if there is evidence of metastatic disease or the patient is medically unfit. This was the case in 12 of 59 patients whose tumour was successfully recanalized in one series (Kiefhaber et al 1987), these patients were well palliated without needing open surgery. The use of laser has much to recommend it if the equipment and expertise are available.

Resection and delayed anastomosis

At full laparotomy the tumour is resected and in the usual variant, the proximal bowel is brought to the surface as an end colostomy, while the distal stump is closed intra-abdominally (Hartmann's operation). The results of representative series are shown in Table 1.2. The mortality of this procedure can be as high as 30% in some series (Vidger et al 1985), although in the 10 series in Table 1.2, the combined mortality of Hartmann's operation for obstruction was 19%. In contrast to the deaths following initial decompression that are usually related to cardiorespiratory complications, in these patients death is often related to intra abdominal sepsis (Waldron & Donovan 1986). Stump dehiscence or retraction of the distal stoma causes complications in up to 10%

Table 1.2 The results of primary resection and delayed anastomosis of obstructing colorectal cancer

Reference	Number of patients	Number of deaths	Number reversed
Fielding et al 1979	24	8	–
Koruth et al 1985b	29	1	17
Vidger et al 1985	22	6	16
Kronborg 1986	27	5	15
Waldron & Donovan 1986	18	9	–
Huddy et al 1988	15	1	12
Dixon & Holmes 1990	32	3	21
Stephenson et al 1990	15	2	2
Gandrup et al 1992	18	3	8
Allen-Mersh 1993	35	6	22
Total	235	44	113

of patients (Stephenson et al 1990). As well as the inconvenience imposed by a stoma, it is a potential source of complications with necrosis and retraction occurring in up to 20% of patients (Stephenson et al 1990, Allen-Mersh 1993).

Reversal of Hartmann's operation is a major task with a higher morbidity and mortality than closure of a loop stoma (Mosdell & Doberneck 1991). Major morbidity occurs in about 30% of patients, including an anastomotic leak rate of about 10% (Mosdell & Doberneck 1991, Roe et al 1991). In those patients who have had a Hartmann's operation and are selected to undergo reversal, the mortality rate is in the region of 2–3% (Roe et al 1991, Wigmore et al 1995).

Although the complications associated with Hartmann's reversal are a significant constraint, the major disadvantage of this strategy is that reversal is frequently not considered appropriate. This means that between one- and two-thirds of patients die with their colostomy *in situ* (Mealy et al 1988, Dixon & Holmes 1990, Stephenson et al 1990, Wigmore et al 1995). The data in Table 1.2 are representative, only 50% of these patients had reversal of their colostomy. Further surgery is not performed because of patient age, advanced disease, poor general health or patient choice. Many of these patients could have been treated by techniques that would have avoided a stoma (Koruth et al 1985a).

Resection and immediate anastomosis

Conceptually, the ideal management of malignant large bowel obstruction would be to remove the tumour and restore bowel continuity at a single operation. This approach has, in the past, been discarded because of a mortality rate from anastomotic leakage of up to 50% (Irvin & Greaney 1977). However, recent data indicate that more acceptable results can be achieved. Segmental resection of left-sided lesions involves anastomosis of unprepared, dilated and oedematous bowel, and traditional teaching is that this is to court disaster (Irvin & Goligher 1973). To minimize these risks, early reports of successful resection and immediate anastomosis employed per-operative bowel preparation by on-table lavage. The use of this technique is demonstrated in Figure 1.3. Initially the colon is fully mobilized, usually involving taking down of both flexures. A large Foley catheter is inserted into the caecum via the appendix stump or terminal ileum. A large bore tube (such as anaesthetic scavenger tubing) is secured into the colon just proximal to the obstruction, but distal to the proposed site of anastomosis. Warm saline is run in antegrade fashion between these tubes, and the surgeon kneads the bowel to ensure mixing of fluid and faeces. It is important to use a short length of scavenger tubing, otherwise the resistance of the tube to the viscous fluid can impede forward flow causing back pressure on the caecum.

These manoeuvres undoubtedly add about 30–40 min to the length of the operation (Koruth et al 1985b, Thomson & Carter 1986, Allen-Mersh 1993) and may, in fact, be unnecessary. Although many surgeons are reassured if the

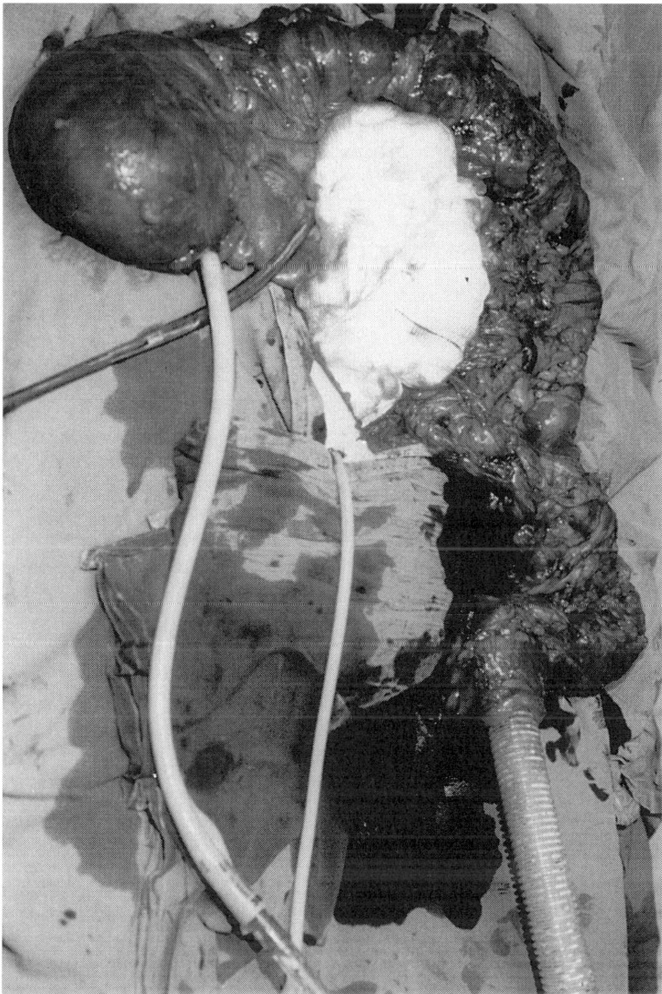

Fig. 1.3 On-table antegrade colonic lavage in progress. There is a large Foley catheter in the caecum and anaesthetic scavenger tubing in the descending colon. Note a suprapubic catheter is also seen.

bowel is emptied of faeces prior to anastomosis, the importance of bowel preparation has been challenged. While experimental data indicate that anastomotic leakage is increased by faecal loading (Smith et al 1983), the clinical data are conflicting with some authorities finding a correlation between leakage and faecal loading (Irvin & Goligher 1973) while others do not (Schrock et al 1973). In recent series good results have been obtained by simple decompression of flatus and extrusion of solid faeces into a bowl (Amsterdam & Krispin 1985, White & Macfie 1985, Mealy et al 1988, Dorudi et al 1990), or even by ignoring the faecal load entirely (Irving & Scrimgeour 1987). Surveys indicate that of surgeons performing resection and primary anastomosis

Table 1.3 Results of primary segmental resection and immediate anastomosis for obstructing colorectal cancer (number of patients expressed as number treated by resection and anastomosis over total number of patients with obstruction treated during series)

Reference	Number of patients	Number of deaths deaths	Number of leaks
Koruth et al 1985b	47/52	4	4
Vidger et al 1985*	18/80	5	3
Thomson & Carter 1986*	20/45	1	1
Pollock et al 1987*	41/44	7	4**
Naraynsingh & Ariyanayagam 1990	30/32	1	0
Murray 1991	29/31	0	0
Allen-Mersh 1993*	15/15	1	0
Stewart et al 1993	60/73	4	4
Total	260/372	23	16
Decompression and extrusion of solid faeces			
Amsterdam & Krispin 1985	25/147	3	1
White & Macfie 1985	33/35	3	4
Mealy et al 1988	25/31	3	2
Dorudi et al 1990	18/18	1	0
Total	101/231	10	7
Intraluminal bypass tube			
Keane et al 1988	6	0	0
Rosati et al 1992	29/31	1	2
Total	35	1	2
No attention to faecal load			
Irving & Scrimgeour 1987	14	1	0

*Series in which caecostomy was used routinely; **radiological leaks only

between one- and two-thirds advise lavage (Pain & Cahill 1991, Carty & Corder 1992), while the remainder simply decompress the colon. The results from 15 recent series, where these techniques have been employed, are shown in Table 1.3. In these series, about two-thirds of all patients who presented with obstruction were treated by resection and anastomosis, while in some of the reports all of the patients were treated in this way. This suggests that patient selection was not a major factor in producing the good results illustrated. The combined mortality rate for these series is only 9% with an anastomotic leak rate of 6%. However, some authors, whose results are not included in Table 1.3, have had a less favourable experience in the treatment of small numbers of patients by these techniques. In three recent series, there were a total of seven anastomotic leaks, two of which were fatal, in the treatment of only thirteen patients (Huddy et al 1988, Stephenson et al 1990, Gandrup et al 1992) and therefore this option must still be exercised with caution. Table 1.3 demonstrates that good results can be obtained with the careful use of either form of bowel preparation and so which approach is used becomes a matter of personal choice. The authors feel that simple extrusion and decompression of the bowel is adequate if there is a load of solid faeces, which may be made fluid and more difficult to manage by lavage. Lavage remains of value if the faecal loading is initially of the viscous fluid variety.

Amongst surgeons who perform resection and immediate anastomosis, there is no consensus on the value of proximal defunctioning. Although diversion is known not to reduce the incidence of dehiscence (Irvin & Goligher 1973, Fielding et al 1979, Mealy et al 1988) it is particularly tempting to leave a tube caecostomy following on-table lavage (Vigder et al 1985, Allen-Mersh 1993). However, caecostomies, unlike colostomies, are known not to reduce the consequences of a leak (Schrock et al 1973) and most authors remove the caecostomy tube at the end of the operation. Certainly if the appendix has been removed at a previous operation and the caecum is entered via an enterotomy, the tube should always be removed at the end of the procedure (Pollock et al 1987). Conceptually similar defunctioning, but without the inconvenience of a stoma, can be achieved using an intraluminal bypass tube. These soft latex tubes are secured to the inside of the bowel proximal to the anastomosis and carry the faecal stream past the anastomosis. This technique has been used to good effect in small series (Keane et al 1988, Rosati et al 1992). However, once again there is need for some caution in view of experimental evidence that defunctioning is associated with a reduction in anastomotic collagen and bursting strength, although there was no apparent effect on healing in this model (Uden et al 1988).

Subtotal colectomy

An alternative strategy for avoiding a stoma in patients with large bowel obstruction is to extend the conventional wisdom of resection and anastomosis of right-sided lesions to the left with performance of a subtotal colectomy. This has several theoretical attractions. The dilated, unprepared proximal bowel is removed and this constitutes in effect a surgical bowel preparation (Klatt et al 1981). An anastomosis between ileum and undilated distal colon can then be constructed. This may be preferable to the colo-colic anastomosis that follows a segmental resection since the leak rate of ileo-colic anastomoses (10%) has been reported to be lower than that from colo-colic anastomoses (18%) (Phillips 1985). In those patients who present with obstruction, it is not usually possible to screen the proximal bowel for neoplasms pre-operatively and assessment of the bowel at operation is poor. This limitation becomes more important since synchronous lesions appear to be more common in patients presenting with obstruction. In seven series including 296 patients with an obstructing carcinoma there were 21 (7.1%) synchronous carcinomas (Bat et al 1985, Kiefhaber et al 1987, Wilson & Gollock 1989, Stephenson et al 1990, Antal et al 1991, Kluger et al 1993, Arnaud & Bergamaschi 1994), while synchronous carcinomas occur in about 3% of all colorectal cancer patients (Hughes et al 1985). Many of these lesions are removed by subtotal colectomy and subsequent screening for metachronous lesions is facilitated.

There are, however, several potential disadvantages of subtotal colectomy. The first is frequency of defaecation and the risk of faecal incontinence, es-

Table 1.4 Results of subtotal colectomy for obstructing colorectal cancer (number of patients expressed as number treated by subtotal colectomy over total number of obstructions treated during series)

Reference	Number of patients	Number of deaths	Number of leaks	Daily stool frequency
Hughes et al 1985	52	6	–	–
Huddy et al 1988	10/42	3	–	–
Halevy & Levy 1989	22/22	1	1	1–3
Wilson & Gollock 1989	18/18	2	0	1–3
Stephenson et al 1990	31/60	1	0	1–4
Antal et al 1991	40/40	0	0	2–3
Brief et al 1991	23	1	0	1–5
Kluger et al 1993	20/20	1	0	2–3
Arnaud & Bergamaschi 1994	44/118	3	2	1–4
Total	260	18	3	

pecially in elderly patients. Although diarrhoea is often a problem in the early postoperative period (Antal et al 1985), it invariably settles to 1–5 motions per day (Table 1.4) and few patients require anti-diarrhoeal medication. The frequency of defaecation is higher after ileo-rectal than ileo-sigmoid anastomosis (Stephenson et al 1990, Arnaud & Bergamaschi 1994) and it has also been suggested that the risk of diarrhoea is related to resection of more than 10 cm of ileum (Brief et al 1991). Secondly, subtotal colectomy is a major operation, that can take over 200 min to perform (Halevy et al 1989). Hughes et al (1985) have stressed that this is a technically demanding operation, which for this and other reasons is appropriate only 'in some cases of obstruction'. The final disadvantage of removing a major part of the colon is the sacrifice of its, largely undetermined, contribution to nutrition. In addition to its well known role in salt and water absorption, the human colon has a functional capacity in nutrient absorption similar to that of 50 cm of jejunum and also has a role in nitrogen metabolism (Moran & Jackson 1992).

Table 1.4 shows that in several small series excellent results have been obtained using subtotal colectomy. In several of these reports the majority of patients who have presented with obstruction have been treated by subtotal colectomy. These series include 250 patients who have been treated with an operative mortality rate of only 7% and a clinical anastomotic leak rate of only 1%. The role of subtotal colectomy in the management of colorectal cancer has recently been addressed. Subtotal colectomy is of value in patients with synchronous carcinomas and patients less than about 50 years of age who present with obstructing carcinomas, especially if they have a positive family history (Brief et al 1991). Subtotal colectomy is also of value in those patients who have serosal tears of the caecum and, particularly, in those with caecal perforation (Pain & Cahill 1991, Arnaud & Bergamaschi 1994).

The operations of immediate resection and anastomosis are certainly more technically demanding than the alternatives, and this is particularly the case for subtotal colectomy. Within a motivated and enthusiastic unit, the peri-operative mortality of operations performed by consultants and trainees may be very similar (White & Macfie 1985, Thomson & Carter 1986, Mealy et al 1988), even for subtotal colectomy (Stephenson et al 1990). However, a more accurate reflection of practice in general probably emerges from the findings of the Large Bowel Cancer Project (Phillips et al 1985). In this survey, the mortality rate of operations performed by trainees (24%) was almost twice that of those managed by a consultant (13%). Surgical experience was found to be particularly important in the selection of patients for resection (Phillips et al 1985) and this will be especially true if immediate anastomosis is contemplated (Koruth et al 1985b). As well as the seniority of the surgeon, their field of special interest is also of relevance. Colorectal surgeons are more likely to perform resection and anastomosis than their non-colorectal colleagues (Carty & Corder 1992, Darby et al 1992). Since specialist surgeons cannot manage all of these patients, it becomes vitally important to encourage the 'dissemination of the more recent advances in surgery to surgeons in training' (Darby et al 1992).

SPECIAL CASES

Perforation

Perforation occurs in a minority (11–18%) of patients with obstruction (Umpelby & Williamson 1984, Phillips et al 1985). The perforation occurs with similar frequency either through the tumour or more proximally secondary to back pressure. This complication is an absolute indication for at least resection, since decompression alone is associated with a high mortality. Resection with anastomosis is safe unless the patient displays circulatory instability or has established sepsis with intra-loop abscesses (Koruth et al 1985b). For left-sided lesions with caecal perforation, subtotal colectomy is probably the most appropriate option (Arnaud & Bergamaschi 1994), while for juxtalesional perforation either subtotal or segmental resection can be performed according to preference.

Rectal cancer

Despite the high proportion of unobstructed cancers that are situated in the rectum, obstruction at this site is an infrequent problem (Phillips et al 1985, Kyllonen 1987). These patient have been treated successfully by resection with or without immediate anastomosis (Dorudi et al 1990, Murray 1991). However, patients with low rectal cancer may be better treated initially by decompression. This allows assessment of tumour resectability, which may well improve in the period after diversion. In those patients with locally advanced lesions, pre-operative radiotherapy can then be delivered. It is in those patients with rectal lesions that decompression across the tumour by a stent or laser seems to be particularly appropriate.

PROGNOSIS

There are several reasons why patients who present with obstructed colorectal carcinomas have a poorer outlook than those who undergo elective surgery.

Primary operative mortality

The immediate mortality associated with the treatment of obstructing carcinomas is higher, at over 20%, than for elective resection in whom mortality is 5–11% (Phillips et al 1985, Kyllonen 1987). The excess mortality is, in part, a reflection of the age of the patients: a quarter of patients presenting with obstruction are over 80 years old compared to only one tenth of patients having elective treatment (Phillips et al 1985, Kyllonen 1987). The mortality rate is higher amongst these elderly patients and is frequently related to cardiorespiratory disease rather than surgical factors (Waldron & Donovan 1986).

Tumour stage

Tumours that present with obstruction tend to be more advanced than other bowel carcinomas. There is a lower proportion of Dukes' A lesions (2–7.5%) than in non-obstructed patients (11–18%) (Phillips et al 1985, Kyllonen 1987, Serpell et al 1989). Furthermore, a higher proportion of patients with obstruction have distant metastases (25–39%) compared to those without obstruction (15–25%) (Kyllonen 1987, Serpell et al 1989). The net result is that potentially curative treatment is possible in a smaller percentage of patients with obstructing lesions (47–60%) than in non-obstructed patients (66–73%) (Kyllonen 1987, Serpell et al 1989, Runkel et al 1991, Ohman 1982).

Those patients who survive the perioperative period have an unfavourable long-term outlook with a crude 5 year survival of 18–32% compared to 35–59% for unobstructed patients (Phillips et al 1985, Kyllonen 1987, Serpell et al 1989). These differences are explicable largely by virtue of the more advanced stage of disease at presentation (Ohman 1982, Phillips et al 1985) and there is little evidence that obstructing lesions are intrinsically more aggressive (Runkel et al 1991). The survival curves of obstructed and non-obstructed cohorts run parallel from 6–18 months after surgery (Phillips et al 1985, Kyllonen 1987). This suggests that the early excess mortality, with consequent worsening of long-term outlook, is secondary to the residual effects of prolonged illness and morbidity.

Delay in resection

There was evidence that primary resection of obstructing tumours improved the long-term outlook compared to staged resection (Fielding & Wells 1974, Irvin & Greaney 1977). This was rationalized on the basis of delay in the performance of definitive surgery with the latter strategy. While some series support this view (Umpleby & Williamson 1984, Vidger et al 1985), others have found evidence to the contrary (Ohman 1982) and most recent data indicate that the initial treatment has little impact on prognosis (Phillips et al 1985, Serpell et al 1989).

CONCLUSIONS

Those patients who present with large bowel obstruction represent a high risk group and they deserve careful evaluation by a suitably trained surgeon. There are circumstances when each of the above treatment options may be appropriate (Stewart et al 1993) and these decisions require fine judgement. The data indicate that primary resection and immediate anastomosis can be performed with a similar mortality rate to the other options. Resection and immediate anastomosis has the advantages of a short postoperative hospital stay and the patient does not have the burden of a stoma, even temporarily. These are major advantages since the prognosis in these patients is generally poor. These arguments would indicate that resection and immediate anastomosis should be the preferred management option in patients with malignant large bowel obstruction.

KEY POINTS FOR CLINICAL PRACTICE

- The surgical treatment of large bowel obstruction is only urgent if there are signs of local peritonitis or if the diameter of the caecum is such that there is a high risk of rupture. In other circumstances the patient should be carefully resuscitated to allow operation by experienced personnel.

- The clinical diagnosis of large bowel obstruction should always be confirmed by a single contrast enema. The characteristic plain radiographic appearance of a volvulus may, however, be a reasonable exception to this rule.

- The use of decompression procedures alone is appropriate only if the primary tumour is unresectable. An internal bypass should also be considered if there are signs of extensive distant spread.

- Resection without anastomosis remains the best option in patients with a left-sided lesion and circulatory instability during operation.

- The aim in management should now be to avoid surgery that entails the formation of a stoma in the majority of patients and there are a range of options from which to choose.

- Segmental resection, with or without per-operative bowel preparation, can be performed with similar morbidity and mortality to less optimal surgery, but with the advantages of minimizing hospital stay and avoidance of a stoma. The value of additional proximal decompression remains unproven.

- Subtotal colectomy has similar advantages to segmental resection and is the procedure of choice if there has been a proximal perforation, in patients with multiple bowel neoplasms and should be considered in young patients (<50 years) presenting with an obstructing carcinoma.

- Recently, techniques to relieve obstruction by trans-tumoral stent or laser recanalization have been developed. These techniques may be particularly useful in the management of those few rectal carcinomas that present with obstruction.

REFERENCES

Allen-Mersh TG 1993 Should primary anastomosis and on-table colonic lavage be standard treatment for left colon emergencies? Ann R Coll Surg Engl 75: 195-198

Amsterdam E, Krispin M 1985 Primary resection with colocolostomy for obstructive carcinoma of the left side of the colon. Am J Surg 150: 558-560

Antal SC, Kovacs ZG, Feigenbaum V et al 1991 Obstructing carcinoma of the left colon: treatment by extended right hemicolectomy. Int Surg 76: 161-163

Arnaud J-P, Bergamaschi R 1994 Emergency subtotal/total colectomy with anastomosis for acutely obstructed carcinoma of the left colon. Dis Col Rect 37: 685-688

Bat L, Neumann G, Shemesh E 1985 The association of synchronous neoplasms with occluding colorectal cancer. Dis Col Rect 28: 149-151

Brewer MS, Brewer J 1993 Tube cecostomy for obstructing carcinoma of the left colon. J Kansas Med Assoc 91: 14-16

Brief DK, Brener B, Goldenkranz R et al 1991 Defining the role of subtotal colectomy in the treatment of carcinoma of the colon. Ann Surg 213: 248-252

Campling EA, Devlin HB, Hoile RW et al 1993 The report of the national confidential enquiry into perioperative deaths 1991/1992. Nuffield Provincial Hospitals Trust and the Kings Fund for Hospitals, London

Carty NJ, Corder AP 1992 Which surgeons avoid a stoma in treating left-sided colonic obstruction? Results of a postal questionnaire. Ann R Coll Surg Engl 74: 391-394

Clark J, Hall AW, Moossa AR 1975 Treatment of obstructing cancer of the colon and rectum. Surg Gynecol Obstet 141: 540-544

Darby CR, Berry AR, Mortensen N 1992 Management variability in surgery for colorectal emergencies. Br J Surg 79: 206-210

Dixon AR, Holmes JT 1990 Hartmann's procedure for carcinoma of rectum and distal sigmoid colon: 5-year audit. J R Coll Surg Edinb 35: 166-168

Dorudi S, Wilson NM, Heddle RM 1990 Primary restorative colectomy in malignant left-sided large bowel obstruction. Ann R Coll Surg Engl 72: 393-395

Eckhauser ML, Mansour AG 1992 Endoscopic laser therapy for obstructing and/or bleeding colorectal neoplasms. Am Surg 58: 358-363

Fielding LP, Wells BW 1974 Survival after primary and after staged resection for large bowel obstruction caused by cancer. Br J Surg 61: 16-18

Fielding LP, Stewart-Brown S, Blesovsky L 1979 Large-bowel obstruction caused by cancer: a prospective study. BMJ 2: 515-517

Gandrup P, Lund L, Balslev I 1992 Surgical treatment of acute malignant large bowel obstruction. Eur J Surg 158: 427-430

Halevy A, Levi J, Orda R 1989 Emergency subtotal colectomy. A new trend for treatment of obstructing carcinoma of the left colon. Ann Surg 210: 220-223

Hoffmann J, Jensen H-E 1984 Tube cecostomy and staged resection for obstructing carcinoma of the left colon. Dis Col Rect 27: 24-32

Huddy SPJ, Shorthouse AJ, Marks CG 1988 The surgical treatment of intestinal obstruction due to left sided carcinoma of the colon. Ann R Coll Surg Engl 70: 40-43

Hughes ESR 1966 Mortality of acute large-bowel obstruction. Br J Surg 53: 593-594

Hughes ESR, McDermott FT, Polglase AL et al 1985 Total and subtotal colectomy for colonic obstruction. Dis Col Rect 28: 162-163

Irvin TT, Goligher JC 1973 Aetiology of disruption of intestinal anastomoses. Br J Surg 60: 461-464
Irvin TT, Greaney MG 1977 The treatment of colonic cancer presenting with intestinal obstruction. Br J Surg 64: 741-744
Irving AD, Scrimgeour D 1987 Mechanical bowel preparation for colonic resection and anastomosis. Br J Surg 74: 580-581
Keane PF, Ohri SK, Wood CB et al 1988 Management of the obstructed left colon by the one-stage intracolonic bypass procedure. Dis Col Rect 31: 948-951
Keen RR, Orsay CP 1992 Rectosigmoid stent for obstructing colonic neoplasms. Dis Col Rect 35: 912-913
Kiefhaber P, Huber F, Kiefhaber K 1987 Palliative and pre-operative endoscopic neodynium-YAG laser treatment of colorectal carcinoma. Endoscopy 19: 43-46
Klatt GR, Martin WH, Gillespie JT 1981 Subtotal colectomy with primary anastomosis without diversion in the treatment of obstructing carcinoma of the left colon. Am J Surg 141: 577-578
Kluger Y, Shiloni E, Jurim O et al 1993 Subtotal colectomy with primary ileocolonic anastomosis for obstructing carcinoma of the left colon: valid option for elderly high risk patients. Isr J Med Sci 29: 726-730
Koruth NM, Hunter DC, Krukowski ZH et al 1985a Immediate resection in emergency large bowel surgery: a 7 year audit. Br J Surg 72: 703-707
Koruth NM, Krukowski ZH, Youngson GG et al 1985b Intra-operative colonic irrigation in the management of left-sided large bowel emergencies. Br J Surg 72: 708-711
Kristiansen VB, Sorensen C, Kjaergaard J et al 1990 Cokostomi kan ikke anbefales sm rutinemetode ved akut venstresidig obstruktiv coloncancer. Ugeskr Laeger 152: 101-103
Kronborg O 1986 The missing randomized trial of two surgical treatment for obstruction due to carcinoma of the left colon and rectum: an interim report. Int J Colorect Dis 1: 162-166
Kyllonen LEJ 1987 Obstruction and perforation complicating colorectal cancer: an epidemiologic and clinical study with special reference to incidence and survival. Acta Chir Scand 153: 607-614
Matheson NA 1989 Management of obstructed and perforated large bowel carcinoma. Baillieres Clin Gastroenterol 3: 671-697
Mealy K, Salman A, Arthur G 1988 Definitive one-stage emergency large bowel surgery. Br J Surg 75: 1216-1219
Mosdell DM, Doberneck RC 1991 Morbidity and mortality of ostomy closure. Am J Surg 162: 633-637
Murray JJ 1991 Nonelective colon resection: alternatives to multistage resection. Surg Clin North Am 71: 1187-1194
Naraynsingh V, Ariyanayagam DC 1990 Obstructed left colon: one-stage surgery in a developing country. J R Coll Surg Edinb 35: 360-361
Ohman U 1982 Prognosis in patients with obstructing colorectal carcinoma. Am J Surg 143: 742-747
Pain J, Cahill J 1991 Surgical options for left-sided large bowel emergencies. Ann R Coll Surg Engl 73: 394-397
Phillips RKS, Hittinger R, Fry JS et al 1985 Malignant large bowel obstruction. Br J Surg 72: 296-302
Pollock AV, Playforth MJ, Evans M 1987 Peroperative lavage of the obstructed left colon to allow safe primary anastomosis. Dis Col Rect 30: 171-173
Roe AM, Prabhu S, Ali A et al 1991 Reversal of Hartmann's procedure: timing and operative technique. Br J Surg 78: 1167-1170
Rosati C, Smith L, Dietel M et al 1992 Primary colorectal anastomosis with the intracolonic bypass tube. Surgery 112: 618-623
Runkel NS, Schlag P, Schwarz N et al 1991 Outcome after emergency surgery for cancer of the large intestine. Br J Surg 78: 183-188
Salim AS 1991 Percutaneous decompression and irrigation for large bowel obstruction: new approach. Dis Col Rect 34: 973-980
Schrock TR, Deveney CW, Dunphy JE 1973 Factors contributing to leakage of colonic anastomoses. Ann Surg 177: 513-518
Serpell JW, McDermott FT, Katrivesis H et al 1989 Obstructing carcinomas of the colon. Br J Surg 76: 965-969
Sjodahl R, Franzen T, Nystrom PO 1992 Primary versus staged resection for acute obstructing colorectal carcinoma. Br J Surg 79: 685-688
Smith SRG, Connolly JC, Gilmore OJA 1983 The effect of faecal loading on colonic anastomotic healing. Br J Surg 70: 49-50
Stephenson BM, Shandall AA, Farouk R et al 1990 Malignant left-sided large bowel obstruction managed by subtotal/total colectomy. Br J Surg 77: 1098-1102
Stewart J, Finan PJ, Courtney DF et al 1984 Does water soluble contrast enema assist in the management of acute large bowel obstruction: a prospective study of 117 cases. Br J Surg 71: 799-801

Stewart J, Diament RH, Brennan TG 1993 Management of obstructing lesions of the left colon by resection, on-table lavage, and primary anastomosis. Surgery 114: 502-505
Tejero E, Mainar A, Ferandez L et al 1995 New procedure for relief of malignant obstruction of the left colon. Br J Surg 82: 34-35
Thomson WHF, Carter SStC 1986 On-table lavage to achieve safe restorative rectal and emergency left colonic resection without covering colostomy. Br J Surg 73: 61-63
Uden P, Blomquist P, Jiborn H et al 1988 Influence of proximal colostomy on the healing of a left colon anastomosis: an experimental study in the rat. Br J Surg 75: 325-329
Umpleby HC, Williamson RCN 1984 Survival in acute obstructing colorectal carcinoma. Dis Col Rect 27: 299-304
Vigder L, Tzur N, Huber M et al 1985 Management of obstructive cancer of the left colon: comparative study of staged and primary resection. Arch Surg 120: 825-828
Waldron RP, Donovan IA 1986 Mortality in patients with obstructing colorectal cancer. Ann R Coll Surg Engl 68: 219-221
White CM, Macfie J 1985 Immediate colectomy and primary anastomosis for acute obstruction due to carcinoma of the left colon and rectum. Dis Col Rect 28: 155-157
Wigmore SJ, Duthie GS, Young IE et al 1995 Restoration of intestinal continuity following Hartmann's procedure: the Lothian experience 1987–1992. Br J Surg 82: 27-30
Wilson RG, Gollock JM 1989 Obstructing carcinomas of the left colon managed by subtotal colectomy. J R Coll Surg Edinb 34: 25-26

2

Aortic aneurysm update

M. M. Thompson   P. R. F. Bell

An abdominal aortic aneurysm (AAA) may be defined as a 50% increase in diameter compared to the expected normal diameter of the aorta (Johnston et al 1991). Abdominal aortic aneurysms are increasing in number (Fowkes et al 1989), and are responsible for 10,000 deaths per year in Britain (Greenhalgh 1990). At present, the only treatment for an AAA is operative repair, which is performed to prevent or deal with aneurysm rupture. This chapter presents a brief review of the current elective management of infra-renal AAA, and then discusses four recent advances: aneurysm pathogenesis, screening, thoracoabdominal aneurysms and endovascular aneurysm repair.

INFRA-RENAL ABDOMINAL AORTIC ANEURYSM – TREATMENT AND OUTCOME

The peri-operative mortality of elective AAA repair has decreased over the last 10 years with rates of less than 5% being reported in selected series, although population based studies often suggest double this figure (Katz et al 1994). Many studies claiming low complication rates have been retrospective with incomplete follow up. However, the Canadian Aneurysm Study has recently reported results from a prospective analysis of 680 patients undergoing AAA repair in 1986 (Johnston 1994b, Johnston 1994a, Johnston & Scobie 1988). The 30-day mortality for patients reaching hospital with a ruptured aortic aneurysm was approximately 50%, with pre-operative creatinine < 1.25 mg/dl, intra-operative urine output > 200 ml and infrarenal clamp site being predictive of early survival. The 5-year survival for this cohort was 26% with late survival being predicted by age and total urine output during aneurysm repair.

The hospital mortality for elective aneurysm repair in the same study was 4.8%, with cardiac events causing death in 69%. The 5-year survival of patients undergoing elective surgery was 68%. Multiple regression analysis identified age, ECG abnormalities and serum creatinine as factors influencing late survival.

Indications for operative repair

The decision to repair an AAA must be made on an individual basis, as the risks of operation must be balanced against the risk of death from ruptured aneurysm. The general consensus of opinion suggests that symptomatic, rapidly expanding or ruptured aneurysms should be repaired as long as medical conditions do not preclude operation (Ernst 1993). The decision to repair asymptomatic aneurysms is more difficult, but repair should be undertaken when the risk of rupture exceeds the risk of surgery. As the rate of aneurysm growth and rupture is directly related to aneurysm size (Darling 1970), most surgeons would repair an AAA larger than 6 cm.

However, for patients with aneurysms between 4–6 cm opinion varies widely, with some surgeons advising operative repair whereas others advocate routine ultrasound surveillance. To resolve this dilemma, the UK small aneurysm trial is randomising 1000 patients with small aneurysms (4–5.5 cm), to operation or surveillance. The results of this trial will allow better informed decisions to be made on patients with small asymptomatic aneurysms (The UK Small Aneurysm Trial Participants 1995).

Conventional repair

Operative technique depends upon the ease of aortic exposure, the extent of the aneurysm and the presence of complications or associated occlusive disease. In general, infra-renal aortic clamping and graft replacement using an inlay technique is the preferred technique. Tube repair is usually possible in 60–70% of aneurysms (Crawford & Crawford 1975). Repair is usually performed under balanced general anaesthesia, and the use of vasodilators and epidural anaesthesia has been suggested to reduce cardiac and metabolic stress (Smith 1992).

Controversy surrounds the use of intra-operative heparin in uncomplicated AAA repair. A recent randomised controlled trial performed by the Joint Vascular Research Group demonstrated that heparinisation did not influence the number of thrombotic complications or the degree of blood loss during aneurysm repair, but did significantly reduce the myocardial infarction rate (Thompson & Clyne 1994). Aprotonin has been utilised to reduce blood loss in cardiac surgery, but had no effect when used as an adjunct to elective aortic procedures (Ranaboldo et al 1994). Peri-operative blood loss may be excessive in complicated aneurysm repair, and it has been suggested that the use of haemodilution techniques or intraoperative blood salvage may reduce transfusion requirements (Tulloh et al 1993, Kelley-Patteson et al 1993).

Cardiac risk assessment and revascularisation

Cardiac related events account for the majority of deaths following AAA repair. Johnston (1994b) has suggested that if all cardiac abnormalities were detected and treated pre-operatively, the resultant improvement in 5-year survival would approach 10–20%. In general, a selective approach to cardiac screening is advocated (Suggs et al 1993). Patients without any clinical or family history of cardiac disease do not necessarily require any investigation. A clinical history of cardiac impairment should be investigated with non-invasive techniques (e.g. dipyridamole-thallium scintigraphy), whereas patients with marked cardiac dysfunction require cardiac catheterisation. Cardiac revascularisation may be required in up to 10% of patients (Cambria et al 1992), but following coronary artery bypass grafting or percutaneous transluminal coronary angioplasty, peri-operative mortality is minimal.

Retroperitoneal or transperitoneal approach

The aorta may be approached transperitoneally or retroperitoneally, with the superiority of each incision being the subject of contention. The retroperitoneal approach is indicated in patients with juxta-renal aneurysms, inflammatory aneurysms, recurrent aneurysms, or in cases with multiple previous abdominal operations. However, this approach remains less popular than the transperitoneal approach for uncomplicated infra-renal aneurysms.

The potential advantages of retroperitoneal exposure include a reduction in blood loss and in the extent of surgical dissection, in addition to the absence of postoperative gastrointestinal dysfunction. A recent randomised controlled trial concluded that the retroperitoneal approach was associated with a lower incidence of gastrointestinal complications, a shorter hospital stay, and a lower total cost, but a significant increase in long-term wound pain (Sicard et al 1995). Interestingly, in this trial the incidence of pulmonary and cardiac complications was similar in the two groups. However, an earlier randomised study suggested that there was no advantage of the retroperitoneal approach (Cambria et al 1990), and therefore no support for its routine introduction.

Inflammatory aneurysms

Inflammatory AAAs are characterised by a grossly thickened laminated wall, which contains a widespread white cell infiltrate. Inflammatory AAAs represent up to 10% of all infra-renal aneurysms, and are macroscopically recognised by their encasement in a white fibrotic layer which envelops the duodenum and retroperitoneum. Inflammatory aneurysms are typically larger and more symptomatic than non-specific AAAs, whilst involvement of the ureters, which are drawn towards the midline, is described in 25%.

Inflammatory aneurysms have a typical appearance on computed tomography (CT) or magnetic resonance imaging (MRI), and the diagnosis may be confirmed by an elevated erythrocyte sedimentation rate. Treatment of these aneurysms is by graft replacement which may be easier using a retroperitoneal approach (Metcalf & Rutherford 1991).

PATHOGENESIS

The integral structural proteins of the aortic wall, elastin and collagen, combine with medial vascular smooth muscle cells to form a series of concentric elastic lamellae which accommodate the haemodynamic stresses imposed by

Fig. 2.1(a)

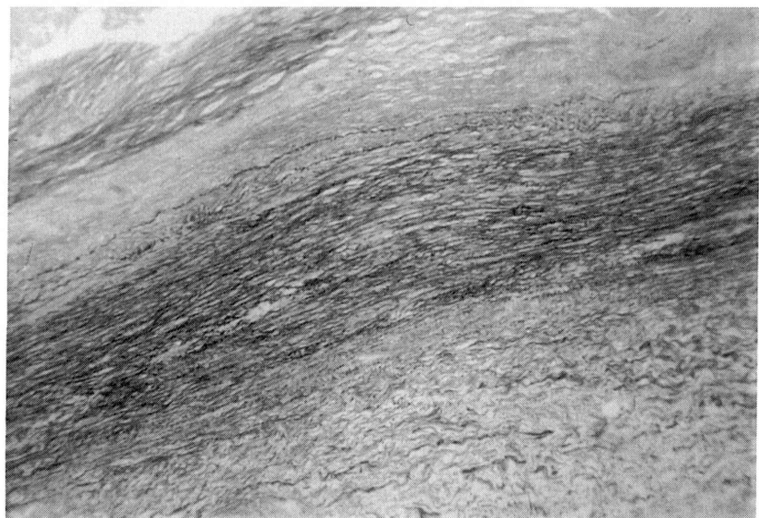

Fig. 2.1(b)

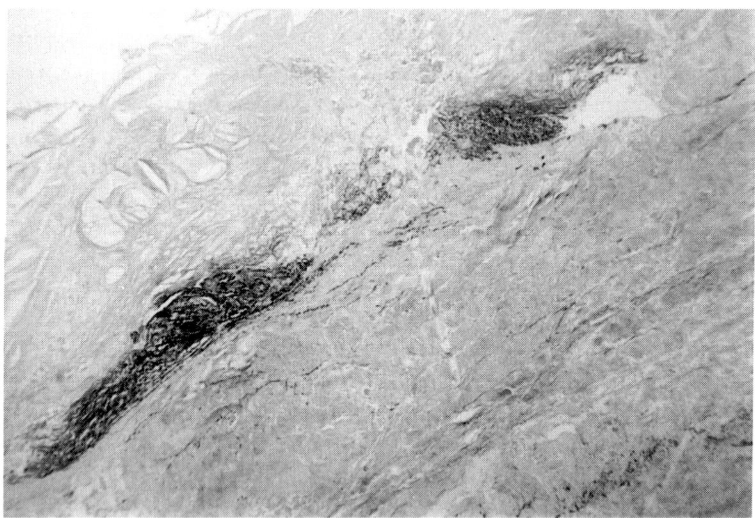

Fig. 2.1 Transverse section of atherosclerotic (a) and aneurysmal (b) aorta stained with elastic van Geison. The orderly elastic lamellae of the normal aorta contrast with the disorganised, fragmented medial structure of an abdominal aortic aneurysm.

cardiac contraction. Non-specific AAAs develop when this architecture becomes fragmented and offers little tensile resistance to the intraluminal pressure (White et al 1993) (Fig. 2.1). The infra-renal aorta is at particular risk of aneurysm development, as the number of elastic lamellae are reduced in comparison with the thoracic aorta (Zatina et al 1984), and medial nutrition may be compromised due to a sparsity of vasa vasorum (Wolinsky & Glagov 1967).

In addition, the infra-renal aorta is exposed to increased haemodynamic stress as the pulse pressure in the aorta is maximal in this segment (McDonald 1968).

Proteolysis and changes in the extracellular matrix

The expansion and thickening of infra-renal AAAs is characterised by an increase in total protein, microfibrillar protein and collagen content, together with a marked reduction in elastin concentration, and in the number of medial smooth muscle cells (Baxter et al 1992). These changes may be secondary to increased collagen turnover, elastin degradation or a combination of both processes. Interestingly, the matrix abnormalities are not confined to the aneurysmal segment, but are found throughout the arterial tree, which suggests that infra-renal aneurysmal disease may be a localised manifestation of a systemic dilating process (Baxter et al 1994).

Several investigators have suggested that elastolysis is the primary event in aneurysm pathogenesis. It has now been conclusively demonstrated that aneurysmal aortic wall has a considerably increased elastase and collagenase activity when compared to atherosclerotic or normal aorta. This increased capacity reflects both an increased expression of serine proteases and metalloenzymes (Cohen et al 1991, Newman et al 1994), and also a reduction in normal inhibitor activity within the aortic wall (Brophy et al 1991). Evidence that proteolysis has an important aetiologic role is strengthened by a strong correlation between AAA size and elastase activity (Louwrens & Pearce 1994), and from the fact that an infusion of elastase is capable of inducing aneurysms in an animal model (Halpern et al 1994).

Abnormal collagen biosynthesis has also been implicated in aneurysm progression, as the concentration and turnover of collagen increases in aneurysmal tissue. The ratio of collagen types I/III is increased in the aneurysmal aortic wall (Deak et al 1992), which may be partly explained by a paracrine mediated overexpression of the Iα pro-collagen gene (Minion et al 1993). Type III collagen metabolism is currently attracting considerable interest as it appears that mutations in the type III collagen gene may cause familial aneurysms, and these may be amenable to DNA screening (Kontusaari et al 1990).

Aneurysms and the immune response

Recent attention has focused on the role of white blood cells and the immune response in the genesis of AAAs. There is a widespread inflammatory infiltrate in the adventitia and media of an AAA that is absent in normal aortic tissue. The infiltrate consists of T cells, polyclonal B cells and macrophages (Koch et al 1990) which appear to be actively participating in an ongoing immune response (Lieberman et al 1992).

Macrophages secrete a number of metalloproteinases which have the ability to degrade the extracellular matrix (Newman et al 1994). In addition, stimulated macrophages may activate latent metalloenzymes through a plasminogen dependent pathway, thus enhancing proteolytic capacity within the aortic wall (Reilly et al 1994). The cellular infiltrate also secretes various growth factors that stimulate angiogenesis and chemotaxis within the arterial adventitia and media (Szekanecz et al 1994). Growth of new vessels is accompanied by destruction of the surrounding extracellular matrix with further turnover of elastin and collagen (Mignatti, 1993).

White cell infiltration obviously plays a central role in aneurysm development. However, it remains debatable as to whether the primary aetiological factor in aneurysmal development is an immune response (possibly autoimmune) or whether the chronic inflammatory infiltrate occurs secondary to pre-existing proteolysis.

Aneurysms and atherosclerosis

Non specific AAAs are conventionally described as 'atherosclerotic', which implies a causative relationship between aortic atherogenesis and aneurysm formation. This traditional perspective has now been challenged on the basis that AAA disease has differing biochemistry, epidemiology and genetics to occlusive disease (Tilson 1992). The peak age of onset of stenosing atherosclerotic disease is 15 years earlier than aneurysmal disease (55 years vs 70 years), and this lag period is difficult to explain if a direct causal relationship between atheroma and aneurysm formation is postulated (Deak et al 1992). It seems more likely that atheroma and aneurysmal disease co-exist as many of the risk factors for the two disease processes are shared (MacSweeney et al 1994).

Future developments

Aneurysmal disease is characterised by changes in the extracellular matrix proteins, excessive proteolytic activity and chronic inflammation. Despite the accumulation of basic physiological and molecular data, the factors which initiate aneurysm development remain uncertain. Future research initiatives are likely to concentrate on gene expression within aneurysmal tissue and on fundamental characteristics of the immune response. The ultimate aim must be to use basic knowledge of aneurysm pathogenesis to identify individuals at risk of aneurysm formation and lessen the risk of aneurysm rupture by specifically targeted medical therapy.

SCREENING

The mortality rate of AAA primarily reflects the rate of aneurysmal rupture, which carries a dire prognosis. The central principle underlying aortic screening is the detection of asymptomatic individuals within the community, which increases the proportion of AAAs that are repaired electively. Screening programmes rely on portable B mode ultrasonography which appears to be safe, well tolerated and repeatable.

Community based screening programmes

Community based screening programmes attempt to identify AAAs in a population old enough to have a significant prevalence of the disease, but young enough to benefit from elective repair (Collin 1993). Established screening programmes have concentrated on the elderly male population (Collin et al 1988, Lucarotti et al 1993, Bengtsson et al 1993), as the incidence of significant aortic dilatation appears to increase with age (Morris et al 1994). Most studies have reported that approximately 8% of individuals had an aortic diameter of greater than 3 cm and that only 2.5% had an aneurysm greater than 4 cm. It has been suggested that a single ultrasound scan in men aged 65 years would exclude 90% of the population from risk of aneurysm development (Emerton et al 1994), and would reduce deaths from ruptured AAA by two-thirds (Lucarotti et al 1993). Screening programmes obviously rely upon a high patient uptake for their effectiveness: compliance over 80% has been reported for some suburban populations (Smith et al 1993).

Is screening worthwhile? – cost/benefit analyses

On the basis of preliminary screening studies, there have been calls for the introduction of a national screening programme (Harris 1992). However, the decision to introduce widespread community based screening depends primarily upon a cost/benefit analysis. The extra costs of screening and subsequent elective treatment need to be balanced against the potential saving in treating ruptured aneurysms. In 1990, Collin suggested that a national aneurysm screening programme could be implemented at a cost of £1 million per year and that 20,000 life-years would be saved annually, at a lower cost per quality life year than the established UK breast screening programme. This opinion was supported by Frame et al (1993) who reviewed all available data and concluded that single examination screening may offer modest benefits, at a relatively high cost per life year.

In contrast to these views, Mason et al (1993) performed an economic analysis which suggested that population based screening should not be introduced. Unfortunately, the benefits of a screening programme can only be conclusively answered by a randomised prospective trial, with death from ruptured aneurysm as the end point. Such a study is virtually impossible in the UK due to the low autopsy rate, which makes the recorded cause of death unreliable. However, strong evidence for the benefits of community screening has recently been presented by Scott et al (1995), who randomised patients in Chichester to screening or control groups. The incidence of aneurysm rupture in the screened group was reduced by 85%.

Selective screening programmes

The introduction of a national screening programme appears unlikely at present. However, several authors have suggested that selective screening programmes, based on high risk groups may be more rational. The incidence of AAA is increased in patients with existing atherosclerotic disease, hypertension, a first degree relative with AAA, and chronic airways disease. Screening tailored to these individuals may detect aneurysms in over 10% of the screened population (MacSweeney et al 1993). Additionally, screening programmes will detect a number of small aneurysms which may not require immediate surgical treatment. Although these aneurysms need serial follow up, preliminary data have suggested that it may be possible to reduce the rate of aneurysm expansion and subsequent rupture by β-adrenergic blockade (Gadowski et al 1994).

THORACOABDOMINAL ANEURYSMS

The first successful treatment of a patient with a thoracoabdominal aneurysm was reported by Etheredge and colleagues in 1955. Despite advances in anaesthetic and surgical technique, thoracoabdominal aneurysms still present a formidable challenge to the surgeon, as they involve the origin of all the major visceral arteries. Thoracoabdominal aneurysms may be classified according to the extent of aortic involvement (Fig. 2.2). In contrast to infra-renal AAAs, approximately 20% of thoracoabdominal aneurysms are secondary to aortic dissection (Svensson et al 1993). The prevalence of thoracoabdominal aneurysms is less than of infra-renal AAA, but nevertheless, approximately one quarter of deaths due to aneurysmal rupture involve complex thoracic or thoracoabdominal aneurysms (Ingoldby et al 1986).

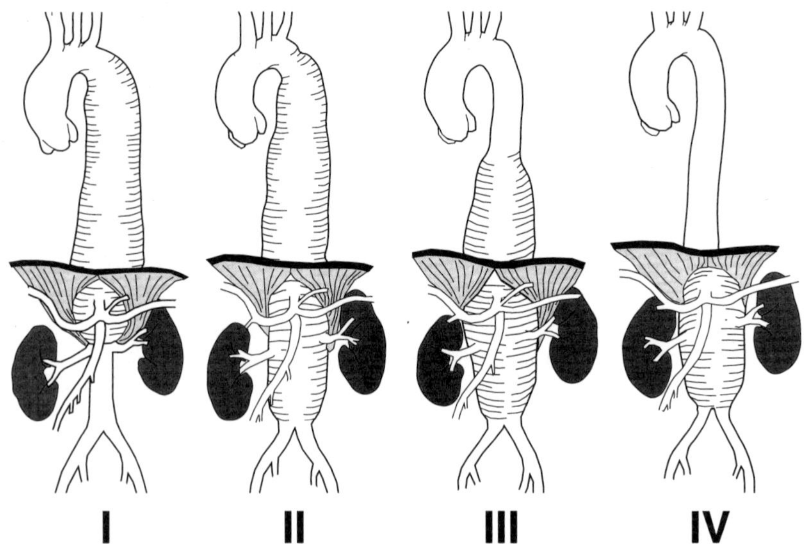

Fig. 2.2 Classification of thoracoabdominal aneurysm based on the extent of aortic involvement (after Crawford et al 1986).

Surgical management

Most patients with thoracoabdominal aortic aneurysms are symptomatic (Crawford et al 1986), and many complain of back pain which often precedes aortic rupture or intramural dissection (Money & Hollier 1994). The incidence of pressure symptoms or those of lower limb ischaemia are commoner than for infra-renal aneurysms (Gilling-Smith & Mansfield 1995). The natural history of untreated thoracoabdominal aneurysms was determined by Crawford and DeNatale (1986) who reported that only 24% of patients were alive at two years and that 50% of these deaths were due to aneurysm rupture. This poor prognosis contrasted with the 59% five-year survival of patients who underwent operative repair. Thoracoabdominal aneurysm surgery therefore, clearly offers improved long-term survival to these patients.

Before operation, all patients should undergo CT or MRI to determine the extent of the aneurysm and its relationship to the visceral arteries. Cross sectional imaging is then followed by arteriography, to delineate any visceral artery stenoses that will need simultaneous surgical correction (Money & Hollier 1994). Patients frequently have associated atherosclerotic coronary artery disease which should be corrected before aortic replacement.

Aneurysm repair uses a thoracoabdominal incision, and is often performed without heparinisation or left heart bypass. The abdominal aorta may be exposed transperitoneally or retroperitoneally, and the diaphragm is divided cirumferentially. The thoracic incision is placed through the ninth or tenth intercostal space for low (Type IV) aneurysms and through the fourth space for higher (Types I and II) lesions. Following exposure, the aneurysm is clamped proximally and distally and a vertical arteriotomy is made in the lateral aneurysm wall. Using a low porosity graft, the proximal anastomosis is fashioned to include adjacent intercostal arteries, whilst any remaining intercostals are directly reimplanted into the graft using an endoaneurysmal inclusion technique (Crawford 1974). The visceral arteries are then directly reimplanted into elliptical openings in the graft with the coeliac, superior mesenteric and right renal arteries being taken on one patch. As the intercostal and visceral arteries are reimplanted, the proximal clamp is moved distally to allow restoration of flow (sequential clamping). The reconstruction is completed by anastomosing the distal graft to the aortic bifurcation or iliac arteries (Hollier 1992). The procedure is often complicated by bleeding from the retroperitoneum or the anastomotic lines. In these cases, disseminated intravascular coagulation (DIC) must be considered, and, if present, should be corrected by the administration of clotting factors and platelets.

The operative mortality varies according to the extent of the aneurysm and the experience of the surgeon, but has been reported to be from 10–35% (Cox et al 1992, Hollier et al 1988). Mortality is increased in ruptured or dissecting aneurysms, elderly patients, patients with concurrent renal or cardiorespiratory disease, and with prolonged aortic clamp times (Svensson et al 1993). The UK experience of thoracoabdominal aneurysm repair is limited in comparison to some of the larger series from the USA. However, the St Mary's group recently reported a series of 110 patients operated on within the past 10 years. The factors associated with high postoperative mortality were Type II aneurysms, aortic dissections, impaired renal or pulmonary function and emergency procedures (Gilling-Smith et al 1995).

Complications

Although repair of thoracoabdominal aneurysms may be accomplished with acceptable mortality rates, the associated morbidity remains high, with renal and respiratory failure occurring in 5.5% and 8%, respectively (Svensson et al 1989, 1991). One of the most feared complications is damage to the spinal cord resulting in paraplegia or paraparesis, which may complicate 20% of reconstructions. The incidence of spinal cord damage is increased in more proximal aneurysms (Crawford Types I & II), and with elongated total clamp time, renal impairment, advanced age and emergency presentations (Svensson et al 1993). The pathogenesis of spinal cord damage is multifactorial, with the most important factors being division of spinal cord arteries, prolonged spinal cord ischaemia, reperfusion injury and postoperative hypotension (Kieffer et al 1994).

The blood supply to the spinal cord is derived from the intercostal arteries, and particularly from the artery of Adamkiewicz, which may be identified on arteriography (Kieffer 1992). Maintenance of spinal cord blood supply may be achieved by reimplantation of patent intercostal arteries, and by distal aortic perfusion, which have been demonstrated to reduce the incidence of neurologic deficits (Svensson et al 1994). Spinal cord pressure increases during aortic clamping, and cerebrospinal fluid drainage has been suggested as a means of reducing paraplegia. The only controlled trial of this technique failed to demonstrate any benefit (Crawford et al 1990), but more recent encouraging reports suggest that the issue remains unresolved (Archer et al 1994). Deep hypothermic circulatory arrest and administration of intrathecal vasodilators have also been investigated, but evaluation of these methods awaits further clinical data.

ENDOVASCULAR ANEURYSM REPAIR

The trend towards endoluminal techniques in vascular surgery has recently been applied to AAA with the advent of endovascular aneurysm repair. This technique was devised in an attempt to treat patients with a large or symptomatic AAA who had severe co-existent cardiac, respiratory or renal disease that precluded conventional aneurysm resection (Nasim et al 1995a, Yusef & Hopkinson 1995). The prognosis of such patients denied elective surgery is dire: 43% die within 24 months from aneurysmal rupture (Szilagyi et al 1972)

Graft design and deployment

The concept of endovascular repair is the introduction of an intraluminal stented graft into an aortic aneurysm from a remote arterial site. The endovascular stented graft is anchored to normal artery above and below the aneurysm sac by self-expanding or balloon-expandable metallic stents, which exclude the aneurysm from the circulation, thus eliminating the risk of rupture. Endoluminal stented grafts are still relatively primitive in design, but may be categorised into two basic types: an unsupported prosthetic graft incorporating a stent at each end (Parodi et al 1991) (Fig. 2.3); or an endoprosthesis consisting of an expansile metallic frame completely covered by ultra-thin graft material (White et al 1994). Initial graft design and experimental work concentrated on straight grafts (Balko et al 1986, Mirich et al 1989, Parodi et al 1991), but more recently both aorto-bi-iliac (Chuter et al 1993), and aorto-uni-iliac grafts have been described (May et al 1994a). In the latter technique, a tapered aorto-iliac or aorto-femoral graft is deployed endovascularly, the contralateral common iliac artery is occluded using endoluminal techniques (coil embolisation or detachable balloon) to prevent blood reflux into the aneurysm sac, and the contralateral limb is then revascularised by a crossover graft.

As a consequence of current size limitations (most aortic prostheses require a 20–28 F sheath), the endograft is usually introduced into the circulation via a femoral arteriotomy or a temporary conduit anastomosed to the iliac artery (Parodi 1993). The graft is manipulated over a guide wire and is deployed under fluoroscopic control. Endovascular aneurysm repair is a complex technique requiring numerous intraluminal 'salvage' manoeuvres, and it is essential that there is close co-operation between vascular surgeons and interventional radiologists during the procedure (Veith 1994).

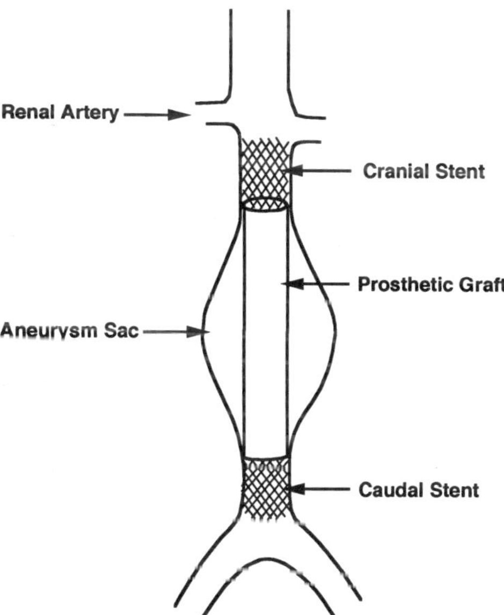

Fig. 2.3 Diagrammatic representation of a straight endograft consisting of an unsupported prosthetic conduit, anchored by metallic stents at either end (after Parodi et al 1991).

Theoretical advantages and disadvantages

The two principal advantages of endovascular as compared to conventional aneurysm repair are the avoidance of intra-abdominal manipulation, and the absence of aortic clamping. Conventional exposure of the infra-renal aorta necessitates a large abdominal incision, mobilisation of the abdominal viscera and retroperitoneal dissection. These procedures are associated with predictable pulmonary and gastrointestinal complications which may be reduced by endovascular repair. The avoidance of aortic dissection will also reduce damage to the para-aortic autonomic nervous system, with elimination of iatrogenic impotence.

Infra-renal aortic clamping during conventional aneurysm repair is associated with a marked reduction in cardiac stroke volume and a rise in left ventricular end diastolic volume (Vandermeer et al 1993; Her et al 1990; Galt et al 1991) which have been implicated in cardiac related deaths. Peri-operative myocardial dysfunction is responsible for 70% of peri-operative aneurysm deaths (Johnston 1994b). In addition, unclamping the aorta and subsequent reperfusion causes a marked fall in mixed venous saturation and the generation of oxygen-free radicals which have been associated with the development of multiple organ failure (Roumen et al 1993, Soong et al 1993, Parry-Billings et al 1992, Murphy et al 1992, Bishop & Sottile 1992). During endovascular repair, the aorta is not clamped, but may be temporarily occluded by devices which use balloon inflation during stent deployment. The reduction or absence of aortic occlusion during endovascular repair may abolish the haemodynamic changes associated with aortic clamping and may reduce both cardiac and systemic complications.

Along with the theoretical, physiological and metabolic advantages, endovascular aneurysm repair, like many 'minimally invasive' techniques, may be associated with earlier discharge from hospital and return to work.

However, despite the numerous theoretical advantages, there are some potential concerns over endoluminal aneurysm repair. As an endoluminal exclusion technique is used, lumbar and patent inferior mesenteric vessels may continue to backbleed into the space between the graft and aneurysm sac. This may lead to a rise in intra-aneurysmal pressure, continued aneurysm expansion and eventual rupture (Sayers et al 1993). Recent experimental evidence however, suggests that small patent lumbar arteries may thrombose following endovascular grafting (Sayers et al 1994), and preliminary clinical results demonstrate that thrombosis of the intra-aneurysmal space occurs after placement of an endograft.

Patient selection

The design of most current endografts imposes rigorous anatomical constraints on the patients that are suitable for endovascular aneurysm repair. The main requirement is a suitable length of 'normal' aorta between the renal arteries and cranial extent of the aneurysm sac, to allow effective proximal fix-

Table 2.1 Current criteria for endovascular aortic aneurysm repair

Criteria for endovascular tube graft	Criteria for endovascular bifurcated graft	Criteria for tapered aorto-iliac graft
Infra-renal aneurysm (no supra -renal extension)	Infra-renal aneurysm (no supra-renal extension)	Infra-renal aneurysm (no supra-renal extension)
Proximal aneurysm neck > 1.5 cm (distance between renal arteries and proximal aneurysm sac)	Proximal aneurysm neck > 1.5 cm	Proximal aneurysm neck > 1.5cm
Distal aneurysm neck > 1.0 cm (distance between distal aneurysm sac and aortic bifurcation)	No distal neck required	No distal neck required
Patent non-diseased superior mesenteric artery (SMA)	Patent non-diseased SMA	Patent non-diseased SMA
Minimal aneurysm tortuosity	Minimal aneurysm tortuosity	Minimal aneurysm tortuosity
Iliac arteries > 8 mm diameter	Iliac arteries > 8 mm diameter	Iliac arteries > 8 mm diameter
Absence of iliac aneurysms	Iliac arteries < 14 mm diameter	Iliac aneurysms acceptable, but one iliac artery must be less than 14 mm
Minimal iliac tortuosity (change in direction < 60°)	Absence of iliac aneurysms	
	Minimal iliac tortuosity	Minimal iliac tortuosity

ation of the endograft. The design of endograft employed also depends on the distal extension of the aneurysm. Patients with a cuff of aorta between the distal extent of the aneurysm and the aortic bifurcation may be suitable for placement of a straight graft, whereas aneurysms extending into the iliac system necessitate a bifurcated or tapered aorto-iliac graft. The current criteria in use in our department are shown in Table 2.1.

Unlike conventional repair, where prosthetic grafts may be tailored to fit the required dimensions, only very limited adjustments may be made to the length and diameter of endovascular grafts during deployment. The requirement for precise determination of aneurysm morphology and size prior to operation has led to renewed interest in aortic imaging. Standard B mode ultrasonography is unable to provide sufficient detailed information to allow planning of endovascular repair. Attention has therefore focused on cross-sectional imaging techniques.

Several trials are in progress to compare the ability of CT turbo-flash MRI (TF-MRI) (Cherryman et al 1994) (Fig. 2.4), colour duplex scanning and

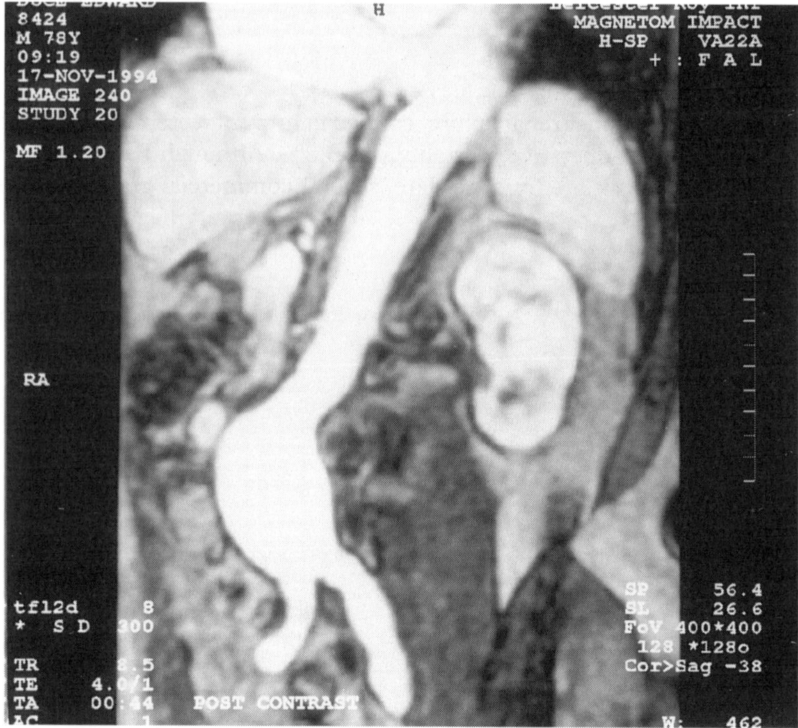

Fig. 2.4 Magnetic resonance angiogram of an abdominal aortic aneurysm.

intra-arterial digital subtraction arteriography (DSA) to determine accurate aneurysm morphology. Early results suggest that TF-MRI provides the best resolution of the proximal aneurysm neck and aortic bifurcation whereas duplex scanning gives good resolution of the iliac arteries.

Clinical results

Endovascular aneurysm repair has been enthusiastically adopted by vascular surgeons throughout the world, and the numbers of patients treated are increasing rapidly (May et al 1994a, Nasim et al 1994, Scott & Chuter 1994, Yusef et al 1994, Moore & Vescera 1994). Although the application of stented grafts was initially suggested by Charles Dotter in 1969, the 'father' of endovascular aneurysm repair is Juan Carlos Parodi, who treated 50 patients between 1990 and 1994 (Parodi, 1994). In his series the success rate of tube endografts was 84% and 75% for tapered aorto-iliac reconstructions. There were four early deaths, 2 from massive microembolism. Five patients had continued blood leakage around the graft into the aneurysm sac (peri-graft extravasation), and one late death occurred due to aneurysm rupture in one of these cases.

May et al (1994b) recently reported a 79% success rate in 43 endovascular repairs, which comprised 28 tube grafts, 11 tapered aorto-iliac reconstructions and 4 bifurcated procedures. Interestingly, 25% of these patients had severe systemic complications (renal failure, cardiac failure and cerebrovascular accident), and the peri-operative mortality was 3.8%. Although Parodi and May have the largest personal series to date, several commercial grafts have been used in multi-centre trials. The Endovascular Technologies EGS system, the Stentor graft and the Chuter bifurcated system have all been deployed in over 50 patients each, and trial results are awaited with interest.

In our unit, endovascular repair has been attempted in 12 patients: seven patients underwent straight graft repair using the Endovascular Technologies EGS system (Moore & Vescera 1994), whilst 5 patients had tapered aorto-iliac reconstructions using a graft constructed from modified Palmaz stents and expanded PTFE (Fig. 2.5). Two patients required conversion to conventional procedures because of access difficulties in one and failure of stent deployment in the other. Complications included one postoperative death from bronchopneumonia, and one episode of transient renal failure that resolved within 30 days. There was a high incidence of synchronous vascular procedures. Access problems necessitated the construction of a temporary iliac conduit in 7 patients and iliac angioplasty in a further two. One patient required a simultaneous femoro-distal bypass and bilateral femoral aneurysm repairs.

Fig. 2.5(a)

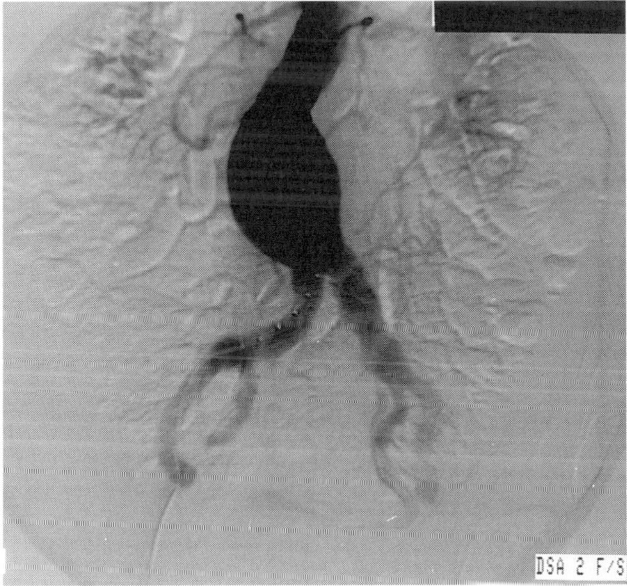

Fig. 2.5 Tapered endovascular aneurysm repair. The pre-operative arteriogram (a) demonstrates an infra-renal aneurysm with an adequate 'neck' between the renal arteries and cranial extent of the aneurysm.

Fig. 2.5(b)

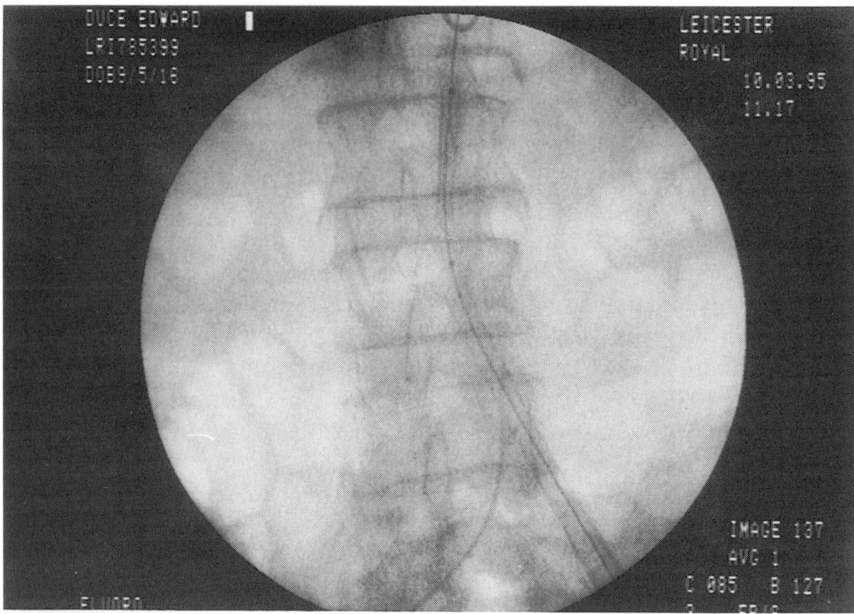

Fig. 2.5(c)

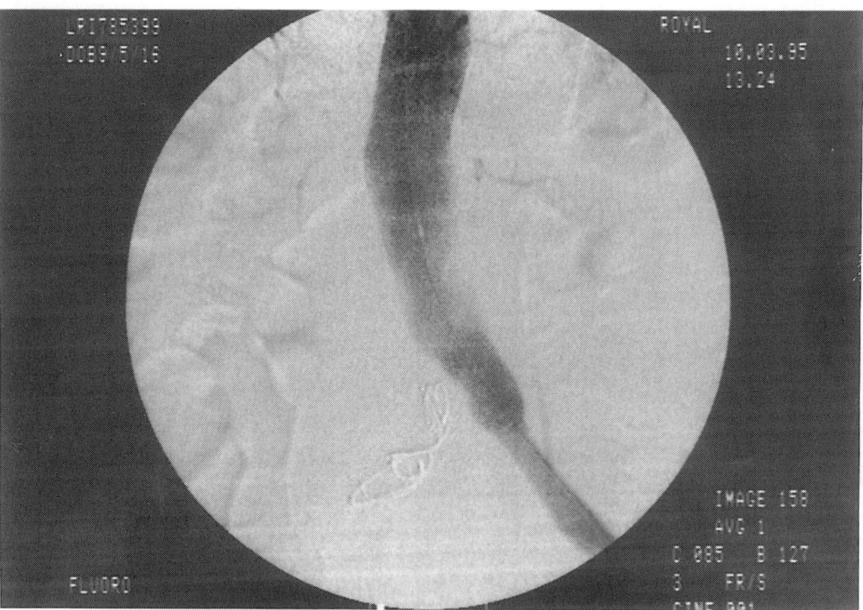

Fig. 2.5 Tapered endovascular aneurysm repair. The pre-operative arteriogram (b) The endograft packaged in a delivery sheath is passed through the aorta to the proximal aneurysm neck. (c) Arteriogram after deployment demonstrating the tapered endograft. (d) Post-operative CT illustrating the cranial aortic stent. (e) Post-operative CT after endovascular repair of AAA. Flow is seen within the endograft which lies inside a thrombosed aneurysm sac.

Fig. 2.5(d)

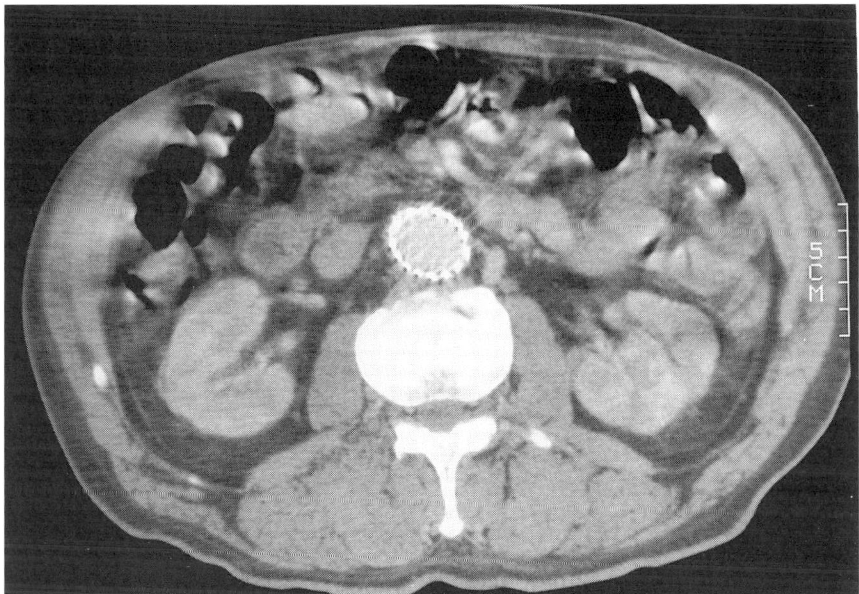

Fig. 2.5(e)

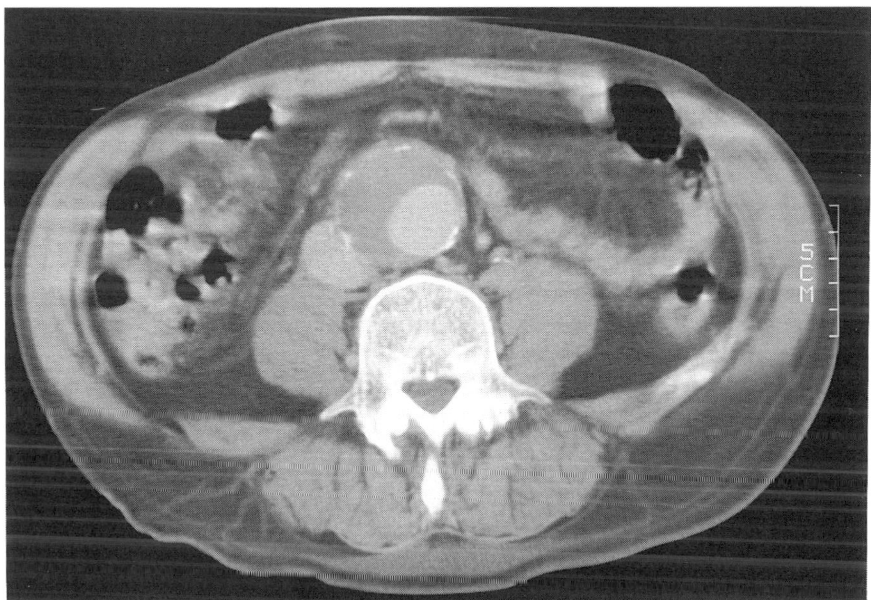

Comment and future directions

There is certain to be marked improvement in endograft manufacture and design over the next few years. Developments in nitinol-based stents and ultra-thin graft material should ensure smaller delivery systems, with an expansion in the number of patients suitable for endovascular repair. Prospective studies will further define the criteria for endovascular grafting, and the majority of aneurysms may be treated by this technique if stents may be placed safely over the renal arteries (Nasim et al 1995b).

Endovascular aneurysm repair has been introduced into clinical practice with some degree of success. However, despite initial enthusiasm for this technique, all early studies have demonstrated a high complication rate. The occurrence of massive microembolism appears to be unpredictable and is associated with a poor prognosis. Obviously, further studies are required to define the physiological and metabolic consequences of endoluminal therapy. Endovascular aneurysm repair offers exciting therapeutic possibilities for elective and emergency treatment (Yusef et al 1995). However, it is essential that the technique is not introduced into widespread practice without careful evaluation, that should include randomised prospective trials.

KEY POINTS FOR CLINICAL PRACTICE

- The retroperitoneal approach to infra-renal AAA has not been universally adopted, but recent evidence suggests that this approach may decrease gastrointestinal complications. Specific indications for retroperitoneal dissection include juxta-renal aneurysms, recurrent aneurysms, inflammatory aneurysms, multiple previous abdominal operations or specific co-existent urological conditions (horseshoe kidney).
- Cardiac related events are responsible for over 50% of deaths following AAA repair. Selective cardiac screening with dipyridamole-thallium scans and subsequent cardiac catheterisation may identify up to 10% of patients who would benefit from coronary revascularisation. Peri-operative mortality appears to be reduced following cardiac revascularisation.
- Abdominal aortic aneurysms are characterised by abnormalities in collagen and elastin concentration associated with increased proteolysis and a marked inflammatory infiltrate within the aortic wall. Further elucidation of aneurysm pathogenesis at the molecular level may allow development of effective medical treatment.
- Community based ultrasound screening for abdominal aortic aneurysms is feasible and appears to reduce the rate of aneurysm rupture. However, clear economic advantages of such programmes have not been conclusively demonstrated and screening of selected, high-risk groups may be more feasible.
- Thoracoabdominal aneurysms are common, and have a high mortality if untreated. Surgical repair prevents death and may be performed with acceptable peri-operative mortality. However, complications are common and techniques to prevent paraplegia are still evolving.

- Endovascular aneurysm repair may be associated with fewer complications than conventional procedures due to the absence of intra-peritoneal manipulation and the avoidance of aortic cross clamping. This procedure may thus be suitable for elderly, unfit patients who are not suitable for conventional surgery.
- Endovascular aneurysm repair is only suitable for a limited number of patients with a length of 'normal' aorta between the renal arteries and the cranial extent of the aneurysm. Cross sectional imaging is required to define aneurysm morphology.
- Endovascular repair is a complex procedure that requires close co-operation between vascular surgeons and interventional radiologists.
- Initial trials of endovascular aneurysm repair have demonstrated a high incidence of complications. The procedure should not be introduced into widespread clinical practice until randomised clinical trials have taken place.

REFERENCES

Archer CW, Wynn MM, Hoch JR, Popic P, Archibald J, Turnipseed WD 1994 Combined use of cerebrospinal fluid drainage and naloxone reduces the risk of paraplegia in thoracoabdominal aneurysm repair. J Vasc Surg 19: 236-248

Balko A, Piasecki GJ, Shah DM, Carney WI, Hopkins RW, Jackson BT 1986 Transfemoral placement of intraluminal polyurethane prosthesis for abdominal aortic aneurysm. J Surg Res 40: 305-309

Baxter BT, McGee GS, Shively VP et al 1992 Elastin content, cross links and mRNA in normal and aneurysmal human aorta. J Vasc Surg 16: 192-200

Baxter BT, Davis VA, Minion DJ, Wang YP, Lynch TG, McManus BM 1994 Abdominal aortic aneurysms are associated with altered matrix proteins of the nonaneurysmal aortic segments. J Vasc Surg 19: 797-802

Bengtsson H, Nilsson P, Bergqvist D 1993 Natural history of abdominal aortic aneurysm detected by screening. Br J Surg 80: 718-720

Bishop RL, Sottile FD 1992 Continuous monitoring of mixed venous saturation during aortic operations. Crit Care Med 20: 332-336

Brophy CM, Marks WH, Reilly JM, Tilson MD 1991 Decreased tissue inhibitor of metalloproteinases (TIMP) in abdominal aortic aneurysm tissue: a preliminary report. J Surg Res 50: 653-657

Cambria RP, Brewster DC, Abbott WM et al 1990 Transperitoneal versus retroperitioneal approach for aortic reconstruction: a randomised prospective study. J Vasc Surg 11: 314-325

Cambria RP, Brewster DC, Abbott WM et al 1992 The impact of selective use of dipyridamole-thallium scans and surgical factors on the current morbidity of aortic surgery. J Vasc Surg 15: 43-51

Cherryman GR, Moody AR, Rodgers P 1994 New imaging techniques and arterial disease. Vasc Med Rev 5: 107-120

Chuter TA, Green RM, Ouriel K, Fiore WM, DeWeese JA 1993 Transfemoral endovascular aortic graft placement. J Vasc Surg 18: 185-195

Cohen JR, Parikh S, Sarfati I, Danna D 1991 Neutrophil elastase mRNA transcripts in abdominal aortic aneurysm patients. Surg Forum 42: 358-359

Collin J, Araujo L, Walton J, Lindsell D 1988 Oxford screening programme for abdominal aortic aneurysm in men aged 65 to 74 years. Lancet ii: 613-615

Collin J 1990 The value of screening for abdominal aortic aneurysm by ultrasound. In: Greenhalgh RM, Mannick JA (eds) The cause and management of aneurysms. WB Saunders, London, pp 447-456

Collin J 1993 Screening for abdominal aortic aneurysm. Br J Surg 80: 1363-1364
Cox GS, O'Hara PJ, Hertzer NR, Piedmonte MR, Krajewski LP, Beven EG 1992 Thoracoabdominal aneurysm repair: a representative experience. J Vasc Surg 15: 780-788
Crawford ES (1974) Thoracoabdominal and abdominal aortic aneurysm involving renal, superior mesenteric and celiac arteries. Ann Surg 179: 763-772
Crawford ES, Crawford JL, Safi HJ et al 1986 Thoracoabdominal aortic aneurysms: preoperative and interoperative factors determining immediate and long term results of operation in 605 patients. J Vasc Surg 3: 389-404
Crawford ES, DeNatale RW 1986 Thoracoabdominal aortic aneurysm: observations regarding the natural course of the disease. J Vasc Surg 3: 578-582
Crawford ES, Svensson LG, Hess KR et al (1990) A prospective randomised study of cerebrospinal fluid drainage to prevent paraplegia after high-risk surgery on the thoracoabdominal aorta. J Vasc Surg 13: 36-46
Crawford ES, Crawford JL 1975 Diseases of the aorta: including an atlas of angiographic and surgical technique. Williams and Williams, Baltimore, USA
Darling RC 1970 Ruptured arteriosclerotic abdominal aortic aneurysms. A pathologic and clinical study. Am J Surg 119: 397-401
Deak SB, Ricotta JJ, Mariani TJ et al 1992 The role of abnormal type III collagen in the development of common aneurysms. J Vasc Surg 15: 926-927
Dotter CT 1969 Transluminally-placed coilspring endarterial tube grafts: long term patency in canine popliteal artery. Invest Radiol 4: 329-332
Emerton ME, Shaw E, Poskitt K, Heather BP 1994 Screening for abdominal aortic aneurysm: a single scan is enough. Br J Surg 81: 1112-1113
Ernst CB 1993 Abdominal aortic aneurysm. N Engl J Med 328: 1167-1172
Etheredge SN, Yee J, Smith JV, Schonberger S, Goldman MJ 1955 Successful resection of a large aneurysm of the upper abdominal aorta and replacement with homograft. Surgery 38: 1071-1075
Fowkes FGC, MacIntyre CCA, Ruckley CV 1989 Increasing incidence of aortic aneurysms in England and Wales. BMJ 298: 33-35
Frame PS, Fryback DG, Patterson C 1993 Screening for abdominal aortic aneurysm in men ages 60 to 80 years. A cost-effectiveness analysis. Ann Intern Med 119: 411-416
Gadowski GR, Pilcher DB, Ricci MA 1994 Abdominal aortic aneurysm expansion rate: effect of size and beta-adrenergic blockade. J Vasc Surg 19: 727-731
Galt SW, Bech FR, McDaniel MD et al 1991 The effect of ibuprofen on cardiac performance during abdominal aortic cross-clamping. J Vasc Surg 13: 876-883
Gilling-Smith GL, Mansfield AO 1995 Thoracoabdominal aortic aneurysm. Br J Surg 82: 148-149
Gilling-Smith GL, Worswick L, Knight PF, Wolfe JHN, Mansfield AO 1995 Surgical repair of thoracoabdominal aortic aneurysm: 10 years' experience. Br J Surg 82: 624-629
Greenhalgh RM 1990 Prognosis of abdominal aortic aneurysm. BMJ 301: 136
Halpern VJ, Nackman GB, Gandhi RH et al 1994 The elastase infusion model of experimental aortic aneurysms: synchrony of induction of endogenous proteinases with matrix destruction and inflammatory cell response. J Vasc Surg 20: 51-60
Harris PL 1992 Reducing the mortality from abdominal aortic aneurysms: need for a national screening programme. BMJ 305: 697-699
Her C, Kizelshteyn G, Walker V, Hayes D, Lees DE 1990 Combined epidural and general anaesthesia for abdominal aortic surgery. J Cardiothorac Anaesth 4: 552-557
Hollier LH, Symmonds JB, Pairolero PC, Cherry KJ, Hallett JW, Gloviczki P 1988 Thoracoabdominal aortic aneurysm repair: analysis of post-operative morbidity. Arch Surg 123: 871-875
Hollier LH 1992 Technical aspects in the repair of thoracoabdominal aortic aneurysms. In: Bell PRF, Jamieson CW, Ruckley CV eds Surgical management of vascular disease. WB Saunders, London, pp 835-842
Ingoldby CJH, Wujanto R, Mitchell JE 1986 Impact of vascular surgery on community mortality from ruptured aneurysms. Br J Surg 73: 551-553
Johnston KW, Scobie TK 1988 Multicenter prospective study of nonruptured abdominal aortic aneurysms. I. Population and operative management. J Vasc Surg 7: 69-81
Johnston KW, Rutherford RB, Tilson DM, Shah DM, Hollier L, Stanley JC 1991 Suggested standards for reporting on arterial aneurysms. J Vasc Surg 13: 444-450
Johnston KW 1994a Ruptured abdominal aortic aneurysm: six-year follow-up results of a

multicenter prospective study. Canadian Society for Vascular Surgery Aneurysm Study Group. J Vasc Surg 19: 888-900

Johnston KW 1994b Nonruptured abdominal aortic aneurysm: six year follow up results from the multicentre prospective Canadian aneurysm study. J Vasc Surg 20: 163-170

Katz DJ, Stanley JC, Zelenock GB 1994 Operative mortality rates for intact and ruptured abdominal aortic aneurysms in Michigan: an eleven-year statewide experience. J Vasc Surg 19: 804-815

Kelley-Patteson C, Ammar AD, Kelley H 1993 Should the Cell Saver Autotransfusion Device be used routinely in all infrarenal abdominal aortic bypass operations? J Vasc Surg 18: 261-265

Kieffer E 1992 The role of spinal cord arteriography before descending thoracic/thoracoabdominal aneurysmectomy. Semin Vasc Surg 5: 141-145

Kieffer E, le Blevec D, Koskas F, Bahnini A, Godet G, Chiras J 1994 Spinal cord protection in surgical repair of thoracoabdominal aneurysm: preoperative and intraoperative measures. In: Yao JST, Pearce WH eds Aneurysms: new findings and treatments. Appleton and Lange, Norwalk, Connecticut, pp 195-205

Koch AE, Haines GK, Pearce WH 1990 Human abdominal aortic aneurysms: immunophenotypic analysis suggesting an immune-mediated response. Am J Pathol 137: 1199-1215

Kontusaari S, Tromp G, Kuivaniemi H, Romanic AM, Prockop DJ 1990 A mutation in the gene for type III procollagen (COL3A1) in a family with aortic aneurysms. J Clin Invest 86: 1465-1473

Lieberman J, Scheib JS, Googe PH, Ichiki AT, Goldman MH 1992 Inflammatory abdominal aortic aneurysm and the associated T-cell reaction: a case study. J Vasc Surg 15: 569-572

Louwrens H, Pearce WH 1994 Role of inflammatory cells in aortic aneurysms. In: Yao JST, Pearce WH eds Aneurysms: new findings and treatments. Appleton and Lange, Norwalk, Connecticut, pp 11-23

Lucarotti M, Shaw E, Poskitt K, Heather B 1993 The Gloucestershire Aneurysm Screening Programme: the first 2 years' experience. Eur J Vasc Surg 7: 397-401

MacSweeney ST, O'Meara M, Alexander C, O'Malley MK, Powell JT, Greenhalgh RM 1993 High prevalence of unsuspected abdominal aortic aneurysm in patients with confirmed symptomatic peripheral or cerebral arterial disease. Br J Surg 80: 582-584

MacSweeney STR, Powell JT, Greenhalgh RM 1994 Pathogenesis of abdominal aortic aneurysm. Br J Surg 81: 935-941

Mason JM, Wakeman AP, Drummond MF, Crump BJ 1993 Population screening for abdominal aortic aneurysm: do the benefits outweigh the costs? J Public Health Med 15: 154-160

May J, White G, Waugh R, Yu W, Harris J 1994a Treatment of complex abdominal aortic aneurysms by a combination of endoluminal and extraluminal aortofemoral grafts. J Vasc Surg 19: 924-933

May J, White GH, Yu W et al 1994b Endoluminal grafting of abdominal aortic aneurysms: causes of failure and their prevention. J Endovasc Surg 1: 44-52

McDonald DA 1968 Regional pulse wave velocity in the arterial tree. J Appl Physiol 24: 73-78

Metcalf RK, Rutherford RB 1991 Inflammatory abdominal aortic aneurysm: an indication for the retroperitoneal approach. Surgery 109: 555-557

Mignatti P 1993 The fibrinolytic system and angiogenesis. Fibrinolysis 7 (Suppl I): 20-21

Minion DJ, Wang Y, Lynch TG, Fox IJ, Prorok GD, Baxter BT 1993 Soluble factors modulate changes in collagen gene expression in abdominal aortic aneurysms. Surgery 114: 252-256

Mirich D, Wright KC, Wallace S et al 1989 Percutaneously placed endovascular grafts for aortic aneurysms: feasibility study. Radiology 170: 1033-1037

Money SR, Hollier LH 1994 The management of thoracoabdominal aneurysms. Adv Surg 27: 285-294

Moore WS, Vescera CL 1994 Repair of abdominal aortic aneurysm by transfemoral endovascular graft placement. Ann Surg 220: 331-341

Morris GE, Hubbard CS, Quick CR 1994 An abdominal aortic aneurysm screening programme for all males over the age of 50 years. Eur J Vasc Surg 8: 156-160

Murphy ME, Kolvenbach R, Aleksis M, Hansen R, Sies H 1992 Antioxidant depletion in aortic crossclamping ischemia, increase of the plasma alpha-tocopheryl quinone/alpha-tocopherol ratio. Free Radical Biol Med 13: 95-100

Nasim A, Sayers RD, Thompson MM, Bell PR, Bolia A 1994 Endovascular repair of abdominal aortic aneurysms. Lancet 343: 1230-1231

Nasim A, Sayers RD, Thompson MM, Bell PRF 1995a Endovascular repair of abdominal aortic aneurysm. Hosp Update 21: 131-135
Nasim A, Thompson MM, Sayers RD, Bell PRF 1995b Investigation of the relationship between aortic stent position and renal function. Br J Surg: in press
Newman KM, Jean-Claude J, Li H et al 1994 Cellular localisation of matrix metalloproteinases in the abdominal aortic aneurysm wall. J Vasc Surg 20: 814-820
Parodi JC, Palmaz JC, Barone HD 1991 Transfemoral intraluminal graft implantation for abdominal aortic aneurysms. Ann Vasc Surg 5: 491-499
Parodi JC 1993 Endovascular repair of abdominal aortic aneurysms. In: Advances in vascular surgery, vol 1. Moseby, St Louis, pp 85-106
Parodi JC 1994 Personal communication
Parry-Billings M, Baigrie RJ, Lamont PM, Morris PJ, Newsholme EA 1992 Effects of major and minor surgery on plasma glutamine and cytokine levels. Arch Surg 127: 1237-1240
Ranaboldo C, Thompson JF, Davies JN et al 1994 Aprotonin in elective aortic reconstruction: a double blind randomised controlled trial (Abstract). Br J Surg 81: 611
Reilly JM, Sicard GA, Lucore CL 1994 Abnormal expression of plasminogen activators in aortic aneurysmal and occlusive disease. J Vasc Surg 19: 865-872
Roumen RM, Hendriks T, van der Ven-Jongekrijg J et al 1993 Cytokine patterns in patients after major vascular surgery, hemorrhagic shock, and severe blunt trauma. Relation with subsequent adult respiratory distress syndrome and multiple organ failure. Ann Surg 218: 769-776
Sayers RD, Thompson MM, Bell PR 1993 Endovascular stenting of abdominal aortic aneurysms. Eur J Vasc Surg 7: 225-227
Sayers RD, Thompson MM, Nasim A, Bell PRF 1994 Endovascular repair of abdominal aortic aneurysms: limitations of the proximal stent technique. Br J Surg 81: 1107-1110
Scott RA, Chuter TA 1994 Clinical endovascular placement of bifurcated graft in abdominal aortic aneurysm without laparotomy (letter). Lancet 343: 413
Scott RAP, Wilson NM, Ashton HA, Kay DN 1995 The five year results of a control study of screening for AAA. Br J Surg: in press
Sicard GA, Reilly JM, Rubin BG et al 1995 Transabdominal versus retroperitoneal incision for abdominal aortic surgery: report of a prospective randomised trial. J Vasc Surg 21: 174-183
Smith FC, Grimshaw GM, Paterson IS, Shearman CP, Hamer JD 1993 Ultrasonographic screening for abdominal aortic aneurysm in an urban community. Br J Surg 80: 1406-1409
Smith G 1992 Anaesthesia for vascular surgery. In: Bell PRF, Jamieson CW, Ruckley CV eds Surgical management of vascular disease. WB Saunders, London, pp 291-308
Soong CV, Blair PH, Halliday MI et al 1993 Endotoxaemia, the generation of the cytokines and their relationship to intramucosal acidosis of the sigmoid colon in elective abdominal aortic aneurysm repair. Eur J Vasc Surg 7: 534-539
Suggs WD, Smith RB, Weintraub WS, Dodson TF, Salam AA, Motta JC 1993 Selective screening for coronary artery disease in patients undergoing elective repair of abdominal aortic aneurysms. J Vasc Surg 18: 349-355
Svensson LG, Coselli JS, Safi HJ, Hess KR, Crawford ES 1989 Appraisal of adjuncts to prevent acute renal failure after surgery on the thoracic or thoracoabdominal aorta. J Vasc Surg 10: 230-239
Svensson LG, Hess KR, Coselli JS, Safi HJ, Crawford ES 1991 A prospective study of respiratory failure after high risk surgery on the thoracoabdominal aorta. J Vasc Surg 14: 271-282
Svensson LG, Crawford ES, Hess KR, Coselli JS, Safi HJ 1993 Experience with 1509 patients undergoing thoracoabdominal aortic operations. J Vasc Surg 17: 357-370
Svensson LG, Hess KR, Coselli JS, Safi HJ 1994 Influence of segmental arteries, extent, and atriofemoral bypass on postoperative paraplegia after thoracoabdominal aortic operations. J Vasc Surg 20: 255-262
Szekanecz Z, Shah MR, Harlow LA, Pearce WH, Koch AE 1994 Interleukin-8 and tumour necrosis factor alpha are involved in human aortic endothelial cell migration. Pathobiology 62: 134-139
Szilagyi DE, Elliott JP, Smith RF 1972 Clinical fate of the patient with asymptomatic abdominal aortic aneurysm and unfit for surgical treatment. Arch Surg 104: 600-606
The UK Small Aneurysm Trial Participants 1995 The UK small aneurysm trial: design, methods and progress. Eur J Vasc Surg 9: 42-48
Thompson JF, Clyne CAC 1994 Intraoperative heparinisation reduces the risk of myocardial infarction during elective aortic surgery (Abstract). Br J Surg 81: 614-615

Tilson MD 1992 Aortic aneurysms and atherosclerosis. Circulation 85: 378-379
Tulloh BR, Brakespear CP, Bates SC et al 1993 Autologous predonation, haemodilution and intraoperative blood salvage in elective abdominal aortic aneurysm repair. Br J Surg 80: 313-315
Vandermeer TJ, Maini BS, Hendershott TH, Sottile FD 1993 Evaluation of right ventricular function during aortic operations. Arch Surg 128: 582-584
Veith FJ 1994 Presidential address: transluminally placed endovascular stented grafts and their impact on vascular surgery. J Vasc Surg 20: 855-860
White GH, Yu W, May J, Stephen MS, Waugh RC 1994 A new nonstented balloon-expandable graft for straight or bifurcated endoluminal bypass. J Endovasc Surg 1: 16-24
White JV, Hass K, Phillips S, Comerota AV 1993 Adventitial elastolysis is a primary event in aneurysm formation. J Vasc Surg 17: 371-381
Wolinsky H, Glagov S 1967 Nature of species differences in the medial distribution of aortic vasa vasorum in mammals. Circ Res 20: 409-421
Yusef SW, Baker DM, Chuter TAM, Whitaker SC, Wenham PW, Hopkinson BR 1994 Transfemoral endoluminal repair of abdominal aortic aneurysm with bifurcated graft. Lancet 344: 650-651
Yusef SW, Hopkinson BR 1995 Endovascular repair of aortic aneurysm. Br J Surg 82: 289-290
Yusef SW, Whitaker SC, Chuter TAM, Wenham PW, Hopkinson BR 1995 Emergency endovascular abdominal aortic aneurysm repair. Lancet 344: 1645
Zatina MA, Zarins CK, Gewertz BL, Glagov S 1984 Role of medial lamellar architecture in the pathogenesis of aortic aneurysms. J Vasc Surg 1: 442-448

3

Recent advances in cardiopulmonary support

A. A. Majid

Techniques of cardiopulmonary support were introduced into clinical practice in the early 1950s. Cardiopulmonary bypass (CPB), pioneered by Gibbon (1954) was initially a risky and technically demanding procedure which could only be attempted in a few highly specialised centres (Aird et al 1954). The mortality rate was high and the procedure might never have become popular but for the work of Kirklin to refine and enhance its safety (Kirklin et al 1955). The procedure has since been further improved and simplified and is now performed routinely all over the world. Further research in the field of cardiopulmonary support has resulted in an expansion of its scope and many new cardiac and pulmonary support devices and procedures have been devised. This chapter will attempt to provide an overview of developments and highlight topics of current interest in the areas of CPB, cardiac support and pulmonary support.

CARDIOPULMONARY BYPASS

Perfusion

During CPB, a pump takes over the mechanical functions of the heart and an oxygenator performs the ventilatory functions of the lungs. Using special cannulae, venous blood is withdrawn from the right atrium, vena cava or a large vein such as the femoral vein. It then enters the CPB circuit where it is oxygenated, cooled or rewarmed and then returned to the aorta or a large artery such as the femoral artery. Although a number of different pumps have been used, the roller pump, based on a design by DeBakey, remains the most popular. In this pump, blood within a plastic tube is squeezed forward by rotating rollers against a back plate and non-pulsatile flow is generated. Flow rate is dependent on the speed of rotation of the rollers and a large range of flow rates can be provided by using tubing of various sizes. Besides the roller pump, the centrifugal pump introduced in 1978, is now also being used in a number of centres. There are two types of centrifugal pump, one that uses an impeller to generate flow and another that uses rotating cones to create a controlled vortex. The flow rate in these pumps is greatly influenced by the afterload and unlike the roller pump is not necessarily related to pump speed. Special flow meters are therefore required to measure flow rate.

With regard to perfusion, three factors need to be considered – flow rate, perfusion pressure and pressure waveform (laminar or pulsatile flow). Although the normal resting adult cardiac output at normothermia is 2.8 $l/min/m^2$, perfusion flow rates of this order result in high pressures within the pump tubing, increased blood trauma and an increase in collateral blood flow which may interfere with the intracardiac procedure. Hypothermia decreases metabolic rate and demand for substrates and allows a lower flow rate to be tolerated. Some degree of hypothermia is therefore employed during CPB so that the perfusion flow rate can be reduced. The flow rates used must however match metabolic demand. Flow rates of 2.2–2.5 $l/min/m^2$ are used for paediatric or adult CPB at normothermia or moderate hypothermia (Kirklin & Kirklin 1990) and there is evidence that these flow rates are more than adequate for the anaesthetised patient. Whole body oxygen consumption as indicated by mixed venous oxygen saturations (Kirklin & Kirklin 1981) is commonly used as a guide to adequacy of perfusion. However, because of regional differences in oxygen consumption as well as shunting to skeletal muscle during CPB (Lazenby et al 1992), mixed venous saturation will not be able to detect inadequate perfusion to specific organs. This factor becomes important if flow rates are reduced during the operative procedure. Since certain situations may require reduction in flow rate, recent investigations have been directed at determining the minimum flow rates that can be used at different depths of hypothermia. A flow rate of 1.6–1.8 $l/min/m^2$, has been identified as being essential to provide adequate oxygenation during moderate hypothermia (Tominaga et al 1993). For deep hypothermia, a minimum flow rate of 0.8 $l/min/m^2$ has been reported (Matsuda et al 1992). Other indices for minimal acceptable low flow CPB have been suggested (Kern et al 1993). Interestingly, patients on long-term beta-blockade have a lower than normal oxygen consumption on CPB (Karzai et al 1994) and infusion of prostaglandin E_1 increases oxygen extraction during low flow CPB (Tominaga et al 1993). These findings offer alternative approaches to alteration of metabolism which may have possible future clinical applications.

The perfusion pressure during CPB should be monitored and controlled. Too high a perfusion pressure raises the pressure within the CPB circuit with the risk of rupture of the circuit, and too low a perfusion pressure may compromise flow through vital organs. It has been demonstrated that autoregulatory mechanisms to maintain organ perfusion may not operate below certain pressures (Sadahiro et al, 1994) and may be abolished in children by moderate or deep hypothermia (Taylor et al 1992). Thus, although some degree of hypotension may be tolerated by adults (Slogoff et al 1990), a perfusion pressure in excess of 50 mmHg is probably advisable, especially in patients with pre-existing organ dysfunction.

Pulsatile flow was fashionable in the 1980s. It was thought that this mode of perfusion would provide better flow through the microcirculation than laminar flow. Roller pumps were thus modified to generate pulsatile flow but, despite extensive studies, no significant benefit could be ascribed to its use. In addition, because of the risk of damage to membrane oxygenators as a result of the high pressures generated within the CPB circuit, pulsatile flow became less popular. Wright (1994) in an important review has drawn attention to the difference in pulsatile power generated by the left ventricle (LV) compared to the pulsatile power generated by modified roller pumps. The LV generates 111 ± 14 mW per stroke, whereas the pulsatile power provided by pulsatile flow systems in clinical practice is only 2 mW. Thus, although arterial waveforms may appear to be pulsatile, they do not impart the same amount of energy to the circulation as the left ventricle. Since the difference in power between laminar flow and pulsatile flow systems is negligible, it is not surprising that few differences have been observed between 'pulsatile' and laminar flow. Future attempts to simulate pulsatile flow as well as investigations into the physiology and benefits of true pulsatile flow must also take into consideration haemodynamic power and impedance.

Oxygenation

Oxygenators available today are a vast improvement on earlier models. There are two types in use, bubble oxygenators and membrane oxygenators.

Bubble oxygenators

These consist of an oxygenating column, a defoaming compartment and an arterial reservoir. In the oxygenating column, oxygen is bubbled through fine holes and mixes with the deoxygenated blood so that oxygenation and carbon dioxide removal occur. Next, a sponge or mesh coated with antifoaming agents removes the remaining bubbles in the defoaming compartment. The blood then enters the reservoir where it collects before being pumped back to the patient.

Membrane oxygenators

The materials used for the early membrane oxygenators were generally unsatisfactory because of poor gas exchange and excessive plasma and fluid losses. A silicone polymer, polydimethylsiloxane (PDMS) was then found to allow gas transfer to occur by diffusion and as such to behave like a true semipermeable membrane. It was also not associated with plasma and fluid leakage and an oxygenator using this material was developed (Kolobow & Bowman 1963) and is still in use. More recently microporous polypropylene with pore sizes in the range of 0.3–0.7 μm has been introduced. Gases pass through the micropores in the form of microbubbles and do not diffuse across as in a true membrane. Oxygenators which use this material are thus not strictly 'membrane' oxygenators although this term is used when referring to them. Unlike PDMS oxygenators, polypropylene oxygenators cannot be used for extended periods because permeability to plasma and fluid occurs after a few hours.

Membrane oxygenators are designed to maximise gas transfer as well as to limit resistance to blood flow. Three principal designs are currently available:

the spiral coil, plate and screen and hollow fibre designs. The hollow fibre configuration consists of capillary tubes with an internal diameter of the order of 200–400 μm and in current models oxygen is passed through the fibres whilst the blood flows outside them. Compared to bubble oxygenators, membrane oxygenators are known to cause less platelet destruction, less microembolism and less complement activation. In addition, they allow independent control of pO_2 and pCO_2 levels, something that is not possible in bubble oxygenators because CO_2 removal depends on oxygen flow rate. As a result, the newer more competitively priced 'membrane' (polyethylene) oxygenators are replacing bubble oxygenators.

Oxygen carriers

The possibility of perfluorocarbons (PFC) being used as a chemical oxygenator by mixing oxygenated PFC with deoxygenated blood is currently under investigation. Oxygenation is achieved by passage of droplets of oxygenated PFC through a blood column or by agitation of a mixture of blood and the oxygenated PFC (Sueda et al 1993). The PFC is subsequently separated from the blood and the oxygenated blood is reinfused. Although results in experimental animals are encouraging, peripheral microemboli are a problem and more efficient separation techniques are required.

Pathophysiology of cardiopulmonary bypass

Systemic inflammatory response

We are just beginning to understand the many pathophysiological effects caused by cardiopulmonary bypass. It is now realised that CPB provokes a systemic inflammatory response, largely initiated by exposure of blood to abnormal surfaces. This exposure is thought to cause activation of the coagulation, fibrinolytic, kallikrein and complement cascades which then interact with each other and amplify their respective effects. The coagulation cascade is activated despite anticoagulation with heparin and subclinical intravascular coagulation occurs. The activated fibrinolytic system results in hyperfibrinolysis (Teufelsbauer et al 1992). The activated kallikrein-bradykinin system increases vascular permeability and dilates arterioles. The complement system produces the anaphylatoxins c3a, c4a and c5a which cause cell lysis and altered vascular permeability (Chenoweth et al 1981). It also activates leukocytes which release damaging elastases and oxygen free radicals. Several cytokines are now thought to be involved in mediating this systemic inflammatory response. Interleukin-6 levels may be a major mediator of the acute phase response to CPB (Butler et al 1992) and interleukin-1, by activating interleukin-8, may be involved in the recruitment and activation of leucocytes (Finn et al 1993, Kalfin et al 1993). Endotoxins may also enter the circulation as a result of the reduced splanchnic flow associated with CPB (Rocke et al 1987). The net result of all these changes is panendothelial injury, tissue oedema and some degree of multiorgan dysfunction (Moat et al 1993). Although many patients withstand these effects very well, deterioration may occur in patients with pre-existing organ dysfunction.

Hormonal changes

The massive release of catecholamines associated with CPB has been well documented. Other hormones are also affected. Thyroid hormone metabolism is altered resulting in the 'euthyroid sick syndrome' (Holland et al 1991) in which there is depression of T3 and free T3 concentrations with a concomitant increase in reverse T3. There is transient suppression of the pituitary-thyroid axis in the neonate (Mainwaring et al 1994). Subtle changes in hormone levels can be difficult to interpret, especially where hormones have a short half-life or when there are complex interactions with receptors (Majid & Ch'ng 1994).

Blood trauma

Blood trauma is another undesirable effect of CPB. Haemolysed cells release free haemoglobin, damaged white cells release enzymes, platelets lose their granules and plasma proteins, including clotting factors, are denatured. Prolonged periods of CPB are thus not well tolerated and CPB times of 4 h or more are associated with significant morbidity and mortality. Cavitation, shear stress, exposure to abnormal surfaces and direct physical trauma result in damage to the formed and soluble components of blood. The pumps, oxygenators (especially bubble oxygenators), cardiotomy suckers and the jet effect at the aortic cannula all contribute to blood trauma; the cardiotomy sucker has been identified as the single most damaging agent. Pump induced haemolysis is caused by surface and shear effects within the pumps. The proportion of surface and shear effects varies with the type of pump, flow rate and pressure. There is a relationship between the index of haemolysis, and the pressure, flow rate and the type of pump (Tamari et al 1993). The centrifugal pump causes less haemolysis in high flow, low resistance circuits (used in adult CPB), and the roller pump in low flow high resistance circuits (used in paediatric CPB).

Both a quantitative as well as a qualitative platelet defect occurs with CPB. Haemodilution is largely responsible for the quantitative platelet deficiency. There are two aspects to the qualitative platelet defect. Loss of alpha granules can be demonstrated in 30% of circulating platelets at the end of CPB (Rinder et al 1991a). In addition, all platelets demonstrate changes in their surface adhesion proteins and have a diminished ability to adhere and to aggregate and hence to contribute towards haemostasis (Rinder et al 1991b).

Neurological sequelae

Neurological sequelae have been reported in up to 30% of patients undergoing CPB. In adults, strokes have been documented in 5% and neurological dysfunction has been detected in 20–30% of adult patients (Shaw et al 1985, 1987, Townes et al 1989, Frye et al 1992). In children, detectable neurological deficits have been reported in up to 25% (Ferry 1990). The causes are multifactorial. Hypoperfusion, either deliberate or inadvertent, during CPB may cause global ischaemia. In addition, transient global ischaemia as evidenced by jugular bulb desaturation can occur during the rewarming phase of CPB (Croughwell et al 1992). Its significance in relation to neurological dysfunction however still requires further study. Alterations in cerebral blood flow occur as a result of changes in pH and pCO_2 and these are influenced to a great extent by the strategy chosen to manage these variables during hypothermia (alpha stat or pH stat, see below). Underlying cerebrovascular and carotid artery disease may only become manifest with the institution of CPB, especially in older patients.

Atherosclerotic disease of the ascending aorta as demonstrated by intraoperative ultrasonography is also more common than previously appreciated (Wareing et al, 1992). It is becoming apparent that cannulation, and the application of cross clamps and side clamps may be major causes of strokes after CPB by dislodging atheromatous plaques from the ascending aorta. Patients with an atherosclerotic aorta who have undergone CPB have a much higher incidence of emboli of atherosclerotic material compared to others (Blauth et al 1992).

Besides particulate emboli, gaseous emboli are a recognised cause of neurological morbidity. Massive air embolism as a result of human error or equipment malfunction has been estimated to occur in about 1: 1000 cases (Kurusz & Wheeldon 1990). Gaseous emboli can also be detected during aortic cannulation. Gaseous microemboli detected by ultrasonography have been found to be more frequently present when bubble oxygenators rather than membrane oxygenators are used (Pearson 1986).

Measures aimed at minimising the risk of CPB

Modulation of the systemic inflammatory and hormonal responses

Materials which stimulate the immune response should not be used in the CPB circuit. As an example, the nylon mesh liner in some bubble oxygenators was found to activate complement. Heparin-coated circuits may help to reduce complement activation (Pekna et al 1994). Ultrafiltration techniques to reduce total body water to counteract the capillary leak associated with CPB are beneficial (Elliott 1993). Leucocyte filters have not yet been found to be useful because of difficulties with biocompatibility and efficacy; cellulose filters whilst efficacious, activate the complement cascade, whilst polyester filters are not very efficacious (Gu et al 1993). The 'euthyroid sick syndrome' can be treated by intravenous t3 administration (Clarke 1993). Antithrombin III administered during CPB can prevent subclinical coagulation but also carries a risk of infection because of its origin from many donors (Hashimoto 1994).

Hypothermia: pH stat or alpha stat?

The strategy to be employed with respect to pH and pCO_2 during hypothermia has generated much discussion. Maintenance of an arterial blood pH of 7.4 and a pCO_2 of 40 mmHg at 37°C is necessary to optimise the efficiency of enzyme systems. Hypothermia changes both the rates of activity of enzymes as well as the pH of water which has a pH of 6.8 at 37°C, but becomes more alkaline as it is cooled. Similarly, blood with a pH of 7.4 at 37°C, has a pH of 7.7 at 20°C. It is not clear how the pH of a hypothermic patient should best be managed. In the 'pH stat' strategy, the pH is strictly maintained at 7.4 even as the blood cools. In the 'alpha stat' strategy, the pH is allowed to drift with hypothermia and it is aimed to have a pH of 7.4 on rewarming of the blood to 37°C. At moderate hypothermia (25–28°C), the difference in pH between the two strategies is not wide enough to be of clinical significance (Rogers et al 1992). However in patients undergoing deep hypothermia (20°C) the differences between the two strategies is likely to be more marked and studies are underway to compare the effects of each of these strategies.

Minimising anaesthetic morbidity

The anaesthetic management of CPB patients is undergoing a minor revolution with the introduction of techniques to hasten postoperative recovery. Conventional high dose opiate anaesthesia which has been used to reduce stress in the perioperative period and decrease the risk of perioperative myocardial infarction and ischaemia has led in some cases to prolonged periods of ventilation with all its attendant complications. The new 'fast track' techniques which aim for early extubation, within 8–10 h of completion of the operation, use a combination of low to medium dose opiates, inhalational agents and short acting intravenous agents. Advantages that have been put forward include improved cardiac and respiratory function and patient comfort, as well as reduction in demand for intensive care facilities (Chong et al 1993). Reservations concerning myocardial ischaemia after bypass continue to be expressed and the subject requires further clarification. Central to the success of a 'fast track' approach is the need to identify those patients who might be suitable for early extubation and those who would be better managed by the conventional method of overnight sedation and ventilation with extubation the following day. New risk scoring systems have been described for patients undergoing CPB. Emergency cases, renal dysfunction, age and reoperation have been identified as important risk factors (Tuman et al 1992, Higgins et al 1992). Length of operating time is also a risk factor and so procedures and surgeons who require a long operating time are important variables. All the above factors require careful consideration before a particular anaesthetic technique is chosen.

Blood conservation

Blood conservation strategies can be broadly grouped into those that aim to reduce blood loss and those that aim to salvage blood. Reduced loss can be achieved by the use of a non-blood prime, meticulous surgical technique and short CPB. Pharmacological interventions have been useful. Aprotinin in particular has been very effective in preserving platelet function and reducing postoperative bleeding (Bidstrup et al 1993). Acute normovolaemic haemodilution entails withdrawal of blood before the start of the operation and retransfusion at the end of the procedure. Although attractive in theory, the volume of blood which can be withdrawn and protected from the effects of CPB is small.

Salvage techniques using the haemofilter can be used intraoperatively after CPB to save significant amounts of blood remaining in the extracorporeal circuit. Shed blood from the mediastinum can also be collected and retransfused but since it does not contain clotting factors and has a low haematocrit its value is doubtful.

Minimising neurological injury

Intraoperative ultrasonography can be used to determine the presence of plaques in the ascending aorta so that cannulation can be performed at alternative sites. A 40 μm filter and bubble trap on the arterial side of the CPB circuit may be useful in reducing gaseous microemboli. A membrane oxygenator rather than a bubble oxygenator may also reduce the incidence of gaseous microemboli. However, in the event of accidental emptying of the reservoir, membrane oxygenators cannot prevent significant quantities of air from entering the circulation. A valve incorporated in the reservoir is an effective means of preventing air from entering the circulation (Mehra et al 1994). In the event of a massive air embolus, recent reports indicate that prompt transfer to a hyperbaric oxygen chamber is an effective means of salvage of an otherwise hopeless situation (Kol et al 1993).

Expansion of the indications for CPB

Newer indications for CPB are being investigated. CPB has been found to be useful for the salvage of patients after failed angioplasty (Teirstein et al 1993). The development of portable cardiopulmonary support systems has allowed patients whilst on full CPB to be transferred from one hospital to another by ground ambulance or even by helicopter (Bennett et al 1994). CPB is useful in the treatment of patients with hypothermia and CPB resuscitation is recommended for such patients in cardiac arrest and for all patients whose core temperatures is less than 25°C (Vretenar et al 1994). The place of cardiopulmonary support in acute emergencies is being explored and some interesting results are being obtained (Hill et al 1992). Experimental work is in progress to develop cannulae and techniques to provide CPB support with the eventual aim of supporting minimal access or cardioscopic surgery (Leggett & Shaw 1994).

CARDIAC SUPPORT

Pharmacological support

Rate, rhythm, preload, afterload and myocardial contractility are the well known determinants of cardiac performance. Derangement of these factors depresses cardiac performance which in turn evokes many neuroendocrine reflexes. It is now appreciated that these reflexes may not always be beneficial. Indeed some may even further depress cardiac performances by adversely affecting the abovementioned determinants. An immense amount of effort has been invested in investigating pharmacological means of supporting the circulation. With the above factors in mind, recent attention has focused on the inotropes, vasodilators, angiotensin converting enzyme (ACE) inhibitors and beta blockers.

Inotropes

Inotropes increase cardiac output by increasing contractility through a number of mechanisms. These mechanisms of action are the basis of a new classification system (Feldman 1993). Class I agents increase intracellular cyclic adenosine monophosphate and include the beta-adrenergic agonists and phosphodiesterase inhibitors. Class II agents, of which digoxin is an example, affect sarcolemmal ion pumps or channels. Class III agents, which are largely experimental, modulate intracellular calcium mechanisms. Class IV agents, such as pimobendan or vesnarinone, have multiple mechanisms of action. This system of classification potentially permits a better comparison of inotropes than a generic system.

Increase in contractility, however, is accompanied by increases in myocardial oxygen demand, a factor which may cause further injury to an already failing myocardium. Despite this, in acute heart failure, e.g. after myocardial infarction or after CPB, inotropes may be necessary to maintain tissue perfusion until other supportive measures can be initiated. Under these circumstances, intravenous infusion of inotropes is used. Some authorities advocate starting with less potent inotropes before changing to or adding more powerful agents, such as adrenaline (Barnard & Linter 1993), whilst others have advocated that strong inotropes with the appropriately tailored dosage be used particularly on weaning from CPB. Since inotropes also increase afterload, simultaneous intravenous infusion of a vasodilator (see below) together with close monitoring of haemodynamic parameters is usually necessary.

With regard to the management of chronic heart failure, the development of oral inotropic agents, such as milrinone, was initially greeted with some excitement since it was hoped that they would revolutionise the management of chronic heart failure. Instead, rather alarmingly, prolonged use has been associated with a higher rate of mortality from ventricular arrhythmias and they are now not used. This outcome is perhaps not too surprising given that inotropes make further demands on a failing myocardium. Although some success has been reported with short courses of intravenous infusions of inotropes in patients with severe congestive heart failure, overall, inotropes have not been very useful in the management of chronic heart failure. It is possible that the aims of therapy may have been too ambitious. Newer clinical approaches with more limited objectives, such as a pharmacological bridge to transplantation, as well as newer agents, e.g. vesnarinone, may yet define a role for inotropes in chronic heart failure.

Vasodilators

Vasodilators have recently enjoyed a resurgence of interest. For clinical purposes, they have been classified according to their site of action, i.e. venodilators, arterial dilators or mixed arteriovenous dilators. Venodilators decrease preload and reduce overstretching of the failing myocardium whilst arterial vasodilators decrease afterload and hence decrease myocardial work.

Although the initial therapy of acute heart failure may include careful intravenous infusions of vasodilators to reduce afterload, they are usually used in acute heart failure in combination with inotropes. Close monitoring of haemodynamic parameters, such as atrial filling pressures, blood pressure or cardiac output, is required when inotropes are used together with vasodilators. The need for inotropes and vasodilators varies according to the needs of each patient and thus the infusion rates have to be individually tailored. Short acting drugs with a rapid onset of action, such as sodium nitroprusside, are therefore preferred to facilitate ease of titration. Inhaled nitric oxide is also a useful vasodilator for patients with pulmonary hypertension since it does not affect systemic blood pressure.

In congestive cardiac failure, individual oral vasodilators have been shown to improve haemodynamics and exercise tolerance, whilst a combination of an arterial and venodilator has been shown to improve survival (Cohn 1986).

Angiotensin converting enzyme inhibitors

Although ACE inhibitors were originally introduced as antihypertensive agents, a number of clinical trials have convincingly demonstrated that they are useful in the management of chronic heart failure. They have even been found to be more beneficial than a combination of arterial and venodilators (Cohn 1991). The beneficial effects of ACE inhibitors were initially attributed to arterial vasodilation but other mechanisms which include increase in parasympathetic tone with restoration of autonomic balance, reduction of myocyte necrosis, as well as an increase in tissue bradykinin, may also be important. Better results are obtained when combined with diuretics than when administered as monotherapy.

Beta blockers

Rather surprisingly, small doses of beta blockers have been found to be beneficial in some patients with chronic heart failure. This approach, which was initially greeted with scepticism, has received increasing support from a number of small trials and it is thought that they act by reducing the undesirable effects of excessive adrenergic activity. This line of therapy is still under investigation, since a small but significant proportion of patients will in fact deteriorate with beta blockers.

In summary, for pharmacological support of acute heart failure, infusions of an inotrope with a vasodilator are used, whilst for chronic heart failure, ACE inhibitors and diuretics are to be preferred.

Cardiac support devices

Intra-aortic balloon pump

A number of ingenious devices to completely support the pulmonary, systemic or both circulations have been introduced in recent years. The intra-aortic balloon pump (IABP) is a device which augments the heart's action (Moulopoulos et al 1962). A balloon inserted via the femoral artery and positioned in the descending thoracic aorta is repeatedly inflated in diastole and deflated in systole. This decreases the afterload in systole and augments flow, especially coronary flow in diastole. Highly soluble gases such as helium or CO_2 are used to inflate the balloon to minimise the risk from gas embolism in the event of balloon rupture. In current models the timing of balloon inflation and deflation in relation to the cardiac cycle is quite precise. Aortic valve incompetence is a contraindication to its use and its effectiveness is limited in infants and children because of aortic elasticity, rapid heart rates, small stroke volume and difficulty of insertion. Two recent large reviews (Naunheim 1992, Cresswell 1992) revealed a high mortality rate (32.3–44%) associated with IABP insertion. These were related to six factors, pre-operative New York Heart Association functional class, transthoracic insertion, pre-operative administration of nitro-glycerine, age, female sex and pre-operative balloon insertion. Despite the overall high mortality, a good functional result was obtained in the survivors.

Haemopump

The Haemopump is a device designed to provide ventricular support. It consists of a cannula which is advanced across the aortic valve into the left ventricle; the other end of the cannula consists of an Archimedes screw. The screw is connected by a flexible drive catheter to a motor which rotates at high speed (15–27 000 rpm) and the rotation of the screw draws blood out of the ventricle and into the aorta. The device can be inserted via the femoral artery. Earlier models could generate flows of 4 l/min but the newer models can generate flows of 7–10 l/min. The main disadvantage of this device is platelet damage and this has limited its use to short-term support. A recent report has demonstrated that it can be used to provide support during coronary artery bypass grafting under special conditions (Lonn et al 1994).

Ventricular assist devices

Devices which mimic the design and functions of the ventricle have been created to provide extended cardiac support. Examples include the Thoratec, Novacor and Abiomed devices. In these devices, blood collects in a chamber similar to an atrium before entering the prosthetic ventricle. The prosthetic ventricle is lined by material designed to minimise the risk of thrombosis and has inlet and outlet valves similar to a normal ventricle. The valves may be mechanical (tilting disc), biological or polyurethane trileaflet valves. The 'ventricular contraction' is generated pneumatically or electrically (by a motor or solenoid) to cause a polyurethane sac or pusher plate to eject blood from the ventricle. In the case of a left ventricular assist device, the inlet is connected to the left atrium or the left Apex and the outlet to the aorta, whilst a right ventricular assist device is connected to the right atrium and the pulmonary artery. Two such devices may be used for biventricular support. The device or devices may be located extracorporeally or implanted in the chest or abdomen. Power supply lines connect the device to an external control console and power source in the case of so-called tethered devices. Fully implanted assist devices powered by a battery pack allow full patient mobility. These devices have been used for support after CPB, and as a bridge to transplantation. Improvements in design and clinical management now allow extended periods of support of over 500 days with a good quality of life. A recent editorial (Frazier 1994) argues the case for discharging these patients from hospital and their management as outpatients. Recently, these devices have also been implanted with the aim of permanent support of the left ventricle.

Total artificial heart

The total artificial heart (TAH) was first implanted in a human as a bridge to transplantation (Cooley et al 1969). Subsequently, beginning in 1982, several TAHs were implanted with the aim of permanent replacement of the native heart. The Jarvik 7 was pneumatically driven and had two ventricles each with an inlet and outflow valve. Unfortunately the aim of a permanent replacement could not be met as the patients suffered dreadful complications related to bleeding, infection and thromboembolism. Their use as a permanent heart replacement was thus discarded and they were used as a bridge to transplantation. However, here too, serious infective and thromboembolic complications occurred resulting in much poorer results being obtained compared to those achieved with left ventricular assist devices.

Based on this experience, a more cautious approach is being made to create a TAH. Currently there are 3 groups in the USA supported by the National Heart, Lung and Blood Institute who are developing an implantable electrically powered TAH with the aim of producing a device suitable for use in end stage heart disease by the year 2000. Such a device would have to fulfil some daunting requirements: they must be sufficiently small to fit into the chest, be minimally thrombogenic, must not predispose to infection, and must be able to produce an adequate cardiac output for at least 5 years without need for servicing (McCarthy et al 1994).

Myoplastic procedures

Cardiomyoplasty was first reported by Carpentier & Chachques (1985). In the modified procedure, which is now known as dynamic cardiomyoplasty, the left or right latissimus dorsi is wrapped around the heart and stimulated by a muscle stimulator in synchrony with ventricular contraction. Several weeks of conditioning are needed before it can be useful. The procedure carries an operative mortality of more than 20%. Best results have been obtained in patients with dilated cardiomyopathy as well as patients in New York Heart Association functional Class III (where Class III refers to those patients who have symptoms with less than ordinary activity). The operative mortality in both these groups is less than 10%. In the survivors, improvement in functional class has been noted, although haemodynamic improvement has not been documented. The mechanism of action of the dynamic cardiomyoplasty is more likely to be through prevention of further distension of the failing heart rather than by augmentation of ventricular contraction.

Aortomyoplasty, described by the same group (Chachques et al 1994), is a further development in the use of the latissimus dorsi as a means of cardiac support and has been tested in experimental animals. In their technique, the ascending aorta is first enlarged with a patch and the latissimus dorsi is subsequently wrapped round the 'neoventricle'. This neoventricle is then stimulated to contract during diastole. They report encouraging results in providing long-term diastolic augmentation.

The skeletal muscle ventricle is another experimental approach which is being explored. In this technique, a ventricle is fashioned from the latissimus dorsi and connected to the thoracic aorta and used as a diastolic counterpulsator. Although effective, the technique suffers from a high incidence of ventricular rupture and is not yet ready for clinical use.

Device selection

Now that the number of devices and procedures available for cardiac support has increased, the next few years will see more intense evaluation with the identification of the best devices as well as their most appropriate indications. The reader is referred to The Society of Thoracic Surgeons (STS) Practice Guidelines for transplantation and heart assist devices where the current indications, contraindications, procedure and expected outcome are detailed (Kaiser 1994).

PULMONARY SUPPORT

The limitations of mechanical ventilation have prompted research into alternative methods of pulmonary support. Extracorporeal membrane oxygenation (ECMO) is a term which has been used to refer to a technique in which the membrane oxygenator is used as an artificial lung to provide oxygenation and CO_2 removal in patients with respiratory failure. This technique has been used in adults, neonates and infants. It involves perfusion of the patient's blood through an oxygenator. The technique has been most successful in neonates with respiratory distress syndrome secondary to meconium aspiration and to a lesser extent in infants with congenital diaphragmatic hernia. Perfusion circuits which involve veno-arterial, veno-venous and arteriovenous routes of removal and return have been used. Best results have been obtained using the veno-arterial technique in which the right internal jugular vein and right common carotid artery are cannulated.

By contrast, the results of ECMO in adults with respiratory failure have been poor and alternative approaches have been explored. Gattinoni et al (1980) proposed that, in patients with acute respiratory failure, areas of normal lung should be protected from the effects of barotrauma associated with mechanical ventilation. They used more gentle modes of ventilation and positive end expiratory pressure to achieve oxygenation through the normal alveoli, and used the 'oxygenator' primarily to remove CO_2. The technique which they refer to as extracorporeal CO_2 removal ($ECCO_2R$) gave encouraging results in patients with adult respiratory distress syndrome (ARDS) but haemorrhage was a major problem. Combination of $ECCO_2R$ with low frequency positive pressure ventilation has resulted in improved outcome (Brunet 1994). Haemorrhage remains a problem but there are improved prospects with the newer heparin bonded oxygenator circuits.

The IVOX is another recent innovation for pulmonary support. It is an oxygenator which is implanted intravenously in the inferior vena cava and straddles the right atrium to reach the superior vena cava. It consists of bundles of crimped hollow polyethylene fibres covered with siloxane and bonded heparin. Oxygen is passed through the fibres and gas exchange occurs across the walls of the hollow fibres. Whilst Phase I clinical trials demonstrated its safety, Phase II trials on patients with ARDS have failed to demonstrate significant clinical benefit. Further improvement in gas exchange capability is required and improvements currently being considered include alterations in pattern of crimping, increase in pore density and increase in number of fibres.

CONCLUSIONS

A great deal of progress has been made in the field of cardiopulmonary support since the pioneering days of Gibbon and his contemporaries. Equipment, techniques and drugs have greatly improved but perhaps more importantly, we are beginning to understand a little better the pathophysiological changes which occur when pharmacological and mechanical support systems are initiated. Progress will undoubtedly be accelerated and the next few years will be very exciting indeed.

KEY POINTS FOR CLINICAL PRACTICE

Cardiopulmonary bypass

- Techniques of CPB are now well established and the indications for CPB are expanding.
- The systemic inflammatory response is being increasingly recognised as an important cause of morbidity, which is increased in patients with preexisting organ dysfunction.
- Atherosclerosis of the ascending aorta is a significant cause of neurological deficits particularly in elderly patients. Intraoperative ultrasonography is a more sensitive means of identifying aortic plaques than palpation.

Cardiac support

- The intraaortic balloon pump is still the most widely used cardiac support device. The newer ventricular assist devices are giving improved results and are capable of providing intermediate term support.

Pulmonary support

- Extracorporeal membrane oxygenation is the treatment of choice for neonates with respiratory distress syndrome secondary to meconium aspiration.

REFERENCES

Aird I, Melrose DG, Cleland WP, Lynn RB 1954 Assisted circulation by pump oxygenator during operative dilatation of the aortic valve in man. BMJ 1: 1284-1287

Barnard MJ, Linter SPK 1993 Acute circulatory support. BMJ 307: 35-40

Bennett JB, Hill JG, Long WB et al 1994 Interhospital transport of the patient on extracorporeal cardiopulmonary support. Ann Thorac Surg 57: 107-111

Bidstrup BP, Harrison J, Royston D et al 1993 Aprotinin therapy in cardiac operations: a report on use in 41 cardiac centres in the United Kingdom. Ann Thorac Surg 55: 971-976

Blauth CI, Cosgrove DM, Webb BW et al 1992 Atheroembolism from the ascending aorta. An emerging problem in cardiac surgery. J Thorac Cardiovasc Surg 103: 1104-1112

Brunet F, Mira JP, Belghith M et al 1994 Extracorporeal CO_2 removal combined with low frequency positive pressure ventilation. Am J Resp Crit Care Med 149: 1447-1462

Butler J, Chong GL, Baigrie RJ et al 1992 Cytokine responses to cardiopulmonary bypass with membrane and bubble oxygenation. Ann Thorac Surg 53: 833-838

Carpentier A, Chachques JC 1985 Myocardial substitution with a stimulated skeletal muscle: first successful clinical case. Lancet ii: 1267

Chachques JC, Haab F, Cron C et al 1994 Long term effects of dynamic aortomyoplasty. Ann Thorac Surg 58: 128-134

Chenoweth DE, Cooper WW, Hugli TE 1981 Complement activation during cardiopulmonary bypass; evidence for generation of C3a and C5a anaphylatoxins. N Engl J Med 304: 497-503

Chong JL, Grebenik C, Sinclair M et al 1993 The effect of a cardiac surgical recovery area on timing of extubation. J Cardiothorac Vasc Anaesth 7: 137-141

Clarke RE 1993 Cardiopulmonary bypass and thyroid metabolism. Ann Thorac Surg 56 (Suppl 1): 535-541

Cohn JN, Archibald DG, Ziesche S et al 1986 Effect of vasodilator therapy on mortality and chronic congestive heart failure: results of a veterans administration cooperative study. N Engl J Med 314: 1547-1552
Cohn JN, Johnson G, Ziesche S et al 1991 A comparison of enalapril with hydralazine-isosorbide dinitrate in the treatment of chronic congestive heart failure. N Engl J Med 325: 303-310
Cooley DA, Liotta D, Hallman GL et al 1969 Orthotopic cardiac prosthesis for two-staged cardiac replacement. Am J Cardiol 24: 723-730
Creswell LJ, Rosenbloom M, Cox JL et al 1992 Intraaortic balloon counterpulsation: patterns of usage and outcome in cardiac surgery patients. Ann Thorac Surg 54: 11-20
Croughwell ND, Frasco P, Blumenthal JA et al 1992 Warming during cardiopulmonary bypass is associated with jugular bulb desaturation. Ann Thorac Surg 53: 827-832
Elliott M 1993 Ultrafiltration and modified ultrafiltration in paediatric open heart operations. Ann Thorac Surg 56: 1518-1522
Feldman AM 1993 Classification of positive inotropic agents. J Am Coll Cardiol 22: 1223-1227
Ferry PC 1990 Neurologic sequelae of open heart surgery in children. Am J Dis Child 144: 369
Finn A, Naik S, Klein N et al 1993 Interleukin-8 release and neutrophil degranulation after paediatric cardiopulmonary bypass. J Thorac Cardiovasc Surg 105: 234-241
Frazier OH 1994 Outpatient LVAD: its time has arrived. Ann Thorac Surg 58: 1309-1310
Frye RL, Kronmal R, Schaff HV et al 1992 Stroke in coronary artery graft bypass surgery: an analysis of the CASS experience. Int J Cardiol 36: 213-221
Gattinoni L, Pesenti A, Rossi F et al 1980 Treatment of acute respiratory failure with low frequency positive-pressure ventilation and extracorporeal CO_2 removal. Lancet, ii, 292-294
Gibbon JH 1954 Application of a mechanical heart and lung apparatus to cardiac surgery. Minnesota Med 37: 171-185
Gu YJ, Obster R, Haan J et al 1993 Biocompatibility of leukocyte removal filters during leukocyte filtration of cardiopulmonary bypass perfusate. Artif Organs 17: 660-665
Hashimoto K, Yamagishi M, Sasaki T et al 1994 Heparin and antithrombin III levels during cardiopulmonary bypass: correlation with subclinical plasma coagulation. Ann Thorac Surg 58: 799-805
Higgins TL, Estafanous FG, Loop FD et al 1992 Stratification of morbidity and mortality outcome by preoperative risk factors in coronary bypass patients. A clinical severity score. JAMA 267: 2344-2348
Hill JG, Bruhn PS, Cohen SE et al 1992 Emergent applications of cardiopulmonary support: a multiinstitutional experience. Ann Thorac Surg 54: 699-704
Holland FW, Brown PS, Weintraub BD, Clarke RE 1991 Cardiopulmonary bypass and thyroid function: a 'euthyroid sick syndrome'. Ann Thorac Surg 52: 46-50
Kaiser GC 1994 Practice guidelines in cardiothoracic surgery. Ann Thorac Surg 58: 903-910
Kalfin RE, Engelman RM, Rousou JA et al 1993 Induction of interleukin-8 expression during cardiopulmonary bypass. Circulation 88 (suppl 5Pt2): II401-II406
Karzai W, Gunnicker M, Vorgrimuler-Karzai UM et al 1994 The effects of beta-adrenoceptor blockade on oxygen consumption during cardiopulmonary bypass. Anesth Analg 79: 19-22
Kern FH, Ungerleider RM, Reves JG et al 1993 Effect of altering pump flow rate on cerebral blood flow and metabolism in infants and children. Ann Thorac Surg 56: 1366-1372
Kirklin JW, DuShane JW, Patrick RT et al 1955 Intracardiac surgery with aid of mechanical pump-oxygenator system (Gibbon type) report of 8 cases. Proc Staff Meeting Mayo Clinic 30: 201-207
Kirklin JK, Kirklin JW 1981 Management of the cardiovascular system after cardiac surgery. Ann Thorac Surg 32: 311-319
Kirklin JK, Kirklin JW 1990 Cardiopulmonary bypass for cardiac surgery. In: Sabiston DC, Spencer FC (eds) Gibbon's diseases of the chest. p 1110
Kol S, Ammar R, Weisz G, Melamed Y 1993 Hyperbaric oxygenation for arterial air embolism during cardiopulmonary bypass. Ann Thorac Surg 55: 401-403
Kolobow T, Bowman RL 1963 Construction and evaluation of an alveolar membrane artificial heart-lung. Trans Am Soc Artif Organs 9: 238-243
Kurusz M, Wheeldon D 1990 Risk containment during cardiopulmonary bypass. Semin Thorac Cardiovasc Surg 2: 400-409

Lazenby WD, Ko W, Zelano JA et al 1992 Effects of temperature and flow rate on regional blood flow and metabolism during cardiopulmonary bypass. Ann Thorac Surg 53: 957-964

Legget ME, Shaw DP 1994 Fiberoptic cardioscopy under cardiopulmonary bypass: potential for cardioscopic surgery? Ann Thorac Surg 58: 222-225

Lonn U, Peterzen B, Granfeldt H, Casimir-Ahn H 1994 Coronary artery operation with support of the hemopump cardiac assist system. Ann Thorac Surg 58: 519-523.

Mainwaring RD, Lamberti JJ, Billman GF, Nelson JC 1994 Suppression of the pituitary thyroid axis after cardiopulmonary bypass in the neonate. Ann Thorac Surg 58: 107-182

Majid AA, Ch'ng SL 1994 Atrial natriuretic peptide, diuresis and cardiopulmonary bypass. Ann Thorac Surg 57: 1369-1370

Matsuda H, Sasako Y, Nakano S et al 1992 Determination of optimal perfusion flow rate for deep hypothermic cardiopulmonary bypass in the adult based on distributions of blood flow and oxygen consumption. J Thorac Cardiovasc Surg 103: 541-548

McCarthy PM, Fukamichi K, Fukumura F et al 1994 The Cleveland Clinic-Nimbus total artificial heart. In vivo hemodynamic performance in calves and preclinical studies. J Thorac Cardiovasc Surg 108: 420-428

Mehra AP, Akins A, Maisuria A, Glenville, BE 1994 Air handling characteristics of five membrane oxygenators. Perfusion 9: 357-362

Moat WE, Shore DF, Evans TW 1993 Organ dysfunction and cardiopulmonary bypass; the role of complement and complement regulatory proteins. Eur J Cardiothoracic Surg 7: 563-573

Moulopoulos SD, Topaz S, Kolff WJ 1962 Diastolic balloon pumping (with carbon dioxide) in the aorta. Mechanical assistance of the failing circulation. Am Heart J 63: 669-675

Naunheim KS, Swartz MT, Pennington DG et al 1992 Intraaortic balloon pumping in patients requiring cardiac operations. J Thorac Cardiovasc Surg 104: 1654-1661

Pearson D 1986 Microemboli: gaseous and particulate. In: Taylor KM ed Cardiopulmonary bypass. Chapman & Hall Medical, London, pp 315-330

Pekna M, Hagman L, Halden E et al 1994 Complement activation during cardiopulmonary bypass: effects of immobilised heparin. Ann Thorac Surg 58: 421-424

Rinder CS, Bohnert J, Rinder HM et al 1991a Platelet activation and aggregation during cardiopulmonary bypass. Anesthesiology 75: 388-393

Rinder C, Mathew J, Rinder H et al 1991b Modulation of platelet surface adhesion receptors during cardiopulmonary bypass. Anesthesiology 75: 563-570

Rocke DA, Gaffin SL, Wells MT et al 1987 Endotoxaemia associated with cardiopulmonary bypass. J Thorac Cardiovasc Surg 93: 832-837

Rogers AT, Prough DS, Roy RC 1992 Cerebrovascular and cerebral metabolic effects of alterations in perfusion flow rate during hypothermic cardiopulmonary bypass in man. J Thorac Cardiovasc Surg 103: 363-368

Sadahiro M, Haneda K, Mohri H 1994 Experimental study of cerebral autoregulation during cardiopulmonary bypass with or without pulsatile perfusion. J Thorac Cardiovasc Surg 108: 446-454

Shaw P, Bates D, Cartlidge NEF et al 1985 Early neurological complications of coronary artery bypass surgery. BMJ 291: 1384-1387

Shaw PJ, Bates D, Cartlidge NEF et al 1987 Long term intellectual dysfunction following coronary artery bypass graft surgery: a six month follow-up study. Q J Med 62: 259-268

Slogoff S, Reul GJK, Keats AS et al 1990 Role of perfusion pressure and flow in major organ dysfunction after cardiopulmonary bypass. Ann Thorac Surg 1990; 50: 911-918

Sueda T, Fukunaga S, Matsuura Y, Kajihara H 1993 Evaluation of two new liquid-liquid oxygenators. ASAIO J 39: 923-928

Tamari Y, Lee-Sensiba K, Leonard EF et al 1993 The effects of pressure and flow on haemolysis caused by Bio-Medicus centrifugal pumps and roller pumps; guidelines for choosing a blood pump. J Thorac Cardiovasc Surg 106: 997-1007.

Taylor RH, Burrows FA, Bissonnette B 1992 Cerebral pressure-flow velocity relationship during hypothermic cardiopulmonary bypass in neonates and infants. Anesth Analg 74: 636-642

Teirstein PS, Vogel RA, Dorros G et al 1993 Prophylactic versus standby cardiopulmonary support for high risk percutaneous transluminal coronary angioplasty. J Am Coll Cardiol 21: 590-596

Teufelsbauer H, Proidl S, Havel M, Vukovich T 1992 Activation of hemostasis during cardiopulmonary bypass: evidence for thrombin mediated hyperfibrinolysis. Thromb Haemost 68: 250-252

Tominaga R, Kurisu K, Fukumura F et al 1993 Effects of pump flow rate on oxygen use during moderate hypothermic cardiopulmonary bypass. ASAIO J 39: 126-131
Townes BD, Bashein G, Hornbein TF et al 1989 Neurobehavioural outcomes in cardiac operations. A prospective controlled study. J Thorac Cardiovasc Surg 98: 774-782
Tuman KJ, McCarthy RJ, March RJ et al 1992 Morbidity and duration of ICU stay after cardiac surgery. A model for preoperative risk assessment. Chest 102: 36-44
Vretenar DF, Urschel JD, Parrott JC, Unruh HW 1994 Cardiopulmonary bypass resuscitation for accidental hypothermia. Ann Thorac Surg 58: 895-898
Wareing TH, Davila-Roman VG, Barzilai B et al 1992 Management of the severely atherosclerotic ascending aorta during cardiac operations. A strategy for detection and treatment. J Thorac Cardiovasc Surg 103: 453-462
Wright G 1994 Haemodynamic analysis could resolve the pulsatile blood flow controversy. Ann Thorac Surg 58: 1199-1204.

4

Helicobacter pylori: an update for surgeons

M. M. Ozmen   R. Patankar   C. D. Johnson

Spiral organisms in the human stomach were first noted by Bottcher in 1874. Early in this century, spiral organisms were reported by several investigators and it is possible that the bacterium they observed was *Helicobacter pylori*. Academic interest did not return to a possible bacteriological aetiology of peptic ulcer disease until Steer, almost 100 years after the first description, carefully described a spiral organism with a patchy distribution deep in the layer of mucus covering the gastric cells. Unfortunately attempts to culture the bacterium were unsuccessful (Steer & Colin-Jones 1975).

The starting point of the huge wave of modern interest in *H. pylori* was in 1983, when Marshall & Warren described 'unidentified curved bacilli' which initially were named *Campylobacter pyloridis*. Characterisation of the organism's properties, including fatty acid composition and ribonucleic acid sequencing, indicated that it did not belong to the genus *Campylobacter*, and consequently in 1989, the organism was renamed *H. pylori*, representing the type species of a proposed new genus *Helicobacter* (Goodwin et al 1989). Since its discovery in 1983, overwhelming evidence has become available that *H. pylori* plays an important role in the pathogenesis of gastroduodenal disease. In this chapter, we will focus first on the current understanding of *H. pylori* and gastroduodenal disease and then discuss the effect of the bacterium and its eradication on surgical practice.

MICROBIOLOGICAL CHARACTERISTICS AND PATHOGENIC ASPECTS

H. pylori is a small curved, Gram-negative, microaerophilic rod with multiple polar flagellae. Its normal habitat is in the stomach of human and other primates, where it survives closely apposed to the gastric mucus secreting cells (Goodwin et al 1990). There, the action of bacterial urease creates an ecological niche in which the pH is neutral and the organism is protected from the acidic gastric juice (Lee 1991). Ammonia generated by *H. pylori* urease activity buffers the bactericidal hydrogen ions in gastric acidic juice, and provides a source of nitrogen for *H. pylori* (Blaser 1992). Besides its protective role, ammonia may also alter gastric epithelial permeability, impair the ionic integrity of mucus and cause hydrogen ion back-diffusion towards the gastric mucosa, resulting in mucosal injury (Hazell & Lee 1986).

H. pylori is intensely antigenic and secretes a number of enzymes and chemicals including urease, catalase, mucinase, lipase, phospholipase A_2, haemolysins and alkaline phosphatase, some of which reduce the viscosity of mucus. The production of catalase protects the bacterium against the toxic effects of reactive oxygen metabolites formed in neutrophils from H_2O_2. In fact, cellular damage may result from this host response and not directly from the bacterium itself, which may explain the heterogeneity of outcomes of infection.

The motility of *H. pylori* is probably due to its spiral shape and the presence of 4–6 flagellae; these permit the bacterium to penetrate the mucus layer and migrate to regions of moderate acidity. Adherence of *H. pylori* to gastric epithelial cells (Hessey et al 1990) and vacuolating cytotoxin production (Figura et al 1989) are considered virulence factors as they are associated with degenerative changes in epithelial cells (Hessey et al 1990). It is unclear which of those properties is mainly responsible for damaging the host cells.

Transmission and epidemiology

H. pylori is the commonest bacterial infection in the world, the prevalence increases with age. In the developing world, infection occurs early in childhood and the incidence is extremely high in the first few years of life approaching 10% per annum. The prevalence may rise to over 80% in young adults, whereas in the developed world, the prevalence rises approximately 0.5% with each year of life (Graham et al 1991).

The presence of *H. pylori* appears to be linked to socioeconomic status and an association between infection and lower educational attainment and with ethnic minorities and immigrants is known (Perez-Perez et al 1990). In a study from Texas, blacks had a higher infection rate earlier in life than whites, but after the age of 60, the prevalence was similar (Graham et al 1991).

The current evidence suggests that the only reservoirs for *H. pylori* are man and the rhesus monkey (Baskerwille & Newell 1988).

Although the route of transmission is still unknown, the high rate of infection in children from *H. pylori*-positive parents and the presence of the same strain within members of the same family suggest that close contact is very important for the spread of infection (Megrand 1993). Animal studies to identify the route of transmission failed to show faecal-oral transmission but did reveal oral-oral transmission (Lee 1991). *H. pylori* has been detected in saliva and dental plaque with PCR and has occasionally been cultured (Majmudar et al 1990) although we have been unable to confirm this using nested PCR (Ozmen et al 1995). *H. pylori* DNA has recently been isolated from faeces by PCR (Mapstone et al 1993) and from a source of drinking water in Peru. It is also capable of survival in river water (Shahamat et al 1989). Iatrogenic person to person transmission via endoscopes has been reported (Langenberg et al 1990) and the high prevalence of infection among endoscopists, particularly those who do not use gloves, suggests that transmission occurs through instruments contaminated with gastric secretions.

DIAGNOSIS

The presence of *H. pylori* can be detected by several different methods which can be classified as invasive and non-invasive tests. Rapid-urease tests (CLO-test), histology, cytology, culture and polymerase chain reaction (PCR) are all based on biopsy samples and need endoscopy. Non-invasive tests include serology and urea breath tests.

The main problem with invasive tests are potential sampling errors which may occur due to the patchy distribution of *H. pylori* in the gastric mucosa. This makes endoscopy-dependent tests relatively insensitive especially in the presence of scanty infection. The predictive value of diagnostic tests for *H. pylori* can be improved by taking more than one biopsy sample or by using more than one endoscopy-dependent test at the same time.

Culture

Culture of endoscopic samples is sensitive and specific, viable bacteria are detected and antibiotic sensitivities can be obtained. However, culture takes several days and results are dependent on the expertise of the operator and the laboratory. Failure to culture *H. pylori* may also result from sampling errors or a delay in plating material. Other factors that interfere with the ability to culture *H. pylori* include swallowed local anaesthetics, simethicone, prior treatment with bismuth, antibiotics or H_2-receptor antagonists and contamination of biopsy forceps with disinfectants. On the whole, culture of endoscopic biopsies for *H. pylori* is relatively expensive and unnecessary unless antibiotic sensitivities are required.

Histology

H. pylori can be seen on biopsy specimens stained by various staining processes, such as Warthin-Starry silver stain, Haemotoxylin-eosin, acridine orange, Giemsa and Browns-Hopps staining (Madam et al 1988).

Histology is operator dependent and scanty organisms may be missed by ordinary staining techniques. Diagnosis of the presence of *H. pylori* by histology tends to be inaccurate especially in the presence of scanty infection (Molyneux et al 1993).

Specific fluorescence techniques and *in situ* hybridisation using a biotinylated 109 base pair PCR product of *H. pylori* as the probe can be used for the detection of very scanty organisms persisting after eradication therapy. These techniques are also useful for the demonstration of coccoid forms or for identifying organisms which have gained access to the lamina propria, when conventional staining methods are insensitive (Dixon 1993). Our initial experience with immunofluorescence suggests that this can be a useful technique to increase diagnostic accuracy when numbers of organisms are small

Despite the low diagnostic sensitivity of the test, histology is the only way of investigating the histopathologic processes involved in infection with *H.*

pylori and results are improved using special stains and the services of an enthusiastic histopathologist.

Rapid urease tests

Rapid urease tests (CLO-test, etc.) are simple biochemical tests which involve placing an endoscopic biopsy into a small amount of solution containing urea, a pH indicator (phenol red) and a bacteriostatic agent. If *H. pylori* are present, the bacterial urease hydrolyzes the urea and produces ammonia. Alkalinisation of the medium produces a colour change from yellow to red. Results are read between 1 min and 24 h. The sensitivity and specificity of these methods are in the region of 95% (Tompkins 1993).

^{13}C or ^{14}C urea breath tests

Bacterial urease activity is also the basis for urea breath tests (UBT). The subject drinks a solution containing [^{13}C]- or [^{14}C]-urea along with a liquid fat meal to delay gastric emptying. If *H. pylori* are present in the stomach, urea is hydrolysed and labelled CO_2 appears in the breath. $^{14}CO_2$ is measured using a beta-counter; $^{13}CO_2$ is measured using an isotope ratio mass spectrometer (IRMS). The ^{14}C-UBT involves exposure to a small amount of radioactivity and must be used with caution in pregnant patients and children. UBT are non-invasive and highly sensitive for the diagnosis of *H. pylori* as the whole stomach is sampled; sensitivity and specificity of these tests is 98–99% (Rauws et al 1989, Logan 1992).

Serology

H. pylori infection can be detected by testing antibodies (IgA, IgG) in serum or saliva. Enzyme linked immunosorbent assay (ELISA) is the best method for serology because of its simplicity, reliability and low cost. ELISA has a sensitivity and specificity of over 90%. Performance of the tests is largely dependent on the antigen used, but is also influenced by age, ethnic group and experience and competence of laboratory personnel (Von Wulffen 1992). Seroconversion takes 22–33 days after infection and acute infection prior to detectable circulating antibody production gives false negative results (Morris et al 1987). Antibody tests may take several months to become negative after eradication.

Selection of test

Labelled UBT is the gold standard for assessment of eradication as well as for the initial diagnosis of infection as it samples the whole stomach. Serology appears in most instances to be the best method for epidemiological studies. If a patient is undergoing endoscopic examination, it is best to take samples for invasive tests and to perform rapid urease tests and histology. Histology is not reliable in the presence of atrophic gastritis, intestinal metaplasia and is inaccurate when infection is scanty. Culture should be performed when antibiotic sensitivity is needed. It is not routinely available and may provide false negative results in the early post-treatment period. At present, PCR is essentially a research tool and is a very sensitive way of detecting parts of the *H. pylori* genome and of identifying different subtypes. Specific probes are available for urease genes and 16S ribosomal RNA (Clayton et al 1992).

THE ROLE OF *H. PYLORI* IN GASTRODUODENAL DISEASE

Non ulcer dyspepsia (NUD)

NUD is estimated to occur in around 30% of the population of the US (Talley et al 1991a). NUD is usually defined as intermittent abdominal pain or symptoms centred in the upper abdomen in the absence of peptic ulceration as confirmed by endoscopy. Symptoms of NUD include abdominal pain, heartburn, early satiety, bloating, belching, postprandial fullness, nausea, vomiting, burping, and retching.

The term functional dyspepsia has been used in subjects who have no evidence of an organic cause. A variety of factors such as gastric acid hypersecretion, gastric and small intestinal motor disorders, psychological and neurohormonal factors and *H. pylori*-associated gastritis may play a role in the pathogenesis of NUD. *H. pylori* has been found in 39–87% of subjects with NUD, but no concrete evidence exists that *H. pylori* is commoner in patients with NUD, than in age and sex matched controls (Lambert 1993). There is conflicting evidence to relate *H. pylori*-associated inflammation and symptoms of dyspepsia. This results from poor definition of the term dyspepsia and the lack of appropriate comparable control groups. Nevertheless, improvement of symptoms of NUD has been shown after eradication of *H. pylori* (Van Zanten 1993). This may be more apparent in the long term than in the short term (McCarthy et al 1995). Probably the difference between the short-and long-term effect of eradication in this study occurred as a result of differences in the method of assessment of eradication. Initially, two endoscopy based tests (culture and histology) were used for this purpose but a year later the presence of *H. pylori* was determined by ^{13}C-UBT. It is likely that ^{13}C-UBT picked up more patients with *H. pylori* than the other two tests did. Our own experience of symptom assessment in over 70 NUD patients is that eradication of *H. pylori* relieves the symptoms in the vast majority of patients.

We believe that patients without an organic cause of dyspepsia, but with *H. pylori* infection, will benefit from eradication treatment. Double blind, placebo-controlled studies with long-term assessment of symptoms are needed to clarify the role and the effect of *H. pylori* eradication on symptom relief in patients with NUD.

Gastritis

It is widely accepted that colonisation of gastric surface epithelium by *H. pylori* is commonly associated with type B chronic gastritis and, characteristically, *H. pylori* gastritis predominantly affects the antrum. Antral mucosa shows superficial or full-thickness infiltration with lymphoid follicles. There is a positive correlation between the number of organisms seen and the number of polymorphonuclear leucocytes in infected tissue (Rautelin et al 1993). It has been shown that successful eradication of *H. pylori* leads to a significant improvement in acute and chronic gastritis and in the patient's symptoms (Valle et al 1991). While glandular atrophy is usually absent or mild, intestinal metaplasia is seen in subjects with chronic inflammation. The prevalence of *H. pylori* decreases with increasing degree of atrophy; Karnes et al (1991) showed that 86% of patients with atrophic gastritis were seropositive for *H. pylori*, but only 33% were diagnosed to have *H. pylori* infection on biopsy. *H. pylori* was also less prevalent in patients with intestinal metaplasia; this is easily understood because *H. pylori* cannot colonize intestinal metaplastic epithelium.

The development of atrophy and intestinal metaplasia was also observed in a long-term follow-up study in Finland (Sipponen et al 1992). The high prevalence of *H. pylori* gastritis and intestinal metaplasia in young members of a gastric cancer family has also been reported (Scott et al 1990). Although the link between *H. pylori* and type B gastritis is well established, the hypothesis that *H. pylori*-associated atrophic gastritis and intestinal metaplasia is a risk factor for gastric carcinogenesis still needs to be established and supported by clinical studies.

Duodenal ulcer

Although the prevalence of *H. pylori* in duodenal ulcer patients has been found to be between 95–100%, there is no direct relationship between *H. pylori* and duodenal ulcer and only a minority of individuals with *H. pylori* will develop a duodenal ulcer during their life (Tytgat et al 1990). There is, however, a clear association between duodenal ulcer disease and *H. pylori* gastritis (O'Donnell et al 1993). Eradication of *H. pylori* reduces the rate of ulcer recurrence. Gastritis and *H. pylori* infection appear to have a dual influence on ulcer risk, on protective and aggressive mechanisms, in accordance with the topography and grade of gastritis and atrophy in the stomach. Although gastritis increases ulcer risk, advanced atrophy in the corpus mucosa decreases the risk because of decreased acid secretion (Sipponen & Hyvarinen 1993). The main question in defining the role of *H. pylori* in duodenal ulcer is how *H. pylori* in the stomach can cause local damage in the duodenum.

This is explained by the presence of gastric metaplasia in the duodenum in patients with duodenal ulcer disease (Goodwin 1988). Evidence now exists that gastric metaplasia or the appearance of gastric mucus secreting cells in the duodenum represents an adaptive change of the duodenal mucosa in response to a high acidity in duodenal bulb (Wyatt et al 1990). When these patients are infected with *H. pylori* and develop antral gastritis, the organisms may spread to the metaplastic epithelium and cause duodenitis. As a result of inflammation and impaired mucosal defences, acid peptic attack on the weakened mucosa leads to erosive duodenitis and ulceration.

Exaggerated postprandial gastrin release is seen in duodenal ulcer patients while fasting serum gastrin is normal. It has been shown that *H. pylori* infection causes interruption of the physiologic mechanisms affecting gastrin-hydrochloric acid homeostasis (Bewett et al 1991). Other mechanisms in the production of hypergastrinemia include inflammatory mediators (IL-1, IL-6, TNF, leukotrienes C4 and D4), and impaired feedback of luminal acid to antral G cells as a result of *H. pylori* urease activity, which generates ammonia in the antral mucus layer (Mai et al 1990). Antral somatostatin content is low; this may be responsible for an increased activity of G cells and exaggerated meal-stimulated gastrin release (Kaneko et al 1992).

Though *H. pylori* infection may explain some of the mysteries of peptic ulcer disease, the association also poses the question of why ulcers develop in a very small percentage of people who have the organism.

Other risk factors, such as increased acidity, nature of the host inflammatory response, cigarette smoking and other genetic and environmental factors, probably contribute to ulceration in a subset of the population with *H. pylori* infection (Soll 1990). Alternatively, the ulcerogenic potential of the bacterial strains may be different. A vacuolizing cytotoxin is more likely to be present in *H. pylori* isolates from duodenal ulcer patients (Cover et al 1990). The presence of a 120 kD protein (Cag protein) in *H. pylori* is associated with the development of chronic active gastritis and duodenal ulcer (Crabtree et al 1991).

Overall, *H. pylori* is undoubtedly the dominant factor in the pathogenesis of peptic ulcer disease. There is, however, a small minority of duodenal ulcers where *H. pylori* has no effect, such as ulcers related to use of non steroidal anti-inflammatory drugs, Crohn's disease and in the Zollinger-Ellison syndrome.

Gastric ulcer

The relationship between *H. pylori* and gastric ulcer remains less clear, though it has been shown that gastric ulcer is associated with *H. pylori* in over 70% of patients. If drug induced ulcers are excluded, the prevalence of *H. pylori* approaches 96% (Tytgat et al 1990, Labenz 1994a). Chronic gastritis, which generally accompanies gastric ulceration, is a characteristically diffuse chronic pan-gastritis and exhibits both multifocal glandular atrophy and intestinal metaplasia.

H. pylori cytotoxins, high ammonia concentrations, formation of cross-reacting antibodies and liberation of neutrophil proteases and toxic oxygen radicals have all been suggested as contributors to atrophy (Marshall 1991, Negrini et al 1991). As in duodenal ulcer, a weakening in the mucosal defences may render the gastric wall susceptible to acid peptic attack. It has been shown that eradication of *H. pylori* speeds up gastric ulcer healing with a 6-week healing rate of about 85%, and refractory ulcers heal within 6–10 weeks after eradication of *H. pylori* (Labenz et al 1994a). Eradication also diminishes the recurrence rate of gastric ulcer, indicating that *H. pylori* plays a major aetiological role in gastric ulcer disease (Graham et al 1992).

Effect of H. pylori *on peptic ulcer healing*

The beneficial effect of *H. pylori* eradication on ulcer healing is clear for both duodenal and gastric ulcer. The mucosal damage and inflammatory processes regress following *H. pylori* eradication and rapid restoration of mucosal integrity is seen (O'Connor et al 1995). A number of studies have shown that patients after eradication of *H. pylori* had significantly more healed duodenal ulcers than those who remained *H. pylori* positive (66–95% vs 34–84%) (McCarthy 1993, Hentschel et al 1993). It has also been reported that duodenal ulcers with *H. pylori* will heal without acid suppression if *H. pylori* is eradicated (Hosking et al 1994). Eradication of *H. pylori* speeds up gastric ulcer healing and most refractory ulcers heal within 6–10 weeks after eradication of *H. pylori* on continued acid suppression with omeprazole (Labenz et al 1994a).

Role of *H. pylori* in ulcer relapse

Eradication of *H. pylori* is followed by a dramatic decrease in the rate of duodenal ulcer recurrence. Penston (1994) reviewed 20 studies in which patients were followed for 1 year after eradication. No recurrences were reported in 6 studies and 13 studies reported an ulcer recurrence rate of less than 10%; the overall rate of ulcer recurrence was 9%. The relapse rate in the 2nd year following eradication was 4–6%. Seven years after initial eradication of *H. pylori*, the ulcer relapse rate was found to be 11% proven by endoscopy or a barium study. Clinical relapse (defined as symptoms identical to previous symptoms) occurred in 22% of *H. pylori* negative patients whereas it was 54% in patients who had *H. pylori* infection (Forbes et al 1994).

The effect of eradication of *H. pylori* on gastric ulcer relapse has not been well established. However, in one study with 130 gastric ulcer patients, treated with either omeprazole or triple therapy, the relapse rate was 51% in the omeprazole group whereas only 3% of patients developed recurrent ulcer in the triple therapy group. Seppala et al (1992) also showed that successful eradication of *H. pylori* prevented gastric ulcer relapse, on the other hand 48% of non-eradicated patients developed a relapse. In the light of this evidence, it seems likely that eradication of *H. pylori* substantially reduces the rate of ulcer recurrence in patients with gastric ulcer.

Role of *H. pylori* in peptic ulcer complications

The major complications of peptic ulcer disease are bleeding, perforation, penetration and gastric outlet obstruction. The frequency of *H. pylori* infection in patients presenting with ulcer complications appears to be lower than in those presenting with uncomplicated disease.

Bleeding

Bleeding is the most frequent complication of chronic ulcer disease and 30% of bleeding ulcers bleed massively (Waren 1987). The risk of rebleeding is high and the mortality of first ulcer bleeding is 0.5–4%, rising to 16–29% in patients with rebleeding (Clason et al 1986). It has been reported that *H. pylori* eradication after acute ulcer bleeding prevents further bleeding episodes (Graham et al 1993, Labenz et al 1994b). In Labenz's study the rebleeding rate 17 months following eradication was zero, whereas in patients with *H. pylori* infection the rebleeding rate was 37%. It has also been reported that 3 days' intravenous treatment with omeprazole and amoxycillin followed by 11 days' oral treatment with the same drugs leads to ulcer healing. One month after this treatment, *H. pylori* eradication was seen in all patients with bleeding peptic ulcers who were managed conservatively (Adamek et al 1994). This finding is very important as initial treatment with only omeprazole in *H. pylori* positive patients with bleeding ulcers may reduce eradication rates.

Although these results are encouraging, more data and double-blind, randomised clinical studies with long-term follow-up are needed to elucidate the role of *H. pylori* in bleeding peptic ulcers.

Perforation

The role of *H. pylori* in perforated peptic ulcer disease is not clear. In one study of acute perforated duodenal ulcer, 48% of patients were *H. pylori* positive (Jensen et al 1992). Furthermore, in a study of patients with new duodenal ulcer disease, 26% of those with perforation were infected by *H. pylori* (Reinbach et al 1992). In contrast, it has been reported that 24/29 patients with perforated peptic ulcer were infected with *H. pylori*, diagnosed by ^{13}C-UBT 8 days postoperatively (Sebastian et al 1995). The number of patients in this study is too small to make any definitive comment on the role of *H. pylori* in perforation. Patients with perforated ulcers should undergo surgery and *H. pylori* status should be checked using either serology for anti-*H. pylori* IgG or ^{13}C-UBT. All patients with *H. pylori* infection should be treated with eradication therapy as it speeds up healing and decreases the relapse rate of ulcer disease.

H. PYLORI AND MALIGNANCY

Gastric lymphoma

There appears to be an association between *H. pylori* infection and gastric MALT type lymphomas. In retrospective studies, *H. pylori* is present in up to 92% of patients of gastric MALT type lymphoma compared with 50% of controls (Wotherspoon et al 1991). Prolonged *H. pylori*-induced inflammation may increase the probability of malignant transformation of lymphoid tissue. Hussell et al (1993) have shown that a specific strain of *H. pylori* might promote cellular proliferation in low-grade B-cell gastric MALT lymphoma by stimulating T-cells. Subsequent studies suggest that these tumours are driven by continuing *H. pylori* antigenic stimulus and regress after *H. pylori* eradication (Wotherspoon et al 1993). The German MALT lymphoma study group has shown that eradication of *H. pylori* infection associated with early stage tumour resulted in complete tumour regression in 70% of patients. During 1 year median follow-up, no relapse of MALT lymphoma occurred. Advanced tumour stages or tumours with transition to high-grade malignancy did not respond to *H. pylori* eradication (Bayerdorffer et al 1995). Long-term follow-up is needed to know whether the patients with complete regression are actually cured.

Gastric adenocarcinoma

The prevalence of *H. pylori* infection in gastric cancer is around 70% (Parsonnet 1993). In a cross-sectional study of gastric cancer patients in Finland, 70–80% of the cancers developed in a stomach with *H. pylori* infection, only 10–15% of the gastric cancer cases occurred in a normal stomach (Sipponen et al 1985). In Peru, where *H. pylori* infection is highly prevalent and begins in early childhood, the prevalence of gastric cancer is significantly higher than in the developed world (Burstein et al 1991). Other evidence suggesting that chronic *H. pylori* infection is associated with gastric adenocarcinoma, especially of the distal stomach is presented by Talley et al (1991b). This is supported by observations that *H. pylori* infection results in chronic gastritis which may progress to atrophic gastritis and intestinal metaplasia, and then to gastric cancer (Sipponen et al 1992a). It has also been suggested that early infection with *H. pylori* results in more intense inflammation and early development of atrophic gastritis with a higher risk of both gastric cancer and gastric ulcer (Blaser et al 1995).

H. pylori may act as a cofactor for carcinogenesis due to the metabolic products of the organism itself. In addition, the subsequent inflammation is also a mechanism for tissue damage. Cytotoxins, production of proteolytic and lipolytic enzymes and production of ammonia are some of the features of *H. pylori* infection believed to be important in carcinogenesis (Sipponen & Seppala 1992).

Several immune reactions and effector cells in the host are stimulated by *H. pylori* infection, which result in liberation of cytokines, superoxide and other free radicals, and of various toxins or growth factors, which may influence and modulate the differentiation, growth and function of the mucosal cells and epithelium (Blaser et al 1992). Metabolic products of bacteria induce rapid cell proliferation which increases the risk of DNA damage and may predispose the mucosa to transformation by mutagens. Production of superoxide anion and other reactive free radicals from activated granulocytes or monocytes/macrophages provides a potential risk for endogenous genetic damage with mutation and malignant transformation of epithelial cells.

H. pylori appears to be one of many aetiological factors in gastric cancer. Other causes of gastritis, duodenogastric reflux, previous gastric surgery, pernicious anaemia and dietary and gastric factors may also play a role. It is possible that some of these factors may potentiate the role of *H. pylori* infection, either by inducing atrophy or metaplasia or by acting as a mutagenic agent on already damaged mucosa.

ERADICATION TREATMENT

The ideal treatment regimen for eradication has not yet been identified. The 'gold standard' is triple therapy with bismuth compounds, e.g. colloidal bismuth subcitrate 120 mg/qds, in combination with tetracycline HCl 500 mg/tds (or amoxycillin 500 mg/tds) and metronidazole 400 mg/tds for two weeks (Graham et al 1992).

With this combination, eradication rates of around 90% are achieved. Another commonly used combination is omeprazole 40 mg/od and amoxycillin 500 mg/qds for 14 days, which eradicates *H. pylori* in around 80% of individuals (Ozmen et al 1994). Problems with triple therapy are the high rates of side effects (30%) and consequently poor compliance. Metronidazole resistance is an increasing problem, especially in developing countries (Graham 1992). The advantages of omeprazole and amoxycillin therapy is the lower incidence of side effects, and a simpler treatment regimen, though penicillin allergy may necessitate substitution of amoxycillin with another antibiotic such as clarithromycin (Labenz et al 1994c).

We believe that a combination of a proton pump inhibitor and amoxycillin should be the first line treatment in the eradication of *H. pylori* before trying classical triple therapy. In patients who are penicillin sensitive or have metronidazole resistant organisms, an alternative antibiotic is clarithromycin. We have achieved high eradication rates in a pilot study (approaching 100%) using a combination of lansoprazole 30mg/bd, clarithromycin 500mg/bd and tinidazole or metronidazole 400mg/bd (Ozmen et al 1995), (lansoprazole is currently not licensed in the UK for the eradication of *H. pylori*). In patients in whom *H. pylori* is not eradicated by standard treatment protocols, addition of omeprezole to classical triple therapy for 7 days is often successful (de Boer et al 1995).

Reinfection with *H. pylori*

Reinfection with *H. pylori* coincides with the risk of ulcer relapse. A recent report using ^{14}C-UBT for assessment of *H. pylori* infection 4–6 years after previous *H. pylori* eradication estimates a reinfection rate of 0.36% annually (Borody et al 1994). A 1.2% annual reinfection rate has also been reported at a mean of 7.1 years after eradication of *H. pylori* (Forbes et al 1994). These data indicate that reinfection is uncommon after successful eradication.

CHANGES IN SURGICAL PRACTICE IN THE *H. PYLORI* ERA

The widespread use of antiulcer drugs, increased understanding of the pathophysiology of peptic ulcer disease and a decline in the incidence of the disease have resulted in a dramatic reduction in the numbers of patients requiring surgical treatment for peptic ulcer disease. The effective eradication of *H. pylori* has resulted in an increased rate of ulcer healing, decreased relapse rates and a lower incidence of complications of peptic ulcer disease. The morbidity of major operations and long-term sequelae that accompany gastric resection or vagotomy, have led to a significant decline in elective surgical procedures for peptic ulcer, despite the recent introduction of laparoscopic techniques which have overcome some of these disadvantages. The indications for surgery in peptic ulcer disease are restricted to the treatment of complications such as bleeding, perforation or gastric outlet obstruction.

The management of acute upper gastrointestinal bleeding is also moving away from operative therapy; endoscopic haemostasis is often effective in reducing the rebleeding rate and morbidity. In general, patients with peptic ulcer complications must have the simplest and most rapid procedure performed in order to decrease morbidity and mortality. After the endoscopic procedure or operation, patients should be tested either by a non-invasive test for *H. pylori* infection. Those with *H. pylori* infection must have eradication treatment as this decreases the rate of ulcer relapse and complications. Potential indications for elective operative intervention include failure to respond to eradication therapy, failure of conservative treatment and relapse following attempted eradication of *H. pylori*. Surgery may be a cheaper alternative to prolonged maintenance therapy in the non-compliant or frequently relapsing patient.

KEY POINTS FOR CLINICAL PRACTICE

- *H. pylori* is the most common infection worldwide. *H. pylori* is transmitted from human to human, most likely via the oral-oral route with a high prevalence noted in developing countries, lower socioeconomic groups and family members of infected subjects.

- *H. pylori* causes chronic active gastritis and is associated with duodenal and gastric ulcers. It may play a role in a subset of subjects with NUD and may be involved in the pathogenesis of gastric lymphoma and gastric adenocarcinoma.

- Diagnosis of *H. pylori*: patients undergoing endoscopy should have biopsies taken for histology and rapid urease test. For patients not undergoing endoscopy, and for the assessment of eradication of *H. pylori* infection, ^{13}C- or ^{14}C-UBT is the gold standard.

- *H. pylori* positive patients with duodenal or gastric ulcer should have eradication treatment as this improves healing of ulcers and decreases complications and the relapse rate.

- Patients with *H. pylori* positive non-ulcer dyspepsia should have eradication therapy as this often alleviates symptoms.

- In patients with peptic ulcer complications, the simplest and most rapid procedure should be performed. All patients must be screened for *H. pylori* and those with infection should have eradication treatment.
- The most effective means of eradicating *H. pylori* is triple therapy (two antibiotics plus bismuth or a proton pump inhibitor (PPI)). Triple therapy with a PPI instead of metronidazole has fewer side effects and a high eradication rate.
- Results of treatment should be monitored and eradication should be confirmed.

REFERENCES

Adamek RJ, Freitag M, Opferkuck W, Ruhl GH, Wegener M 1994 Intravenous omeprazole/amoxycillin and omeprazole pretreatment in *H. pylori* positive acute peptic ulcer bleeding. A pilot study. Scand J Gastroenterol 29: 880-883

Baskerwille A, Newell DG 1988 Naturally occurring chronic gastritis and *C. pylori* infection in the rhesus monkey: a potential model for gastritis in man. Gut 29: 465-472

Bayerdoorffer E, Neubauer A, Rudolph B et al 1995 Regression of primary gastric lymphoma of mucosa-associated lymphoid tissue type after cure of *H. pylori* infection. Lancet 345: 1591-1594

Bewett EJ, Smith JTL, Nwokolo CU, Hudson M, Sawyer AM, Pounder RE 1991 Eradication of *H. pylori* abolishes 24 hour hypergastrinemia: a prospective study in healthy subjects. Aliment Pharmacol Ther 5: 283-290

Bottcher 1874 Derpater Medicinische Zeitschrift 5: 148

Blaser MJ 1992 Hypothesis on the pathogenesis and natural history of *H. pylori* induced inflammation. Gastroenterology 102: 720-727

Blaser MJ, Chyou PH, Nomura A 1995 Age at establishment of *H. pylori* infection and gastric carcinoma, gastric ulcer and duodenal ulcer risk. Cancer Res 55: 562-565

Borody T 1994 *Helicobacter* reinfection rate in patients with cured duodenal ulcer. Am J Gastroenterol 89: 529-532

Burstein M, Monge E, Leon-Barcia R et al 1991 Low peptic ulcer and high gastric cancer prevalence in a developing country with a high prevalence of infection by *H. pylori*. J Clin Gastroenterol 13: 154-156

Clason AE, Macleod DA, Elton RA 1986 Clinical factors in the prediction of further haemorrhage or mortality in acute upper gastrointestinal haemorrhage. Br J Surg 73: 985-987

Clayton CL, Kleanthaus H, Coates P et al 1992 Sensitive detection of *H. pylori* using PCR. J Clin Microbiol 30: 192-200

Cover TL, Dooley CP, Blaser MJ 1990 Characterization of human serologic response to proteins in *H. pylori* broth culture supernatants with vacuolizing cytotoxin activity. Infect Immun 58: 603-610

Crabtree JE, Taylor JD, Wyatt JE et al 1991 Mucosal IgA recognition of *H. pylori* 120FDA protein, peptic ulceration and gastric pathology. Lancet i: 332-335

De Boer W, Driessen W, Jansz A, Tytgat G 1995 Effect of acid suppression on efficacy of treatment for *H. pylori* infection. Lancet 345: 817-820

Dixon M 1993 Histological diagnosis. In: Northfield TC, Mendall M, Goggin PM eds *H. pylori* infection. Kluwer, pp 110-115

Figura N, Guglielmeti P, Rossolini A et al 1989 Cytotoxin production by *Campylobacter pylori* strains isolated from patients with peptic ulcers and from patients with chronic gastritis only. J Clin Microbiol 27: 225-226

Forbes GM, Glaser ME, Cullen DJE et al 1994 Duodenal ulcer treated with *H. pylori* eradication: 7 year follow-up. Lancet 343. 258-260

Goodwin CS 1988 Duodenal ulcer, *Campylobacter pylori* and the 'leaking roof' concept. Lancet ii: 1467-1469

Goodwin CS, Armstrong JA, Chilwers T et al 1989 Transfer of *Campylobacter pyloridis* and *C. mustelae* to *Helicobacter* gen. nov. as *Helicobacter pylori* comb. nov and *Helicobacter mustelae* comb. nov. respectively. Int J Systematic Bacteriol 39: 2378-2379

Goodwin CS, Armstrong JA 1990 Microbiological aspects of *H. pylori* (*C. pylori*). Eur J Clin Microbiol Infect Dis 9: 1-3

Graham DY, Adam E, Reddy GT et al. 1991 Sero-epidemiology of *H. pylori* infection in India. Comparison of developing and developed countries. Dig Dis Sci 36: 1084-1088

Graham DY, Hepps KS, Ramirez FC, Lew GM, Saeed ZA 1993 Treatment of *H. pylori* reduces the rate of rebleeding in peptic ulcer disease. Scand J Gastroenterol 28: 939-942

Graham DY, Lew GM, Malaty HM et al 1992 Factors influencing the eradication of *H. pylori* with triple therapy. Gastroenterology 102: 493-496

Hazell SL, Lee A 1986 *Campylobacter pyloridis*, urease, hydrogen ion back diffusion and gastric ulcers. Lancet 2: 15-17

Hentschel E, Brandstatter G, Dragosic SB et al 1993 Effect of ranitidine and amoxycillin plus metronidazole on the eradication of *H. pylori* and the recurrence of duodenal ulcer. N Engl J Med. 328: 308-312

Hessey SJ, Spencer J, Wyatt JI 1990 Bacterial adhesion and disease activity in *Helicobacter* associated chronic gastritis. Gut 31: 134-138

Hosking SW, Ling TKW, Chung SCS 1994 Duodenal ulcer healing by eradication of *H. pylori* without anti-acid treatment: randomised controlled trial. Lancet 343: 508-510

Hussel T, Isaacson PG, Crabtree JE, Spencer J 1993 The response of cells from low grade B cell gastric lymphomas of mucosa associated lymphoid tissue to *Helicobacter pylori*. Lancet 342: 571-574

Jensen DM, You S, Pelayo E, Jensen ME 1992 The prevalence of *H. pylori* and NSAID use in patients with severe upper gastrointestinal haemorrhage and their potential role in recurrence of ulcer bleeding. Gastroenterology 102: A90

Kaneko H, Nakada M, Mitsuma T et al 1992 *Helicobacter pylori* infection induces a decrease in immunoreactive somatostatin concentrations in human stomach. Dig Dis Sci 37: 409-416

Karnes WE, Samhoff JM, Siurola M et al 1991 Positive serum antibody and negative tissue staining for *H. pylori* in subjects with atrophic body gastritis. Gastroenterology 101: 167-174

Labenz J, Borsch G 1994a Evidence for the essential role of *H. pylori* in gastric ulcer disease. Gut 35: 19-22

Labenz J, Borsch G 1994b Role of *H. pylori* eradication in prevention of peptic ulcer bleeding relapse. Digestion 55: 19-23

Labenz J, Leverkus F, Borsch G 1994c Omeprazole plus amoxycillin for cure of *H. pylori* infection. Factors influencing the treatment success. Scand J Gastroenterol 29: 1070-1075

Lambert JR 1993 The role of *H. pylori* in non ulcer dyspepsia. A debate. Gastroenterol Clin N Am 22: 141-151

Langenberg W, Rauws EAJ, Oudbier JH, Tytgat GNJ 1990 Patient to patient transmission of *C. pylori* infection by fibreoptic gastroduodenoscopy and biopsy. J Infect Dis 161: 507-511

Lee A 1991 *Helicobacter pylori*: causal agent in peptic ulcer, microbiological aspects. J Gastroenterol Hepatol 6: 115-120

Logan RPH 1992 Detection of *H. pylori* by the ^{13}C-urea breath test. In: Rathbone BJ, Heathley RV eds *H. pylori* and gastroduodenal disease. Oxford, Blackwell, pp 88-106

Madam E, Kemp J, Westblom TU et al 1988 Evaluation of staining methods in identifying *C. pylori*. Am J Clin Pathol 90: 450-453

Mai UEH, Perez-Perez GI, Wahl LM, Wahl SM, Blaser MJ, Smith PD 1990 Inflammatory and cytoprotective responses by human monocytes are induced by *H. pylori*: possible role in the pathogenesis of type B gastritis. Gastroenterology 98: A662

Majmudar P, Shah SM, Dhunjibhoy KR, Desai HG 1990 Isolation of *H. pylori* from dental plaque in healthy volunteers. Indian J Gastroenterol 9: 271-272

Mapstone NP, Lynch D, Lewis F et al 1993 PCR identification of *H. pylori* in faeces from gastritis patients. Lancet 341: 447

Marshall BJ 1983 Unidentified curved bacilli on gastric epithelium in active chronic gastritis. Lancet i: 1273

Marshall BJ 1991 Virulence and pathogenicity of *H. pylori*. J Gastroenterol Hepatol. 6: 121-124

McCarthy CJ, Collins R, Beattie S, Hamilton H, O'Morain C 1993 Short report: treatment of *H. pylori* associated duodenal ulcer with omeprazole plus antibiotics. Aliment Pharmacol Ther 7: 463-466

McCarthy CJ, Patchett S, Collins RM, Beattie SM, Keane C, O'Morain C 1995 Long term prospective study of *H. pylori* in non-ulcer dyspepsia. Dig Dis Sci 40: 114-119

Megrand F 1993 Epidemiology of *H. pylori* infection. Gastroenterol Clin N Am 22: 73-88

Molyneux AJ, Horris MD 1993 *H. pylori* in gastric biopsies – should you trust the pathology report? J R Coll Phys Lond 27: 119-120

Morris A, Nicholson G 1987 Ingestion of *C. pyloridis* causes gastritis and raised fasting pH. Am J Gastroenterol 82: 192-199
Negrini R, Lisato L, Zanella I et al 1991 *H. pylori* infection induces antibodies crossreacting with human gastric mucosa. Gastroenterology 101: 437-445
O'Connor HJ, Kanduru C, Bhutta AS et al 1995 Effect of *H. pylori* eradication on peptic ulcer healing. Postgrad Med J 71: 90-93
O'Donnell M, Alexander-Williams J, Heathley RV et al 1993 Management issues for debate: the problems in perspective. Aliment Pharmacol Ther 7 (suppl 2): 49-55
Ozmen MM, Patankar RS, Johnson CD 1994 Eradication of *H. pylori* in patients with gastroduodenitis: double vs triple therapy (abstract). Br J Surg 81 (suppl): 56
Ozmen MM, Johnson CD 1995 Is short term triple therapy with lansoprazole, clarithromycin and metronidazole a definitive answer for *H. pylori* eradication? (letter) Am J Gastroenterol 90: 1542-1543
Ozmen MM, Gough A, Johnson CD 1995 Polymerase chain reaction (PCR) for detection of *Helicobacter pylori* DNA in patients with *H. pylori* induced gastritis suggests that dental plaque is not a reservoir. Gut 37 (suppl 2): A31
Parsonnet J 1993 *H. pylori* and gastric cancer. Gastroenterol Clin N Am 22: 89-104
Penston JG 1994 *H. pylori* eradication – understandable caution but no excuse for inertia. Aliment Pharmacol Ther 8: 369-389
Perez-Perez GI, Taylor DN, Bodhodatto L et al 1990 Seroprevalance of *H. pylori* infections in Thailand. J Infect Dis 161: 1237-1241
Rautelin H, Blomberg B, Freudkind H, Jarnerot G, Danielsson D 1993 Incidence of *H. pylori* strains activating neutrophils in patients with peptic ulcer disease. Gut 34: 599-603
Rauws EAJ, Royen EAV, Langenberg W et al 1989 ^{14}C-Urea breath test in *C. pylori* gastritis. Gut 30: 798-803
Reinbach D, Cruickshank G, McColl KEL 1992 Acute perforated duodenal ulcer is not associated with *H. pylori* infection. Gut 33 (suppl 1): S67
Scott N, Diament R, Murday Y et al 1990 *Helicobacter* gastritis and intestinal metaplasia in a gastric cancer family. Lancet 333: 728
Sebastian M, Chandran Prem VP, El Ashaal YIM, Sim AJW 1995 *H. pylori* infection in perforated peptic ulcer disease. Br J Surg 82: 360-362
Seppala K, Pikkorainen P, Karvonen AL, Gormsen M, Finnish Gastric ulcer study group 1992 The role of *H. pylori* eradication in gastric ulcer healing and relapses (abstract). Gastroenterology 102: A162
Shahamat M, Vives-Rego J, Paszko-Kolva C, Pearson AD, Colwell RR 1989 Survival of *C. pylori* in river water: ^{3}H-thymidine uptake and viability under stimulated environmental conditions. Klin Wochenschr 67: 63
Sipponen P, Kekki M, Havapakaski J et al 1985 Gastric cancer risk in chronic atrophic gastritis: statistical calculations of cross-sectional data. Int J Cancer 35: 173-178
Sipponen P, Kosinen T, Valle J et al 1992a *H. pylori* infection and chronic gastritis in gastric cancer. J Clin Pathol 45: 319-323
Sipponen P, Seppala K 1992b Gastric carcinoma: failed adaptation to *H. pylori*. Scan J Gastroenterol 193 (suppl): 33-38
Sipponen P, Hyvarinen H 1993 Role of *H. pylori* in the pathogenesis of gastritis, peptic ulcer and gastric cancer. Scand J Gastroenterol 28 (suppl 196): 3-6
Soll AH 1990 Pathogenesis of peptic ulcer and implications for therapy. New Engl J Med 322: 909-916
Steer HW, Colin-Jones DG 1975 Mucosal changes in gastric ulceration and their response to carbenoxolone sodium. Gut 16: 590-597
Talley NJ, Colin-Jones D, Koch KL et al 1991a Functional dyspepsia: a classification with guidelines for diagnosis and management. Gastroenterol Int 4: 145
Talley NJ, Zinmaster AR, Dimagno EP et al 1991b Gastric adenocarcinoma and *H. pylori* infection. J Natl Cancer Inst 83: 1734-1739
Tompkins D 1993 Microbiological tests. In: Northfield TC, Mendall M, Goggin PM (eds) *H. pylori* infection. Kluwer, pp 116-126
Tytgat GNJ, Axon ATR, Dixon MF et al 1990 *H. pylori*, causal agent in peptic ulcer disease? In: Working Party Report of the World Congress of Gastroenterology, 26-31 August 1990, Sydney, Australia. Oxford, Blackwell, pp 36-45
Valle J, Seppala K, Sipponen P, Kosunen T 1991 Disappearance of gastritis after eradication of *H. pylori*: a morphometric study. Scand J Gastroenterol 26: 1057-1065

Van Zanten VSJO 1993 A systematic overview (meta-analysis of outcome measures in *H. pylori* gastritis trials and functional dyspepsia. Scand J Gastroenterol 28 (suppl 199): 40-43

Von Wulffen H 1992 An assessment of serological tests for detection of *H. pylori*. Eur J Clin Microbiol Infect Dis 11: 577-582

Waren P 1987 Incidence, diagnosis and natural course of upper gastrointestinal haemorrhage. Prognostic value of clinical factors and endoscopy. Scand J Gastroenterol 22 (suppl 137): 26-27

Wotherspoon AC, Ortiz-Hidalgo C, Falzon MR, Isaacson PG 1991 *Helicobacter pylori* associated gastritis and primary B cell gastric lymphoma. Lancet 338: 1175-1176

Wotherspoon AC, Doglioni C, Diss TC et al 1993 Regression of primary low grade B cell gastric lymphoma of mucosa associated lymphoid tissue type after eradication of *Helicobacter pylori*. Lancet 342: 575-577

Wyatt JI, Rathbone BJ, Sobola SM et al 1990 Gastric epithelium in the duodenum: its association with *H. pylori* and inflammation. J Clin Pathol 43: 981-986

5

The management of superficial bladder cancer

T. R. L. Griffiths   D. E. Neal

In England and Wales, 7000 new cases of superficial bladder cancer are diagnosed each year. After primary treatment which usually comprises transurethral resection of the tumour, 60–70% of superficial papillary tumours will recur (Greene et al 1973). In 10–20% of cases, superficial tumours will progress to muscle invasion or metastatic disease (Lutzeyer et al 1982). Follow-up must be life-long. The workload due to superficial bladder cancer is therefore considerable. Repeated hospital admissions cause inconvenience and anxiety to patients.

Recent developments will reduce delays in diagnosis and minimise the number of follow-up cystoscopies, especially those requiring general anaesthesia. New indications for intravesical therapy have been recognised. The availability of orthotopic reconstruction of the bladder has made cystectomy less mutilating. New prognostic factors are being analyzed as a result of advances in the field of molecular biology. This chapter addresses the current management options available in superficial bladder cancer and summarises recent progress in the field of molecular biology relevant to bladder cancer.

CLASSIFICATION OF SUPERFICIAL BLADDER CANCER

At the time of initial diagnosis, 60–70% of bladder tumours are classified as 'superficial'. Superficial tumours are defined by the tumour, node, metastases (TNM) classification (Union Internationale Contre le Cancer 1992) as Ta (papillary carcinoma not invading beneath the basement membrane of the urothelium), T1 (papillary carcinoma invading the connective tissue of the submucosa but not the underlying detrusor muscle) and Tis (Carcinoma *in situ*: 'flat tumour'). The vast majority (90%) are transitional cell in origin. The remainder are typed either as squamous cell carcinoma or adenocarcinoma.

HAEMATURIA CLINICS

Painless haematuria is the main presenting symptom of superficial bladder cancer. Patients with this symptom require a cystoscopy and imaging of the upper tracts either by means of intravenous urography (IVU) or plain abdominal radiography plus ultrasonography. Urine cytology should also be assessed, but a normal cytology report does not exclude malignancy. In addition, any man with a urinary tract infection or frequency, urgency and dysuria and any woman with an intractable urinary tract infection despite antibiotic treatment requires investigation.

Haematuria clinics (Britton 1993) involve organising a special urology outpatient clinic alongside a flexible cystoscopy clinic. Ideally this should be an 'open access' clinic with all investigations including IVU being performed on the same day. This service facilitates early diagnosis and has been shown to work particularly well in the District General Hospital setting (Hasan et al 1994a). Studies have suggested that delay in the diagnosis and treatment of bladder cancer might affect patient survival (Wallace & Harris 1965). Other studies remain inconclusive (Gulliford et al 1991). In reality, probably the only patients who benefit from early treatment are those with T1 tumours that are going to progress to muscle invasion, patients with primary carcinoma *in situ* and T2 or T3 tumours which have not metastasised into the vascular or lymphatic systems.

Flexible cystoscopy under local anaesthesia provides an immediate diagnosis of bladder pathology thereby reducing patient anxiety and identifying those patients who need definitive treatment. It enables better planning of inpatient waiting lists. There is no evidence that flexible cystoscopy is less sensitive than conventional rod lens examination (Walker et al 1993). The procedure is well tolerated (Powell et al 1984) as a diagnostic procedure. However few patients will tolerate biopsy of a tumour or treatment by cystodiathermy.

At the time of initial tumour resection, care should be taken to ensure that biopsies are taken from any suspicious red patches which may indicate carcinoma *in situ*. It is also wise to take biopsies of apparently normal epithelium near to and far from the tumour, again to determine whether underlying carcinoma *in situ* is present. The use of bladder washings can be helpful to study DNA ploidy measurements. A deep resection biopsy taken from the base of the initial primary tumour and sent separately is mandatory to ensure that complete tumour staging is carried out by the histopathologist.

PROGNOSTIC FACTORS

Many workers have reported tumour characteristics which are related to the likelihood of tumour recurrence, progression to muscle invasion or metastatic disease and survival. Tumour stage, grade, size, and number of tumours at presentation (Lutzeyer et al 1982, Heney et al 1983), and the presence of mucosal abnormalities elsewhere in the bladder such as dysplasia (Althausen et al 1976) or carcinoma *in situ* (Smith et al 1986), and abnormal urine cytology and DNA ploidy all provide prognostic information.

Considerable disagreement has been shown among pathologists in the interpretation of the pT category (Abel et al 1988) and histological grade (Ooms et al 1983). In the latter study, an intra-individual variation of 50% was also found when the same pathologists reviewed their slides seven months later. Tumours > 5 cm in diameter are known to have a worse prognosis (Heney et al 1983), but the interpretation of size is subjective. Urologists should be aware of the lack of precision in interpreting biopsies from normal-appearing bladder mucosa. In one study, a consensus was reached on severe dysplasia and carcinoma in situ, but in the milder forms of dysplasia, pathologists only managed to reproduce their own assessment in 62% of cases (Richards et al 1991). Urine cytology may detect carcinoma *in situ* which has not been found by random mucosal biopsies. This is because the surface urothelial cells which are not adherent in carcinoma *in situ* are washed off. In patients with marked irritative symptoms such as bladder pain, urethral irritation and dysuria, but no abnormal clinical findings, the cytological examination of several specimens of urine is recommended. Bladder washings are a useful adjunct to cystoscopy. The yield of cells is often higher in bladder washings than from urine cytology (Mellon et al 1991). When ploidy is compared by multivariate analysis with other prognostic factors, it has no clinical advantage over stage and grade (Lipponen et al 1990). It may have a place in sub-classifying grade 2 tumours.

FOLLOW-UP REGIME

A multivariate analysis has delineated two prognostic factors which are not subjective in nature (Parmar et al 1989). At diagnosis, the urologist notes whether the tumour is solitary or multifocal. At the first follow-up cystoscopy at three months, the presence or absence of tumour is recorded. When combined, these two factors are significantly associated with the interval to subsequent recurrence. These two factors allow classification of patients with superficial bladder cancer into three groups who have different prognoses (Table 5.1).

On the basis of these findings, a proposed follow-up regime has been suggested (Hall et al 1994a).

- Group 1 patients can be followed up safely by means of flexible cystoscopy at annual intervals only.

Table 5.1 The three proposed prognostic groups and their relationship to risk of recurrence

Prognostic groups	Cystoscopic findings
Group 1	Solitary tumour at presentation; no tumour recurrence at three months (20% risk of recurrence at 1 year)
Group 2	Solitary tumour at presentation; tumour recurrence at 3 months Multiple tumours at presentation; no tumour recurrence at 3 months (40% risk of recurrence at 1 year)
Group 3	Multiple tumours at presentation; tumour recurrence at 3 months (90% risk of recurrence at 1–2 years)

- Group 2 patients should be followed up three monthly by flexible cystoscopy for the first year.
- Group 3 patients require three-monthly rigid cystoscopic assessment under general anaesthesia.

THERAPY WITH INTRAVESICAL AGENTS

There are two types of intravesical agents, namely chemotherapeutic agents and immunotherapeutic agents.

Intravesical chemotherapeutic agents

A number of studies using a wide variety of agents have shown that chemotherapeutic agents can be used as an adjunct to transurethral resection (Lum & Torti 1990, Franklin & Benson 1994). The most commonly used agents include thiotepa, mitomycin, doxorubicin (adriamycin) and epirubicin.

Patients are asked to refrain from fluid intake for 4 h before attending for intravesical chemotherapy to reduce dilution by urine output and to aid in retention of the cytotoxic agents. At the time of therapy, a urethral catheter is inserted and the residual urine is drained. The intravesical agent is introduced through the urinary catheter and the catheter is then clamped. The cytotoxic agent is retained in the bladder for about 2 h. In many institutions, the patient is rotated during this period to promote contact of the cytotoxic agent with the entire bladder surface. Significant chemical cystitis is related to the frequency of instillation and the drug concentration in the bladder and affects about 5% of patients.

The incidence of systemic toxicity is related to the molecular weight of the agent (Table 5.2). The greater the molecular weight, the less likely it is to be absorbed and the less the risk of systemic toxicity. Thiotepa has a relatively low molecular weight and leucopenia and thrombocytopenia have been reported irrespective of dose. Haematological side effects are less common in patients undergoing intravesical mitomycin C therapy. Skin rashes can occur with mitomycin C or epirubicin (Oosterlinck et al 1993).

Intravesical immunotherapeutic agents

Immunotherapeutic agents in current use include Bacillus Calmette Guérin (BCG), interferon and keyhole-limpet haemocyanin.

BCG immunotherapy

The intravesical instillation of BCG vaccine for bladder cancer was first reported in 1976 (Morales et al). A variety of BCG strains have been studied (Tice, Pasteur, Connaught, Armand Frappier, Evans (formerly Glaxo), Moreau and RIVM). Differences in efficacy between strains is well docu-

Table 5.2 Intravesical agents and their relative molecular weights

Cytotoxic agent	Molecular weight
Thiotepa	189
Epodyl	262
Mitomycin C	329
Doxorubicin	580
Epirubicin	580

mented. BCG is a biological preparation and is subject to damage in handling and administration. Many studies quote the dose given in milligrams. This does not give an indication of the number of colony forming units. It seems likely that differences between strains may depend more on the number of viable colonies than the type of strain.

The mechanism of action of BCG immunotherapy in the bladder is not entirely clear. BCG must attach to urothelium for there to be an active response and the binding site is probably fibronectin (Ratliff 1989). There may be an element of non-specific response to BCG, but at least some of the immunological response must be specific. Cytokines may be involved in the antitumour activity of BCG immunotherapy. The use of markers which might give a measure of the immune response to BCG is currently being investigated to allow the dose to be titrated. Markers which have been assessed include the level of interleukins and interferon-gamma in the urine, the appearance of human leucocyte antigen on tumour cells and the response of peripheral blood lymphocytes.

Side effects are more common with BCG immunotherapy than with any other form of intravesical therapy (Lamm et al 1992a). Up to 90% of patients complain of cystitis, although in the majority, this symptom is self-limiting and can be improved with phenazopyridine, propantheline bromide or oxybutynin.

Systemic toxicity is a major disadvantage of BCG immunotherapy. Although less common than cystitis, systemic side effects can have serious consequences for the patient. These complications include fever > 39°C (2.9%), granulomatous prostatitis (0.9%), major haematuria (1%), pneumonitis/hepatitis (0.7%), arthritis/arthralgia (0.5%), skin rash (0.3%), orchitis/epididymitis (0.4%), fibrosis of the bladder (0.7%), renal abscess (0.1%) and cytopenia (0.1%). Granulomatous pneumonitis or hepatitis should be treated with combination antituberculous therapy for 6 months. Pyrexias of unknown origin (> 39.5°C) following BCG immunotherapy should be treated intensively in hospital with combination antituberculous chemotherapy. If BCG sepsis develops, cycloserine 500 mg twice daily for 5 days should be added to the above regime. All the complications are responsive to isoniazid 300 mg.

There are active measures which can be taken to reduce the risk of systemic toxicity following BCG immunotherapy. BCG should not be instilled if the catheterisation has been traumatic resulting in haematuria and it should not be given immediately following transurethral resection. Most regimens do not commence BCG immunotherapy for 1 week after transurethral resection. Direct intralesional injection of BCG should be avoided. BCG immunotherapy is contraindicated in immunocompromised patients and in those who are pregnant, lactating or have recurrent urinary tract infections.

Other immunotherapy

Intravesical interferons and keyhole-limpet haemocyanin are at an early stage of assessment of clinical efficacy. The advantage of keyhole-limpet haemocyanin is that it appears to be considerably less toxic than BCG immunotherapy.

Intravesical therapy to reduce the risk of recurrence in newly-diagnosed low risk papillary tumours

The results of two large multicentre randomised clinical trials suggest that a single instillation of intravesical chemotherapy immediately after transurethral resection is worthwhile in low risk patients and can reduce the rate of recurrence by up to 50%.

The Medical Research Council (MRC) Urological Cancer Working Party Trial (Tolley et al 1988) compared transurethral resection alone with transurethral resection plus a single postoperative instillation of mitomycin and instillations at each of the 3-monthly follow-up visits during the first year. 502 patients with newly diagnosed Ta or T1 transitional cell carcinoma of the bladder were assessed. A single dose of 30 mg mitomycin significantly reduced the recurrence rate after a minimum of 3 year follow-up, and the time to first recurrence was lengthened. The EORTC (European Organisation for Research and Treatment of Cancer) trial (protocol 30863) compared the instillation of 80 mg epirubicin with an instillation of sterile water immediately after transurethral resection in 432 patients (Oosterlinck et al 1993). Only solitary new or recurrent Ta and T1 tumours were enrolled. After a mean follow-up of 2 years, it was evident that a single instillation of 80 mg epirubicin had decreased the recurrence rate by nearly 50% compared with water.

European randomised trials comparing BCG with cytotoxic agents in patients at low risk of recurrence have not shown any superiority for BCG. An EORTC GU group randomised prospective trial comparing the RIVM-BCG strain with mitomycin C showed that the two agents were equally effective in preventing recurrence of superficial bladder cancer (DeBruyne et al 1988). The BCG schedule consisted of 6-weekly instillations which was repeated if there was a recurrence at 3 or 6 months. The dose of mitomycin C was 30 mg and it was given as 4-weekly instillations on weeks 1–4 after transurethral resection followed by 5-monthly instillations. A Dutch Southeast Cooperative Group randomised trial compared the efficacy of intravesical mitomycin C with that of RIVM-BCG strain and Tice BCG strain (Vegt et al 1995). The schedules were the same as those used for the EORTC trial. 84 of 387 papillary tumours (22%) were TaG1 and therefore at low risk of recurrence. They concluded that mitomycin C and RIVM-BCG treatments were equally effective. Both were more effective than Tice-BCG therapy. The conclusions from trials reported to date comparing BCG immunotherapy with intravesical chemotherapy are that mitomycin C is better tolerated and is equal to BCG immunotherapy in the prevention of tumour recurrence in low risk patients. The toxicity of single drug instillations of epirubicin or mitomycin C are minimal. The implications to the patient of avoiding cystoscopic assessment and of potential savings in cost should not be ignored (Hall 1994b).

Intravesical therapy to reduce the recurrence rate in rapidly recurring papillary tumours

The evidence to date is not conclusive, but is suggestive that in patients with rapidly recurring tumours, BCG immunotherapy may provide superior protection from recurrence. A North American clinical trial conducted by the Southwest Oncology group (Lamm et al 1993) revealed a highly significant advantage of BCG over mitomycin C which prompted the early closure of the trial. Only patients with rapidly recurring tumours were enrolled and the BCG arm included maintenance therapy. It should be noted that the mitomycin C dose was only 20 mg whereas most European studies of mitomycin C use a dose of 30 mg. Given the systemic side effects of BCG immunotherapy, most European urologists would opt for a trial of intravesical chemotherapy first and reserve BCG for refractory multifocal disease.

Intravesical therapy for carcinoma *in situ*

Small areas of focal carcinoma *in situ* can be treated by transurethral resection in the same manner as papillary Ta and T1 tumours. However, if diffuse carcinoma *in situ* is treated by surgery alone, 60% of these areas will progress to muscle invasion and one-third of the patients will die within 5 years (Utz et al 1970). Similarly carcinoma *in situ* accompanied by severe dysplasia in normal appearing urothelium has a sinister prognosis. These patients require adjuvant intravesical treatment in the form of BCG, adriamycin or epirubicin in the first instance in an attempt to reduce the number of cystoscopies.

In a meta-analysis of the use of mitomycin C and carcinoma *in situ*, a complete response was achieved in 29–100% of the patients with a mean percentage of 38% (Bouffioux 1991). A similar analysis of the use of doxorubicin in a range of studies showed a complete response range of 10–66% with a slightly better mean complete response rate (53%) (Bouffioux 1991).

A Phase II study coordinated by the EORTC GU Group (protocol 30861) was set up to investigate the use of BCG Connaught strain in carcinoma *in situ*. Preliminary results have shown that intravesical BCG treatment yields up to 80% complete remission after 1–6-weekly instillations (Jakse et al 1992). However 10–40% of the initial complete responders recur within 5 years.

North American studies have shown similar initial complete response rates. A meta-analysis of 18 series comprising patients with carcinoma *in situ* found an overall complete response rate of 70% with 6 instillations of BCG at intervals of 1 week, increasing to 82% if an additional 3 instillations were given at 3 months (Lamm et al 1992b). It was also noted that when maintenance treatment was given, 64–75% of patients who responded completely remained free of tumour and retained their bladders for 5 or more years.

At present, intravesical BCG appears to be the treatment of choice in carcinoma *in situ* of the bladder. Maintenance therapy appears to be beneficial in reducing the incidence of recurrence following a complete response. Whether the excellent preservation of a complete response rate with time in the maintenance arm of the Southwest Oncology Group Trial of BCG therapy is confirmed by further studies remains to be seen (Lamm 1992b). The effect of intravesical BCG on survival from bladder cancer is not known. In view of the systemic toxicity associated with BCG, some urologists would advocate intravesical chemotherapy as a first line treatment. BCG would be reserved for those who failed to respond completely to intravesical chemotherapy. However the risk of progression to muscle invasion increases with time. At the present time, an EORTC Phase III trial (protocol 30906) is investigating which intravesical modality should be used first. The poor prognosis of patients with carcinoma *in situ* who fail to respond to intravesical BCG should be remembered as many of them will require early cystectomy.

THE MANAGEMENT OF PT1G3 BLADDER TUMOURS

High grade tumours extending through the lamina propria into the submucosa have a poor prognosis. Approximately 20–50% of these will progress to muscle invasion. Within 2–5 years, one-third will have metastasized (Abel et al 1988, Birch & Harland 1989). Admittedly some cases of subsequent muscle invasion are due to the failure of inclusion of muscle in the initial tumour biopsy. The optimal treatment for pT1G3 tumours is unclear. It is the subject of a current MRC trial which is comparing transurethral resection plus BCG versus transurethral resection and radiotherapy. The policy of determining treatment on the basis of grade is open to question given the inconsistencies in grade interpretation cited earlier in this chapter.

Many urologists would currently recommend cystectomy following diagnosis in these circumstances particularly if the tumour was multifocal and was accompanied by concomitant carcinoma *in situ*. A 5-year cure rate of 85–90% in stage T1 tumours following cystectomy has been reported (Malkowicz et al 1990). The development of orthotopic reconstruction of the bladder has made cystectomy a more attractive option.

In a meta-analysis of 7 series with 309 patients, the risk of progression in T1 disease was reduced from 35% to 13% with intravesical BCG treatment (Cookson & Sarosdy 1992). Maintenance treatment reduced the rate of progression to 7% in their personal series of 86 patients. In this series, the 5-year disease-free rate with an intact bladder was 80%. In contrast, another study reported that 15 of 29 patients (52%) with T1 disease before BCG treatment progressed to muscle invasion within 29 months follow-up. In the group of patients with persistent T1 disease at the 3 month follow-up cystoscopy, 82% progressed to muscle invasion (Herr 1991). To date, no study has convincingly demonstrated that intra-vesical treatment improves survival. Furthermore, randomised trials tend to attract patients with a good prognosis.

Radiotherapy in T1 disease is generally thought to have a poor outcome, although 5-year survival rates of about 60% are quoted by some authors (Duncan & Quilty 1986). Surprisingly, a complete or incomplete response to radiotherapy had no impact on survival. Many urologists would offer immediate cystectomy to fit young patients with multiple or solitary T1G3 tumours and concomitant carcinoma *in situ*. In young patients with T1G3 disease without concomitant carcinoma *in situ*, repeat resection of the primary tumour area should be performed at the first cystoscopic follow-up. Random biopsies should be taken and bladder washings carried out for cytological analysis. If these patients have persistent tumour at this stage they too should be offered cystectomy. In institutions which favour BCG immunotherapy as primary treatment in T1G3 disease, the patient should be assessed after two cycles of therapy. Patients who have recurrent disease after two complete cycles of BCG should be offered cystectomy provided they are fit for a general anaesthetic. Patients who have a complete response to BCG treatment should undergo intensive surveillance with frequent follow-up rigid cystoscopies including regular mucosal biopsies and cytological analysis of bladder washings. Such patients are not suitable for follow up by means of flexible cystoscopy.

URINARY TRACT RECONSTRUCTION AFTER CYSTECTOMY

The development of urinary tract reconstruction of the bladder has made cystectomy a more attractive option for patients with high risk superficial bladder cancer. Provided the urethra is present and the patient is motivated, it is possible to produce a continent bladder (orthotopic reconstruction) of satisfactory capacity. If urethrectomy is necessary, it is possible to construct a continent diversion. The need to perform clean intermittent self catheterisation (CISC) several times a day necessitates a pre-operative trial of manual dexterity.

The indications for urethrectomy in conjunction with cystectomy are controversial. In general, the risk of urethral recurrence is about 5 to 10% at 5 years (Stöckle et al 1990) with the major risk of subsequent urethral recurrence being prostatic involvement (Levinson et al 1990). Other factors include multifocal tumours and carcinoma *in situ* of the bladder. Absolute contraindications to orthotopic reconstruction include urethral tumour and prostatic carcinoma *in situ* or tumour (Skinner et al 1991).

Various sections of bowel have been used in orthotopic reconstruction. One of the commonest symptoms following orthotopic reconstruction is nocturnal incontinence. Urodynamic assessment of reconstructed bladders has shown that detubularised ileum provides a reservoir with the least amount of pressure activity during filling which should in theory reduce the incidence of nocturnal incontinence. Whichever method is used, regular postoperative assessment of the upper tracts by means of ultrasonography is important as high intra-vesical pressures can develop over time. The reconstructive urologist needs to be familiar with several techniques. Sigmoid diverticular disease would preclude the use of sigmoid colon; small bowel with a short mesentery may cause difficulties in mobilisation. Sometimes the caecum may not reach the urethra. An antireflux procedure is recommended for the implantation of the ureters (Leduc et al 1987).

The mechanism of continence in continent diversion includes the Mitrofanoff Principle, narrow efferent limbs (Indiana pouch) and invaginated efferent limbs (Kock pouch). In the Mitrofanoff approach, the urinary reservoir is provided with a narrow conduit which is tunnelled submucosally to achieve a continence mechanism (Hasan et al 1994b). The conduits used include the appendix, ureter, fallopian tube or narrowed sections of bowel. The Kock pouch refined by Skinner and associates is the commonest form of continent diversion performed (Skinner et al 1987). Unfortunately, the technique has a high re-operation rate as a result of problems with the continence mechanism.

ADVANCES IN BASIC SCIENCE

Non-random chromosomal deletions

Early cytogenetic studies with karyotypic analysis have defined numerical and structural changes in several chromosomes (Hopman et al 1991). However karyotyping is time-consuming and reliable results can only be achieved by analysing cells which have been stimulated into mitosis. Although DNA content can be determined by flow cytometric or image analysis, it does not provide information about genetic events which determine tumour evolution. Fluorescence *in situ* hybridisation (FISH) has enabled the rapid characterisation of genetic aberrations in interphase nuclei of individual cells. One study has shown that in aneuploid tumours, there was no discrepancy between FISH and flow cytometry (Matsuyama et al 1994). In contrast, minor chromosomal aberrations were found in 90% of cases by FISH whereas flow cytometry deemed the sample as diploid. Therefore, it would suggest that flow cytometric analysis will fail to detect DNA abnormalities in the presence of minor chromosomal aberrations for one or two chromosomes.

The most frequent non-random chromosomal aberration in low grade superficial tumours is the loss of chromosome 9q (Cairns et al 1993). Monosomy 9 has also been reported in random mucosal biopsies taken adjacent to the primary tumour (Matsuyama et al 1994); it also has been reported in bladder washings taken from patients with a past history of bladder cancer but with no apparent evidence of a recurrence (Wheeless et al 1994). These findings are exciting and suggest that loss of chromosome 9 is an early genetic event in bladder cancer, possibly resulting in the loss of at least one tumour suppressor gene.

Monoclonal origin versus field change in metachronous bladder cancer

One theory for the synchronous or metachronous formation of superficial bladder tumours is that a chemical insult results in a field change in the form of dysplasia or carcinoma *in situ*. *In situ* changes in the urothelium are often found near the base of primary tumours. Such field changes would theoretically result in multiclonal oncogene activation or loss of tumour suppressor genes.

Support for the monoclonal theory has recently come from a genetic study in 4 women who presented with multifocal tumours (Sidransky et al 1992). It was found, using polymorphic markers, that in each individual the same X chromosome was activated in each of the concomitant tumours. Interestingly, each of the tumours in a given patient showed loss of the same chromosome 9q allele. This again gave support to the theory that loss of the chromosome 9q allele is an early event in bladder cancer initiation. The success of single instillation intravesical chemotherapy given immediately after transurethral resection (in terms of an increased time to first recurrence) may be due to prevention of tumour implantation.

New prognostic factors

Epidermal growth factor receptor (EGFR) is emerging as an important prognostic factor. In a recent prospective study, 212 patients with newly diagnosed bladder cancer were followed up for a mean of 26.5 months (Mellon et al 1995). The presence of EGFR was confirmed in multivariate analyses to be an independent predictor of stage progression and mortality. EGFR did not provide independent prognostic information regarding recurrence. EGFR positive patients had a 6-fold increased relative risk of dying from bladder cancer but grade remained a superior predictor of cancer death with an 8-fold relative risk. EGFR was found to be 80% sensitive and 93% specific in predicting stage progression in pT1G3 bladder cancer. EGFR may, therefore, have a role to play in deciding the most appropriate management of high risk patients.

Expression of the tumour suppressor gene p53, has been shown by some authors in multivariate analysis to be an independent prognostic marker for progression in carcinoma *in situ* of the bladder (Sarkis et al 1994). In this retrospective study, p53 expression was the only independent prognostic marker for progression. In another retrospective trial, T1 tumours exhibiting overexpression of p53 have been reported to have a higher probability of disease progression (Sarkis et al 1993, Thomas et al 1994). Cordon-Cardo and associates found that the accuracy of detecting p53 mutations by immunohistochemistry was over 90% (Cordon-Cardo et al 1994). Numerous studies have confirmed that p53 mutation is a late event in bladder cancer. No association has been reported between the presence of p53 mutations and survival in muscle-invasive tumours (Vet et al 1994). However the prognostic significance of p53 mutations in low stage and low grade tumours is not yet known.

Reduced expression of the tumour suppressor gene retinoblastoma (Rb) is associated with high stage and high grade bladder cancer. A significantly reduced tumour-free survival is associated with altered Rb expression (Logothetis et al 1992, Cordon-Cardo et al 1992). To date, no additional significant prognostic information has been derived from studying the oncogenes c-erbB-2 and H-ras in bladder cancer.

KEY POINTS FOR CLINICAL PRACTICE

- The instigation of haematuria clinics and the use of flexible cystoscopy will reduce delays in diagnosis and will allow investigation of patients at a single clinic visit. It is uncertain whether this will improve survival.
- A targeted follow-up policy based on the number of tumours at presentation and the presence or absence of tumour at the 3-month cystoscopy should reduce unnecessary cystoscopies while at the same time concentrating resources on patients with a high risk of recurrence and progression.
- A single instillation of intravesical epirubicin or mitomycin C immediately following transurethral resection in newly diagnosed patients increases the time to recurrence and reduces the recurrence rate by 50% with minimal side effects.
- Intravesical BCG immunotherapy is probably more effective than intravesical chemotherapy in reducing the recurrence rate and risk of progression in high-risk patients with rapidly recurrent tumours.
- In view of its systemic toxicity, BCG immunotherapy is usually reserved for patients with diffuse carcinoma in situ or refractory multifocal disease.
- Orthotopic reconstruction of the bladder following radical cystectomy is now an option in patients at high-risk of progressing to muscle invasion or metastatic disease.
- Young patients with diffuse carcinoma *in situ*, pT1G3 tumours and refractory multifocal disease who might be candidates for urinary tract reconstruction should be referred to specialist centres.
- Cooperation between basic scientists and clinicians has identified new prognostic factors with possible clinical implications.

REFERENCES

Althausen AF, Prout GR, Daly JJ 1976 Non-invasive papillary carcinoma of the bladder associated with carcinoma *in situ*. J Urol 116: 575-580

Abel PD, Henderson D, Bennett MK et al 1988 Differing interpretations by pathologists of the pT category and grade of transitional cell cancer of the bladder. Br J Urol 62: 339-342
Birch BRP, Harland SJ 1989 The pT1G3 bladder tumour. Br J Urol 64: 109-116.
Bouffioux C 1991 Intravesical adjuvant treatment in superficial bladder cancer. Scand J Urol Nephrol Suppl 138: 167-177
Britton JP 1993 Effectiveness of haematuria clinics. Br J Urol 71: 247-252
Cairns P, Shaw ME, Knowles MA 1993 Preliminary mapping of the deleted region of chromosome 9 in bladder cancer. Cancer Res 53: 1230-1232
Cookson MS, Sarosdy MF 1992 Management of stage T1 superficial bladder cancer with intravesical Bacillus Calmette Guérin therapy. J Urol 148: 797-801
Cordon Cardo C, Wortinger D, Petrylak D et al 1992 Altered expression of the retinoblastoma gene product: prognostic indicator in bladder cancer. J Natl Cancer Inst 84: 1251-1256
Cordon-Cardo C, Dalbagni G, Saez GT et al 1994 p53 mutations in human bladder cancer: genotypic versus phenotypic patterns. Int J Cancer 56: 347-353
Debruyne F, van der Meyden A, Schreinecres L et al 1988 BCG RIVM intravesical immunoprophylaxis for superficial bladder cancer. In: Schröder, Klijn, Pinedo, Splinter, de Voogt (eds) Progress and controversies in oncological urology, II, EORTC GU Monograph No V Alan R Liss, New York, p 511
Duncan W, Quilty PM 1986 The results of a series of 963 patients with transitional cell carcinoma of the urinary bladder primarily treated by radical megavoltage X-ray therapy. Radiother Oncol 7: 299-310
Franklin J, Benson MC 1994 New techniques in management and treatment of superficial bladder cancer. In: Neal DE ed Tumours in urology, Springer Verlag, London pp 65-75
Greene LF, Hanash KA, Farrow GM 1973 Benign papilloma or papillary cancer of the bladder. J Urol 110: 205-207
Gulliford MC, Petruckevitch A, Burney PGT 1991 Survival with bladder cancer, evaluation of delay in treatment, type of surgeon and modality of treatment. BMJ 303: 437-440
Hall RR, Parmar MKB, Richards AB, Smith PH 1994a Proposal for changes in cystoscopic follow-up of patients with bladder cancer and adjuvant intravesical chemotherapy. BMJ 308: 257-260
Hall RR 1994b Superficial bladder cancer. BMJ 308: 910-913
Hasan ST, German K, Derry CD 1994a Same day diagnostic service for new cases of haematuria – a District General Hospital experience. Br J Urol 73: 152-154
Hasan ST, Marshall C, Neal DE 1994b Continent urinary diversion using the Mitrofanoff principle. Br J Urol. 74: 454-459
Heney NM, Ahmed S, Flanigan MJ et al 1983 Superficial bladder cancer: progression and recurrence. J Urol 130: 1083-1086
Herr HW 1991 Progression of stage T1 bladder tumours after intravesical Bacillus Calmette-Guérin. J Urol 145: 40-44
Hopman AHN, Moesker O, Smeets AWGB et al 1991 Numerical chromosome 1, 7, 9 and 11 aberrations in bladder cancer detected by *in situ* hybridisation. Cancer Res 51: 644-651
Jakse G, Hall R, Bono A et al 1992 Intravesical BCG in patients with carcinoma *in situ* of the urinary bladder. First results of the EORTC Genitourinary Group protocol 30861. In: Vilavicencio H, Fair WR (eds) Evaluation of chemotherapy in bladder cancer (Societé Internationale d'Urologie reports) Churchill Livingstone, Edinburgh pp 13-24
Lamm DL, van der Meijden APM, Morales A et al 1992a Incidence and treatment of complications of Bacillus Calmette-Guérin intravesical therapy in superficial bladder cancer. J Urol 147: 596-200
Lamm DL 1992b Carcinoma *in situ*. Urol Clin North Am 19: 499-508
Lamm DL, Crawford ED, Blumenstein B et al 1993 SWOG 8795: a randomised comparison of Bacillus Calmette-Guérin and mitomycin C prophylaxis in stage Ta and T1 transitional cell carcinoma of the bladder (abstract). J Urol 149: 282A
LeDuc A, Camey M, Teillac P 1987 An original anti-reflux uretero-ileal implantation technique: long term follow-up. J Urol 137: 1156-1158
Levinson AK, Johnson DE, Wishnow KI 1990 Indications for urethrectomy in an era of continent urinary diversion. J Urol 144: 73-75
Lipponen PK, Collan Y, Eskelinen MJ et al 1990 Comparison of morphometry and DNA flow cytometry with standard prognostic factors in bladder cancer. Br J Urol 65: 589-597
Logothetis CJ, Xu HJ, Ro JY et al 1992 Altered expression of retinoblastoma and known prognostic variables in locally advanced bladder cancer. J Natl Cancer Inst 84: 1256-1261

Lum BL, Torti FM 1991 Adjuvant intravesical pharmacotherapy for superficial bladder cancer. J Natl Cancer Inst 83: 683-695
Lutzeyer W, Rubben H, Dahm H 1982. Prognostic parameter of superficial bladder cancer: an analysis of 315 cases. J Urol 127: 250-252
Malkowicz SB, Nichols P, Lieskovsky G et al 1990 The role of radical cystectomy in the management of high grade superficial bladder cancer. J Urol 144: 641-645
Matsuyama H, Bergerheim USR, Nilson I et al 1994 Nonrandom numerical aberrations of chromosomes 7, 9 and 10 in DNA-diploid bladder cancer. Cancer Genet Cytogenet 77: 118-124
Mellon K, Shenton BK, Neal DE 1991 Is voided urine suitable for flow cytometric DNA analysis? Br J Urol 67: 48-53
Mellon K, Wright C, Kelly P et al 1995 Long-term outcome related to epidermal growth factor receptor status in bladder cancer. J Urol 153: 919-925
Morales A, Eidinger D, Bruce AW 1976 Intracavitary Bacillus Calmette-Guérin in the treatment of superficial bladder tumours. J Urol 116: 180-183
Ooms ECM, Anderson WAD, Alons CL et al 1983 Analysis of the performance of pathologists in the grading of bladder tumours. Hum Pathol 14: 140-143
Oosterlinck W, Kurth KH, Schröder F et al 1993 A prospective European Organisation for Research and Treatment of Cancer Genitourinary Group randomised trial comparing transurethral resection followed by a single intravesical instillation of epirubicin or water in single stage Ta, T1 papillary carcinoma of the bladder. J Urol 149: 749-752
Parmar MKB, Freedman LS, Hargreave TB, Tolley DA 1989. Prognostic factors for recurrence and follow-up policies in the treatment of superficial bladder cancer: Report from the British Medical Research Council subgroup on superficial bladder cancer (Urological Cancer Working Party). J Urol 142: 284-288
Powell PH, Manohar V, Ramsden PD, Hall RR 1984 A flexible cystoscope. Br J Urol 56: 622-644
Ratliff TL 1989 Mechanisms of action of BCG for bladder cancer. Prog Clin Biol Res 310: 107-122
Richards B, Parmar MKB, Anderson CK et al 1991 Interpretation of biopsies of 'normal' urothelium in patients with superficial bladder cancer. Br J Urol 67: 369-375
Sarkis AS, Dalbagni G, Cordon-Cardo C et al 1993 Nuclear overexpression of p53 protein in transitional cell bladder carcinoma: a marker for disease progression. J Natl Cancer Inst 85: 53-59
Sarkis AS, Dalbagni G, Cordon-Cardo C et al 1994 Association of p53 nuclear overexpression and tumour progression in carcinoma in situ of the bladder. J Urol 152: 388-392
Sidransky D, Frost P, Von Eschenbach A et al 1992 Clonal origin of metachronous tumours of the bladder. N Engl J Med 326: 737-740
Skinner DG, Leiskovsky G, Boyd SD 1987 Continuing experience with the continent ileal reservoir (Kock pouch) as an alternative to cutaneous urinary diversion: an update after 250 cases. J Urol: 137 1140-1144
Skinner DG, Boyd SD, Lieskovsky G et al 1991 Lower urinary tract reconstruction following cystectomy: experience and results in 126 patients using the Kock ileal reservoir with bilateral ureteroileal urethrostomy. J Urol 146: 756-760
Smith G, Elton RA, Chisholm GD et al 1986 Superficial bladder cancer: intravesical chemotherapy and tumour progression to muscle invasion or metastases. Br J Urol 58: 659-663
Stöckle M, Gökcebay E, Riedmiller H, Hohenfellner R 1990 Urethral tumour recurrences after radical cystoprostatectomy: the case for primary cystoprostatectomy. J Urol 143: 41-43
Thomas DJ, Robinson MC, Charlton R et al 1994 P53 expression, ploidy and progression in PT1 transitional cell carcinoma of the bladder. Br J Urol 73: 533-537
Tolley DA, Hargreave TB, Smith PH et al 1988 Effect of intravesical mitomycin C on recurrence of newly diagnosed superficial bladder cancer: interim report from the Medical Research Council Subgroup on superficial bladder cancer (Urological Cancer Working Party). BMJ 296: 1759-1761
Union Internationale Contre le Cancer 1992 The TNM classification of tumours. Geneva: UICC
Utz DC, Hanash KA, Farrow GM 1970 The plight of the patient with carcinoma *in situ* of the bladder. J Urol 103: 160-164
Vet JAM, Bringuier PP, Poddighe PJ 1994 p53 mutations have no additional prognostic value over stage in bladder cancer. Br J Cancer 70: 496-500

Vegt PDJ, Witjes JA, Witjes WPJ et al 1995 A randomised study of intravesical mitomycin C, Bacillus Calmette-Guérin RIVM treatment in pTa-pT1 papillary carcinoma and carcinoma *in situ* of the bladder. J Urol 153: 929-933

Walker L, Liston TG, Lloyd-Davies RW 1993 Does flexible cystoscopy miss more tumours than rod-lens examination? Br J Urol 72: 449-450

Wallace DM, Harris DL 1965 Delay in treating bladder tumours. Lancet 2: 332-334

Wheeless LL, Reeder JE, Hans R et al 1994 Bladder irrigation specimens assayed by fluorescence *in situ* hybridisation to interphase nuclei. Cytometry 17: 319-326

6

Trauma centres

R. M. Kirby *J. B. Elder* *J. Templeton*

This chapter examines the background to the concept of Trauma Centres, the set-up of such centres in North America and Europe and the background to the Trauma Centre theory in the UK.

Trauma Centres are an established feature of health care in both North America and Europe. It is generally accepted that they have resulted in improved care of patients following major injuries with a resultant increased survival. The concept of the trauma centre has yet to be established in the UK despite recurrent debates on the subject (Royal College of Surgeons 1988, Earlam 1993, Interdepartmental Committee 1939). A pilot project initiated by the Department of Health in response to a report from the Royal College of Surgeons established a Trauma Centre in a large multi-specialty tertiary hospital and compared the treatment of patients within its catchment area with that of a similar population around two other hospitals not designated as Trauma Centres. The results of this study and the process of evaluation are being assessed at the time of writing.

FEATURES OF TRAUMA

Trauma affects all ages of the population but appears as an epidemic affecting mostly young adults. Each year 545 000 patients suffer an accident, and 850 000 bed nights per year are required for road traffic accidents alone in the UK; 18 000 deaths are caused annually (Royal College of Surgeons 1988). It has been estimated that 205 000 years of life were lost in England and Wales (ages between 15 and 64) in 1990 alone. Violent death is the highest cause of death in young adult males. Death and disability in this age group have major consequences not only on an individual basis and for family groups, but also have an accumulative economic effect nationally both in terms of resources required for treating and rehabilitating these patients and also through loss of employment man hours. The World Health Organization has assessed that 1% of the gross national product in developing and developed countries is used for the management of trauma patients alone and in the UK accidents account for 7% of all NHS expenditure. *Health of the Nation* targets are to reduce death rates of children under 15 and people of 65 and over by 33% and in young people of 15–24 by 25% by the year 2005 (Royal College of Surgeons 1988, Office of Health Economics 1992, Templeton 1994, Department of Health 1993).

TRIMODAL DISTRIBUTION OF TRAUMA DEATHS

Trunkey identified a trimodal distribution of deaths following trauma (Trunkey 1983, 1985). The first peak of deaths occurs within a few seconds to minutes after injury and accounts for over half of all deaths. These deaths are due to overwhelming injury to the brain, heart or great vessels. The second peak occurs between a few minutes and an hour after injury. Brain injuries and haemorrhage are the principal cause of death in this group. Airway obstruction is a common mode of death in patients with potentially treatable head injuries who die at this stage. The third peak occurs several days or weeks after the initial injury, usually due to multi-organ failure or overwhelming sepsis. The second and third peaks should be regarded as potentially preventable.

Prevention of accidents or injury is probably more important than all attempts at dealing with injury. For example, the use of helmets for motorcyclists and cyclists has been shown to be beneficial (Williams 1989). The use of seat belts in cars has been accepted and the limitation of firearms in certain parts of North America has been associated with a lower mortality from trauma. Once serious injury has occurred, however, the problem passes from having a legislative solution to a medical one. The first peak of deaths is virtually inevitable and very little can be done to affect these. The second peak, however, can be reduced by prompt initial care in the pre-hospital phase, by early hospital resuscitation and by prompt and competent definitive care. This period has been labelled as 'The Golden Hour'. Management at this time will affect the third peak of deaths.

GENERAL CATEGORIES OF TRAUMA

Injuries may be divided into three general categories: immediately life-threatening; urgent; and non-urgent. Immediate life-threatening injuries affect 5% of trauma patients in North America but account for 50% of all in-hospital trauma deaths. Urgent injuries are not immediately life-threatening but may become so or result in significant disability. Urgent injuries in North America comprise approximately 10–15% of all patients. Approximately 80% of all injuries fall into the non-urgent category (Committee on Trauma 1989).

The importance of efficient ambulance and para-medic systems is apparent, although debate continues about the economics and efficiency of air transport versus road transport. Para-medic training is gaining ground and organisations such as BASICS (British Association for Immediate Care) have been formed to promote prompt care of patients in the field. More recently in the UK, mostly at the instigation of the Royal College of Surgeons, ATLS (Advanced Trauma Life Support) training has become widespread amongst medical practitioners involved in both the immediate resuscitation and the definitive care of patients. Generally, hospitals concerned with the reception of injured patients in the UK are not organised or networked, whereas the system of Trauma Centres set up in the USA has proven beneficial effects (West et al 1983, 1988).

Measuring severity of trauma

There are two main methods of measuring the severity of injured patients. The Injury Severity Score (ISS) is an index of anatomical injury. It is calculated from the abbreviated injury scale (AIS) where each injury is given a severity score from 1 (minor) to 6 (fatal). The highest AIS in each of 6 defined body regions is identified and the sum of the squares of the largest 3 is the ISS. A score of 6 in any region automatically gives a maximum ISS which is 75. Patients with an ISS of 16 or greater are defined as severely injured. This was devised by the Association for the Advancement of Automotive Medicine of the USA, initially for impact injury assessment, but expanded with the evolution of Trauma systems to include penetrating trauma (Association for the Advancement of Automotive Medicine 1990). The ISS does not allow for multiple injuries in the same body region and takes no account of age or pre-existing disease processes.

The Trauma Score (TS) was developed by Champion and colleagues (1983) to help in the initial assessment of injured patients. This is a physiologically based system. The respiratory rate, respiratory effort, capillary refill, systolic blood pressure and Glasgow Coma Score were each given a coded score. Each was coded 0–4 and the highest score of 16 was therefore seen in the relatively uninjured or in early stages following more severe injuries (Gilpin 1991). Unlike the ISS, the Trauma Score changes as the status of the patient deteriorates. Because the respiratory effort and the capillary refill are not straightforward parameters to measure, a Revised Trauma Score (RTS) has been introduced based on three factors. These are the Glasgow Coma Score, systolic blood pressure and the respiratory rate. Each is coded 0–4. The RTS is created using longitudinal regression analysis. A coded score of less than 8 may be associated with severe injury.

TRISS

The RTS can be plotted against the ISS and the relationship between these two is known as TRISS (Fig. 6.1). A 50% probability of survival for a group can be represented by a diagonal line. Co-ordinates above the line have estimated survival probabilities < 50% and those below the line > 50%. Survivors above the line and deaths below the line are unexpected outcomes and require further review in analysis.

Comparisons between the work of different hospitals may be made by using these methods and by finding both an injury severity match ('M' statistic) and the population outcome comparison ('Z' statistic) which measures the difference between the actual and predicted numbers of deaths or survivors (Boyd et al 1987, Yates et al 1990, 1993, Champion et al 1989, Spence et al 1988).

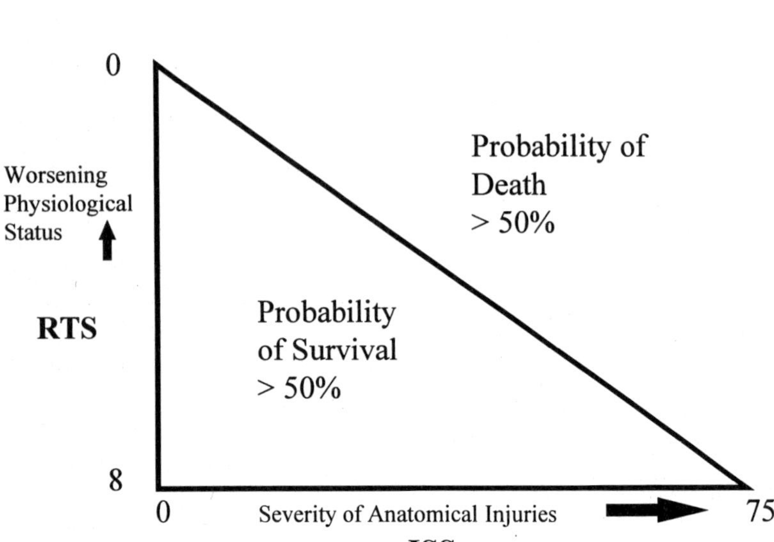

Fig. 6.1 The TRISS plot.

The Committee on Trauma of the American College of Surgeons started a Major Trauma Outcome Study (MTOS) based on TRISS scores and the first results of the UK MTOS were reported in 1992 (Yates et al 1992).

HISTORY OF TRAUMA SERVICES

Although the care of the critically injured is not always perceived to be of prime importance, the concept of caring for victims of trauma in a professional manner is not new. In 1888, Robert Jones was appointed Consulting Surgeon to the Manchester Ship Canal at the time of its construction. In a working population of up to 20 000 men, there were 1292 injuries in 6 years. Of these, 130 were fatal and 165 led to permanent injury. Jones instigated a system of 3 independent hospitals each with a resident doctor, external medical sources and a direct 'overland railway' system running the length of the canal for rapid delivery of trauma victims. The effectiveness of this system was acknowledged to have been beneficial in preventing even more loss of life (Seddon 1961).

In 1939, the Interdepartmental Committee on Persons Injured by Accident referred to 'the serious defects under which injuries are treated in a large number of our hospitals'. Despite this, they concluded that proposals for the institution of general trauma services were not called for. In defiance of this conclusion, the Birmingham Accident Hospital opened in the old Queens Hospital building under the pioneering leadership of William Gissane in April 1941. The hospital was staffed by teams led by resident consultant staff and quickly demonstrated that a professional and experienced approach to the management of trauma patients resulted in increased recovery and survival figures. In June 1944, injured soldiers were transferred to the UK following the Normandy landings. Gissane advocated a National system of about 20 accident hospitals although this view was not widely supported at that time (London 1982).

In 1961, the Accident Services Review Committee of the British Medical Association proposed a three tier service with Minor Injury Units staffed by general practitioners, District General Hospital Units under the supervision of specialists and Regional Trauma Units each serving a population of 1-2 million people. At the same time, the Ministry of Health Standing Medical Advisory Committee was suggesting a two tier system and the recommendations of this latter report were accepted. As a result of this, a two tier system based on small casualty services and Accident and Emergency Departments within District General Hospitals was set up, but there were no proposals for Regional Trauma Units. In 1971, a new type of specialist/consultant in Accident and Emergency Medicine was proposed and appointed.

Trauma services in the USA

In 1979, West and colleagues examined a group of injured patients in the adjoining counties of San Francisco and Orange County. They demonstrated that survival rates for major trauma could be improved by transporting severely injured patients to a Trauma Centre rather than the nearest hospital. In Orange County, two-thirds of non-CNS related deaths and one-third of CNS related deaths were judged to have been potentially preventable. Only one of 92 deaths in San Francisco County was so judged. Trauma victims in Orange County were younger and the magnitude of injuries causing death was less than in San Francisco. Following the creation of Trauma Centres in Orange County, preventable deaths fell from 73% to 4%. Further studies in North America confirmed that there were major survival advantages to treating the severely injured in specialist centres rather than in the nearest hospitals (Cales 1984, West et al 1983, Shackford et al 1986, Kane 1992).

The Committee on Trauma at the American College of Surgeons suggested three levels of trauma services (Committee on Trauma 1989). Level 3 Trauma Centres or Local Trauma Centres are small community hospitals without resident staff able to deal with minor injuries but with protocols for transfer of more seriously injured patients. Level 2 centres or Community Trauma Centres are designated larger hospitals with more facilities available for dealing with a large volume of trauma but without a wide range of specialties being available. Level 1 Trauma Centres or Regional Resource Trauma Centres are designated major hospitals able to deal with major trauma, not only in terms of large numbers but also with a wide range of available specialties. In 1989, there were 638 'certified' Trauma Centres among 5265 general Civilian Hospitals in the US (Howard 1994). Canadian units are operating similar systems (McMurty et al 1989, Pagliarello et al 1992).

Trauma surgery in the USA is a subspecialty of general surgery. Severely injured patients are usually admitted under the care of a Trauma Service unless they have unisystem injuries in which case they are admitted under the care of the appropriate specialty.

Trauma systems in Europe

In Germany, specialised ambulances or helicopters are used for high speed transport of injured patients to a network of specialised Trauma Centres. Any supervising doctor concerned in the transport of patients to these centres is required to have intensive care experience.

France is divided into 95 administrative areas or Départements. By law each Département is required to provide a SAMU (Service d'Aide Médicale Urgente). This is an emergency medical service based in the main hospital in the principal city Départements. A SAMU doctor is available for resuscitation at the scene of an accident and for care of the patient during transport. The controller of the SAMU will decide which local hospital will receive the injured patient. There is, therefore, medical input in the pre-hospital care of injured patients before transport to the definitive unit (RCS 1988).

TRAUMA CARE IN THE UK

Trauma care at present in the UK is a haphazard affair and remains so, despite increasing interest in trauma management. Any hospital with an Accident and Emergency Department may receive major trauma depending on decisions made by the local Ambulance Unit. Patients may, therefore, arrive either in a small department staffed at night only by a Senior House Officer or they may arrive in a larger unit where they may be assessed and treated by experienced staff of either Consultant or Higher Trainee level. The Confidential Enquiry into Peri-operative Deaths (CEPOD) noted, in 1987, that patients had died after being taken into Accident and Emergency Departments which were not geared to the initial management of major trauma. CEPOD proposed a review of the workload and siting of major trauma centres to resolve these problems (Buck et al 1987).

A landmark study instigated by the Royal College of Surgeons Working Party retrospectively analysed 1000 deaths from injury (Anderson et al 1988). Of 1000 deaths, 514 patients had been admitted to hospital alive. Amongst the 514 initial survivors, 102 (20%) deaths were judged to have been potentially preventable by 4 assessors. When cases in which 3 of 4 assessors considered death was preventable were included, the total was rose to 170 (33%). 89 of the 170 patients had multiple injuries and, although 73 apparently needed an operation, 57 did not receive one. In total, two-thirds of all non-central nervous system deaths were judged to have been preventable. The mean age of these patients was 41. The principal cause of death was bleeding, with hypoxia as the second most common cause.

The care of 14 648 injured patients treated in 33 British hospitals was reported in the first report of the UK Major Trauma Outcome Study (MTOS) in 1992 (Yates et al 1992). The conclusions from this report demonstrated the inadequacy of the initial management of major trauma in the UK. A Senior House Officer was in charge of initial hospital resuscitation in 57% of patients with severe injuries. Although senior staff were usually responsible for definitive operations, only 46% of patients judged to require early operation arrived in theatre within 2 h. The mortality for 6 111 patients sustaining blunt trauma and treated in the 14 busiest hospitals was significantly higher than in a comparable North American data set, although the outcome of 597 patients with penetrating injuries was better than that of a comparable group in the US.

An important earlier study in the Report of the Working Party of The Royal College of Surgeons examined unexpected survivors following major trauma. The shared characteristics of these patients were that they had been transferred from the scene of the accident directly and rapidly; resuscitation had been performed by a consultant on arrival, intra-cerebral damage was rapidly excluded by computed tomography and, if operations were required, they were performed without delay and were definitive. Resuscitation was continued in the intensive care unit and was based on measurement of oxygen transport and at no time was transfer to another hospital necessary (Royal College of Surgeons 1988, Spence & Redmond 1988). The clinical messages from these studies painfully echo the findings of West, Trunkey and Lim in 1979 in the Orange County study. Nine years later in a leading article in the *British Journal of Surgery*, Trunkey commented on the 'suboptimal care' offered to trauma patients in the UK and proposed a system of trauma care based around Trauma Centres (Trunkey 1988).

In conclusion to its 1988 report published a few months before Trunkey's leading article, The Royal College of Surgeons Working Party had also proposed the instigation of Trauma Centres on a regional or multi-district basis. They proposed that such Trauma Centres should take patients with life-threatening injury, the management of which was beyond the facilities or capabilities of most District General Hospitals. The Trauma Centre staff should ensure immediate and appropriate care for injured patients, all patients with multiple system or major injury should be evaluated initially by the Trauma Team and the surgeon responsible for overall care of the patient (Team Leader) should be identified. Optimum staff requirements for Trauma Centres were laid out (Table 6.1).

Department of Health project

In 1991, the Department of Health funded a single Trauma Centre on an experimental format to evaluate its cost-effectiveness in the UK. The trial was designed to compare this designated Trauma Centre with comparator sites in similar hospitals with similar facilities not designated as trauma centres. Following submission of bids, the North Staffordshire Hospital was chosen to be the Trauma Centre; Hull Royal Infirmary and the Royal Preston Hospital

Table 6.1 Optimum staff requirements for Trauma Centres as suggested by The Royal College of Surgeons Working Party

Essential specialties	
General Surgery	Orthopaedic Surgery
Anaesthesia	Emergency Medicine
Neurosurgery	Urological Surgery
Ophthalmic Surgery	Maxillo-Facial/Dental Surgery
Plastic Surgery	Otorhinolaryngological Surgery
Paediatric Surgery	Intensive Therapy
Cardiology	Diagnostic and Interventional Radiology
Respiratory Medicine	Nephrology
Chemical Pathology	Haematology
Bacteriology	
Desirable specialties	
Cardiothoracic Surgery	Gastro-enterology
Essential operating theatre requirements	
Fully staffed operating theatres available 24 h/day	
Cardio-pulmonary bypass	
Operating microscope	
Monitoring equipment	
Essential radiological facilities	
Angiography of all types	CT
Ultrasonography	Nuclear medicine

were selected to be the comparator sites. The Department of Health allocated £1 million annually to the North Staffordshire Hospital over the period of this study. Most (88%) of this funding went directly into salaries including those for 4 consultants. The University of Sheffield Medical Care Research Unit was funded to evaluate, independently, the Trauma Centre and the comparator sites. The aim of the study was 'to observe the impact, in terms of changes in clinical outcome and cost, of regionalising trauma care services for patients suffering from severe injury'. They were to measure changes in the 'probability of death' and judge avoidable deaths (Redmond et al 1993, Williams 1990).

Background to Stoke-on-Trent trauma system

North Staffordshire Hospital, Stoke-on-Trent, has over 1 300 beds serving a local population of 500 000. All the specialties in Table 6.1 are on site except paediatric surgery and there is a 10-bedded ICU. There had been a background of Trauma Research based in the Academic Department of Traumatic and Orthopaedic Surgery in the Postgraduate School of Medicine of the University of Keele. An epidemiological study on trauma in the district had been started in 1989. Over a 12-month period, the Accident and Emergency Department treated 89 631 patients. Of these, 60 607 (67.6%) were injured

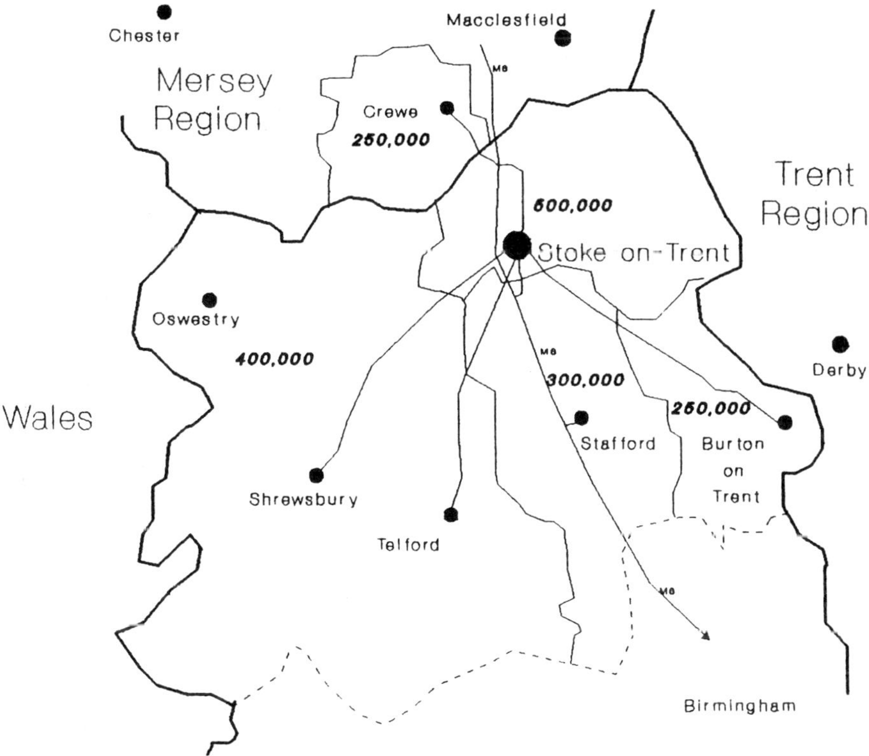

Fig. 6.2 The North West Midlands Trauma System based on the Trauma Centre at the North Staffordshire Hospital, Stoke-on-Trent. The site of main roads are shown, and the populations of the individual districts are displayed.

and 2 506 (4.1%) of the injured required admission to hospital, and 114 patients had major injuries (ISS, Injury Severity Score, > 16); there were an additional 24 injured patients with a revised trauma score (RTS) < 8 who were also considered to be severely injured. There was thus a background to assess the impact of a Trauma System on this trauma service.

The North Staffordshire Trauma System drains a population of approximately 2 million (Fig. 6.2). Five satellite District General Hospitals are at the periphery of the geographical area and Stoke-on-Trent is near the centre. Patients are transferred directly to North Staffordshire Hospital by road or by helicopter either from the site of the accident at the instigation of the ambulance service or from one of the outlying hospitals. Decisions are made depending on physiological features (Revised Trauma Score) or mode of injury (Table 6.2).

Management of the Trauma Centre

A trauma executive, chaired by the Chief Executive of the Trust, supervises the

Table 6.2 Protocol for the admission of seriously injured patients to Trauma Centre

Unconscious or significant history of unconsciousness
Triage RTS < 7.8, GCS < 13
Pedestrian hit by car
Motorcyclist or cyclist (unless accident was stationary or very low speed)
Motor vehicle accident at speed
Death of anyone in that accident
Fall from a height greater than 10 feet (3 m)
Burns of 10% or more of body surface
Inhalation burns
Fractured shaft of femur
More than 1 long bone fracture
Possible cervical spine fracture
More than 1 body compartment involved
Penetrating injury to head, neck, chest or abdomen
Entrapment for more than 20 min
Amputation of a limb

financial costs and spending of the Trauma Centre. Each hospital within the system is represented on a Trauma System Committee which examines the work of the entire system. A multidisciplinary Trauma Centre Committee determined the initial protocols for admission to the Trauma Centre (Table 6.2) and for the initial management of patients including those with possible intra-abdominal injuries (Table 6.3).

Setting up the Trauma Centre

North American and European Trauma Centres had been visited independently by an orthopaedic surgeon, anaesthetist, accident and emergency surgeon and a general surgeon to see different models of Trauma Centres at work. Although North American Trauma Centres are led by general surgeons (trauma surgeons) the previous study carried out at the North Staffordshire Hospital (Trauma Research Group 1991) had demonstrated that general surgical involvement in the management of patients with major injuries in North Staffordshire was low. It was, therefore, agreed that the Trauma Team Leader should be an Accident and Emergency specialist or an anaesthetist with a special interest in trauma and with no conflicting timetabled commitments during the period on duty. Each of the six consultants (2 anaesthetists, 4 A&E surgeons) is on duty for 24 h and is resident in the hospital overnight.

Trauma Team

Initially, the Trauma Team consisted of senior specialists but within a short time it was altered to a more junior team led by the resident consultant Trauma Team Leader although including an anaesthetic registrar/senior registrar in addition to Accident and Emergency Department SHOs. At the discretion of the Trauma Team Leader, the full Trauma Team (including

Table 6.3 Indications for diagnostic peritoneal lavage (DPL) or abdominal ultrasonography

Strong indications

Unconscious patient
Paralysed/ventilated patient
Hypotension of unknown cause

Indications

Evidence of abdominal injury in a patient who was hypotensive prior to resuscitation
Injuries above and below the diaphragm

Contra-indications

Shocked patient with obvious abdominal injury
Penetrating injury to the abdomen

neurosurgery, orthopaedic surgery and general surgery) is summoned. A protocol was written for resuscitation based on ATLS teaching. After resuscitation, patients are referred to the appropriate specialty for admission. Default admissions (i.e. those with no single injury) come under the control of the Traumatic and Orthopaedic Service.

Rehabilitation

Part of the remit of the Department of Health study was to examine those patients surviving major injury. It has been recognised since 1918 that active rehabilitation plays an important role in the management of trauma patients (Jones 1918). A specialised rehabilitation unit which forms part of the North Staffordshire Hospital receives patients following discharge from the acute wards for rehabilitation training.

Results of study

Following the designation of the North Staffordshire Hospital as a Trauma Centre, the number of cases admitted directly from the scene of an accident gradually increased (Table 6.4). At the same time, mortality rates gradually reduced even though the average age of the patients admitted increased.

Table 6.4 Early results from North Staffordshire Trauma Centre (1989–1990 before establishment of the Trauma Centre; 1992–1993 and 1993–1994 Trauma Centre functioning) (Bain 1996)

	1989–1990	1992–1993	1993–1994
A&E admissions	2506	2647	2769
Severely injured (SI)	138	251	227
ISS > 15	114	170	184
RTS < 7.84	24	81	43
General surgical involvement in SI	22	64	59
Operations in SI	65	115	129
General surgical operations in SI	10	26	16
Deaths	38	55	48

The contribution of general surgery was analysed separately. Approximately 25% of the severely injured patients admitted to the Trauma Centre were assessed by general surgeons. The majority of these were seen in the Accident and Emergency Department and many did not require further appraisal. Higher proportions were seen by neurosurgical (70–85%) and orthopaedic teams 34–55%. Fewer than 15% of severely injured patients required general surgical operations with the majority of these being laparotomies. This is undoubtedly a result of the low incidence of penetrating trauma compared to the North American experience (Renz & Feliciano 1995). A separate study of trauma deaths in the district (Hussain & Redmond 1994) identified only 11.2% of pre-hospital trauma deaths due to penetrating injury. The low proportion of patients needing help from general surgery would suggest that there is no place for a 'Trauma Surgeon' in General Surgery in the UK even within a large tertiary hospital/Trauma Centre. This does not deny, however, the importance of the general surgeon in the identification and treatment of major intra-abdominal injuries when intervention has been shown to be vital (Table 6.3).

The conclusions of the Department of Health Study have not been published at the time of writing this chapter. However it is unlikely that large differences will be found between the designated Trauma Centre and the comparator sites because these hospitals are similar in size to the designated Trauma Centre with well-organised A&E departments, supported by a Trauma team and excellent facilities. They are already effectively acting as Trauma Centres. Therefore the awaited report will not necessarily answer the question whether patients should be transferred to large hospitals or treated in small units.

A number of large tertiary hospitals have already set up formal Trauma Units. The Helicopter Emergency Medical Service (HEMS) based at the Royal London Hospital has been bringing trauma patients into a specially converted unit. The Trauma Unit has been under the direction of general surgeons and all multiple trauma patients stay under their care, although patients' injuries may be managed by other specialist teams (Earlam 1992, Kirk et al 1993). Oxford has also set up a unit with resident consultant staff at night to receive and treat injured patients. Many other large tertiary referral hospitals, or those with a substantial trauma workload have organised trauma teams along the lines advocated by the RCS to receive trauma patients and to deal with immediate injury.

FUTURE OF TRAUMA CARE IN THE UK

A Trauma Centre does not need to be a purpose built unit and the designation and terminology, which may be contentious, are unimportant. There are at present 320 hospitals in the UK with Accident and Emergency Units. Of these, 23 have neurosurgery departments on site and only 7 of these also have cardiothoracic surgery on site. The whole of the UK would benefit from approximately 26 trauma systems each serving 5–10 District General Hospitals and each with 1 designated tertiary referral centre with facilities for neurosurgery and cardiovascular surgery which may or may not have the designation of 'Trauma Centre'. A network of this kind including approximately 180 District General Hospitals would greatly facilitate national planning for disasters and would lead to better care of the severely injured.

The Trauma Centre Project in Stoke-on-Trent was initiated with temporary funding of £1 million annually. If this is repeated nationwide through 26 centres it would cost £26 million either to the National Health Service or to the Treasury on top of the present NHS budget. It has been recognised in the US that Trauma Centres, although carrying a certain prestige, represent a drain on resources and are therefore not always encouraged (Eastman et al 1994, Hammond 1990, Thal & Rochon 1991). With the Health Service reforms in Britain leading to a split between purchasers and providers of health care, the initiation of multi-district systems presents extra difficulties. This should not, however, be allowed to postpone any longer the necessary change in the management and control of the trauma epidemic of the UK. It remains to be seen, however, whether there is enough paediatric trauma to justify a separate trauma system to deal specifically with injured children (Teanby et al 1994, Levy et al 1994).

Pre-hospital care

Although Trauma Centres are envisaged as being at the centre of the trauma system, professional pre-hospital care is vital. The ambulance service is crucial to the function of the Trauma System. Severely injured patients should be taken from the scene of the accident to the most appropriate hospital which may not always be the nearest hospital. This places great responsibility on the ambulance crews and communication between crews at the scene of the accident and the Trauma Centre is vital. Trauma team leaders can give advice directly and relieve the burden of responsibility on the ambulance service. Standards of trauma care need to be developed for triage criteria and Trauma Centre designations. A trauma register is required to accumulate relevant data so that trends can be identified and problems addressed.

Quality control

Once a nationwide system is operational, the work will need to be closely monitored. This can be done by using the clinical opinion of independent assessors and, mathematically using the TRISS formula which allows comparisons to be made between different hospitals or trauma systems. In 1987 Shackford and colleagues wrote: 'This is not a fixed target, this must be the start of the new system. The system must be honed and audited'. It is only by fulfilling these criteria that a nationwide trauma system for the UK will be shown to have major benefits in the new millenium.

KEY POINTS FOR CLINICAL PRACTICE

- Trauma is the major cause of death in young adult males.
- Deaths after major trauma follow a trimodal pattern. Deaths within a few minutes are usually inevitable but deaths occurring in the second peak (up to a few hours) should be regarded as potentially preventable.
- Early transfer of patients to a specialised centre has been shown to be associated with a reduced death rate in North America.
- A network of trauma systems based on District General Hospitals and Trauma Centres should be set up in the UK.
- Trauma Centres need not be separate structures but should be designated tertiary hospitals with suitable facilities and major specialties on site including cardiothoracic surgery and neurosurgery.
- The pattern and incidence of trauma in the UK does not require the formation of a specialist discipline of trauma surgery within general surgery.
- General surgical participation in the management of major trauma is vital to reduce unnecessary deaths.

REFERENCES

Anderson ID, Woodford M, de Dombal FT, Irving M 1988 Retrospective study of 1000 deaths from injury in England and Wales. BMJ 296: 1305-1308

Association for the Advancement of Automative Medicine 1990 The Abbreviated Injury Scale 1990 Revision. Des Plainess, Illinois, USA

Bain IM, Kirby RM, Cook AL, Oakley PA, Templeton J 1996 The role of the general surgeon in a British Trauma Centre. BrJ Surg 83: in press

Boyd CR, Tolson MA, Copes WS 1987 Evaluating trauma care: the TRISS method. J Trauma 27: 370-378

Buck N, Devlin HB, Lunn JN 1987 The Report of a Confidential Enquiry into Perioperative Deaths. The Nuffield Provincial Hospitals Trust and The King's Fund, London

Cales RH 1984 Trauma mortality in Orange County: the effect of implementation of a regional trauma system. Ann Emerg Med 13: 15-24

Champion HR, Sacco WJ, Hunt TK 1983 Trauma severity scoring to predict mortality. World J Surg 7: 4-11

Champion HR, Sacco WJ, Copes WS 1989 A revision of the trauma score. J Trauma 29: 623-629

Committee on Trauma, American College of Surgery 1989 Hospital Resources for Optimal Care of the Injured Patient. American College of Surgeons, Chicago, USA

Committee on Trauma, American College of Surgeons 1989 Advanced Trauma Life Support Course. American College of Surgeons, Chicago, USA

Department of Health 1993 Accidents Key Area Handbook. HMSO, London

Earlam RJ ed 1992 The Royal London Hospital Daily Express helicopter emergency medical service. Saldatore, Bishops Stortford

Earlam RJ 1993 Trauma Centres. Br J Surg 80: 1227-1228

Eastman AB, Bishop GS, Walsh JC 1994 The economic status of Trauma Centers on the eve of health care reform. J Trauma 36: 835-844, discussion 844-846

Gilpin DA, Nelson PG 1991 Revised trauma score: a triage team in the Accident and Emergency Department. Injury 22: 35-37

Hammond J, Gomez G, Eckes J 1990 Trauma systems. Economic and political considerations. J Fla Med Assoc 77: 603-605

Howard JM 1994 Trauma – the disease that was neglected. Progress: past and that to be. J R Coll Surg Edinb 39: 335-343
Hussain LM, Redmond AD 1994 Are pre-hospital deaths from accidental injury preventable? BMJ 308: 1077-1080
Interdepartmental Committee 1939 Final report on Rehabilitation of Persons Injured by Accidents. HMSO London
Jones R 1918 Notes on military orthopaedics. British Red Cross Society, Cassels, London
Kane G, Wheeler NC, Cook S et al 1992 Impact of the Los Angeles County trauma system on the survival of seriously injured patients. J Trauma 32: 576-583
Kirk CJC, Earlam RJ, Wilson AW, Watkins ES 1993 Helicopter emergency medical service operating from the Royal London Hospital: the first year. Br J Surg 80: 218-221
Levy EN, Griffith JA, Carvajal HF 1994 Pediatric trauma care is cost effective: a comparison of pediatric and adult trauma care reimbursement. J Trauma 36: 504-507
London PS 1982 Inaugural William Gissane lecture – Man and memorial. Br J Accid Surg 14: 211-234
McMurty RY, Nelson WR, de la Roche MR 1989 Current concepts in trauma. 2. The Sunnybrook Medical Centre trauma progression: the first 11 years. Can Med Assoc J 141: 555-559
North Staffordshire Hospital 1993 Trauma Centre. Stoke on Trent, UK
Office of Health Economics. Compendium of health statistics 1992, 8th edn
Pagliarello G, Dempster A, Wesson D 1992 The integrated trauma program: a model for co-operative trauma triage. J Trauma 33: 198-203
Redmond AD, Johnstone S, Maryosh J, Templeton J 1993 A Trauma Centre in the UK. Ann R Coll Surg Engl 75: 317-320
Renz BM, Feliciano DV 1995 Unnecessary laparotomies for trauma: a prospective study of morbidity. J Trauma Injury Infect Crit Care 38: 350-356
Royal College of Surgeons of England 1988 Report of the Working Party on The Management of Patients with Major Injuries. Royal College of Surgeons, London
Seddon HJ 1961 The Manchester Ship Canal and the colonial frontier. J Bone Joint Surg 43B: 425-443
Shackford SR, Hollingworth-Fridlund P, Cooper GF, Eastman AB 1986 The effect of regionalization upon the quality of trauma care as assessed by concurrent audit before and after institution of a trauma system: a preliminary report. J Trauma 26: 812-820
Shackford SR, Hollingsworth-Fridlund P, Mcardle M, Eastman AB 1987 Assuring quality in a trauma system – the Medical Audit Committee: composition, cost, and results. J Trauma 27: 866-875
Spence MT, Redmond AD, Edwards JD 1988 Trauma audit – the use of TRISS. Health Trends 20: 94-97
Teanby DN, Lloyd DA, Gorman DF, Boot DA 1994 Regional review of blunt trauma in children. Br J Surg 81: 53-55
Templeton J 1994 Organising the management of life-threatening injuries. Br J Bone Joint Surg 76B: 3-5
Thal ER, Rochon RB 1991 Inner-city Trauma Centers—financial burdens or community saviors? Surg Clin North Am 71: 209-219
Trauma Research Group 1991 An incidence study of trauma in the North Staffordshire Health District. University of Keele, UK
Trunkey DD 1983 Trauma. Sci Am 249: 28-35
Trunkey DD 1985 Towards optimal trauma care. Arch Emerg Med 2: 181-195
Trunkey DD 1988 A time for decisions. Br J Surg 75: 937-939
West JG, Trunkey DD, Lim RC 1979 Systems of trauma care. Arch Surg 114: 455-459
West JG, Williams MJ, Trunkey DD, Wolferth CC 1988 Trauma systems: current status—future challenges. JAMA 259: 3597-3600
Williams BT 1990 Regional Trauma Centre evaluation. Department of Health, London, UK
Williams M 1989 The protective performance of bicyclists' helmets in accidents. Royal Melbourne Institute of Technology, Melbourne, Australia
Yates DW 1990 Scoring systems for trauma (ABC of major trauma). BMJ 301: 1090-1094
Yates DW, Woodford M, Hollis S 1992 Preliminary analysis of the care of injured patients in 33 British hospitals: first Report of the United Kingdom Major Trauma Outcome Study. BMJ 305: 737-740
Yates DW, Woodford M, Hollis S 1993 Trauma audit: clinical judgement or statistical analysis? Ann R Coll Surg Engl 75: 321-324

7

Bone metastases

S. E. Downey *N. J. Bundred*

Over 30% of patients with cancer eventually develop bone metastases. Breast, lung and prostate carcinomas account for over 80% of patients with metastatic bone disease, although renal, squamous and thyroid cancers commonly metastasize to this site (Table 7.1). Of the 21 000 people who die from breast and prostate cancer in the UK each year, 75% will develop bone metastases prior to death. The presence of bone metastases not only leads to bone pain, which may be difficult to control, and disability, which significantly impairs quality of life for the patient, but also carries the risk of life-threatening complications such as pathological fracture, cord compression and hypercalcaemia.

NORMAL BONE REMODELLING

Bone consists of a collagenous matrix which is formed by osteoblasts in closely packed lamellae and contains a variety of extracellular proteins, such as osteocalcin, glycosaminoglycans, and growth factors, such as transforming growth factor β (Yoneda et al 1994). This matrix is calcified by the deposition of hydroxyapatite crystals along the collagen fibres. Bone remodelling depends upon the interaction between osteoblasts (bone forming cells) and osteoclasts (bone removing cells). Daily, damaged bone recruits osteoclasts to its surface which dissolve the bone matrix and release calcium via the extracellular fluid into the blood stream (Fig. 7.1). Osteoblasts are attracted into the cavity and produce the collagen matrix in which some remain and differentiate into osteocytes. The osteoblasts are also responsible for calcification of the matrix (min-

Table 7.1 Incidence of bone metastases from different primary cancers and the type of lesions most often produced

Sites of primary	Incidence of bone metastases (%) Median	Range	Type
Breast	73	47–85	lytic (rarely sclerotic)
Prostate	68	33–85	sclerotic
Thyroid	42	28–60	lytic
Kidney	35	33–40	lytic
Bronchus	36	30–55	lytic/sclerotic
Colon/rectum	11	8–13	lytic
Oesophagus	6	5–7	lytic
Stomach/carcinoids	5	3–11	sclerotic

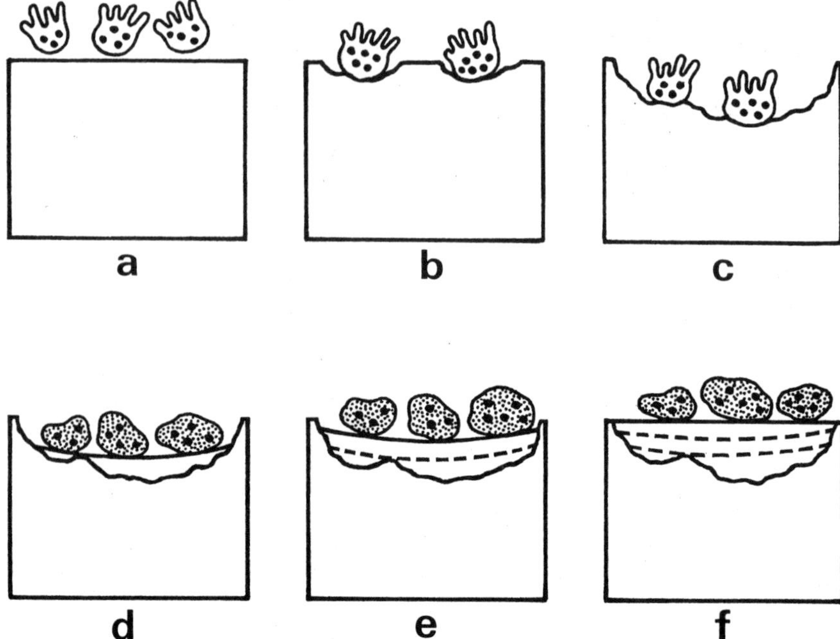

Fig. 7.1 Sequence of events in bone remodelling: multi-nucleated osteoclasts are attracted to the bone surface (a) and dissolve the bone matrix (b) to form a cavity or Howships lacuna (c). Osteoblasts are attracted into the cavity (d), where they produce collagen matrix (e) and mineralise the matrix from the base (f).

eralisation) which occurs 10–15 days after the matrix has been laid down (Fig. 7.1). Each resorption cavity is a dynamic remodelling site and there are an estimated 1–2 million sites in an adult skeleton (Boyce 1991). The association of bone resorption followed by bone formation is termed 'coupling'. Several factors act on osteoclasts either locally (interleukin-1 and tumour necrosis factor), or systemically (parathyroid hormone and 1,25 vitamin D). Bone formation is also influenced by growth factors released locally.

Mechanisms of bone metastasis

Metastasis occurs by invasion of tumour cells into blood vessels, or lymphatics. Tumour emboli are detectable in the circulation of patients at the time of diagnosis, during therapy, and in the terminal stages (Nagy 1965). The majority of tumour cells are destroyed in the circulation by mechanical turbulence (Fidler 1970). Surviving cells attach to and penetrate the endothelium to establish themselves in the stroma of the involved organ. Immunocytochemistry using monoclonal antibodies identifies tumour cells in bone marrow aspirates taken just before surgery in 38% of patients with early breast cancer (Harbeck et al 1994). These micrometastases are present in 19%

of patients with locally recurrent disease, 30% of those with extraskeletal metastases, and 100% of patients with overt bone metastases (Mansi et al 1991). Since only 10–20% of women develop bone metastases within the first 5 years after surgery, many of the cancer cells detected must remain quiescent.

Venous blood from the pelvis and breast flows directly into the valveless vertebral venous plexus (Batson 1940). It is believed that carcinoma may spread via this venous plexus, a theory supported by magnetic resonance imaging findings that the posterior half of the vertebral body, closest to the vertebral venous plexus, is most frequently involved in metastatic disease (Asdourian et al 1990).

Bone metastases start by deposition of tumour cells in the marrow and medium conditioned by bone marrow stromal cells is known to stimulate growth of breast and prostate cancer cell lines (Chackal-Roy et al 1989). The distribution of bone metastases is unrelated to the tissue of origin, most lesions occurring in the axial skeleton, especially the spine, pelvis and ribs (Galasko 1981). This reflects the distribution of red bone marrow which is one of the most metabolically active tissues of the body, and which supports the proliferation and differentiation of the progenitor cells of the haemopoietic system and provides a fertile soil in which the 'seeds' of tumour cells may grow. It may not just be the soil that is important, since in breast cancer, tumours that are well-differentiated, oestrogen receptor positive and produce parathyroid hormone related protein are more likely to develop bone metastases (Elston et al 1980, Powell et al 1991). In animal models, inhibition of bone turnover leads to a reduction in the number of bone metastases which develop when cancer cells are injected intravenously, suggesting that bone resorption itself may produce factors that enhance metastasis (Yoneda et al 1994). Once established, bone metastases cause a local breakdown of normal coupling and in certain cancers, such as breast cancer, osteolysis predominates, whilst in others, such as prostate cancer, osteoblastic bone formation occurs. It should be noted, however, that even when bone formation is stimulated in prostate cancer, the bone that is formed is weaker woven and osteolysis is still a large component of prostate cancer metastases (Clarke et al 1991).

Bone destruction by tumour cells was originally proposed to be due to direct bone resorption. Recent evidence suggests that the major action of tumour cells in bone is to activate osteoclasts by the release of osteoclast activating factors, such as parathyroid hormone related protein (PTHrP), prostaglandins and interleukin-1 from the tumour cells (Mundy 1988) (Fig. 7.2).

Diagnosis of metastases

Patients with bone pain who have previously undergone cancer surgery must be assumed to have skeletal metastases until proven otherwise. The initial investigation of bone pain is controversial. Skeletal radiographs are widely available but for a metastasis to be visible on a radiograph it must be greater

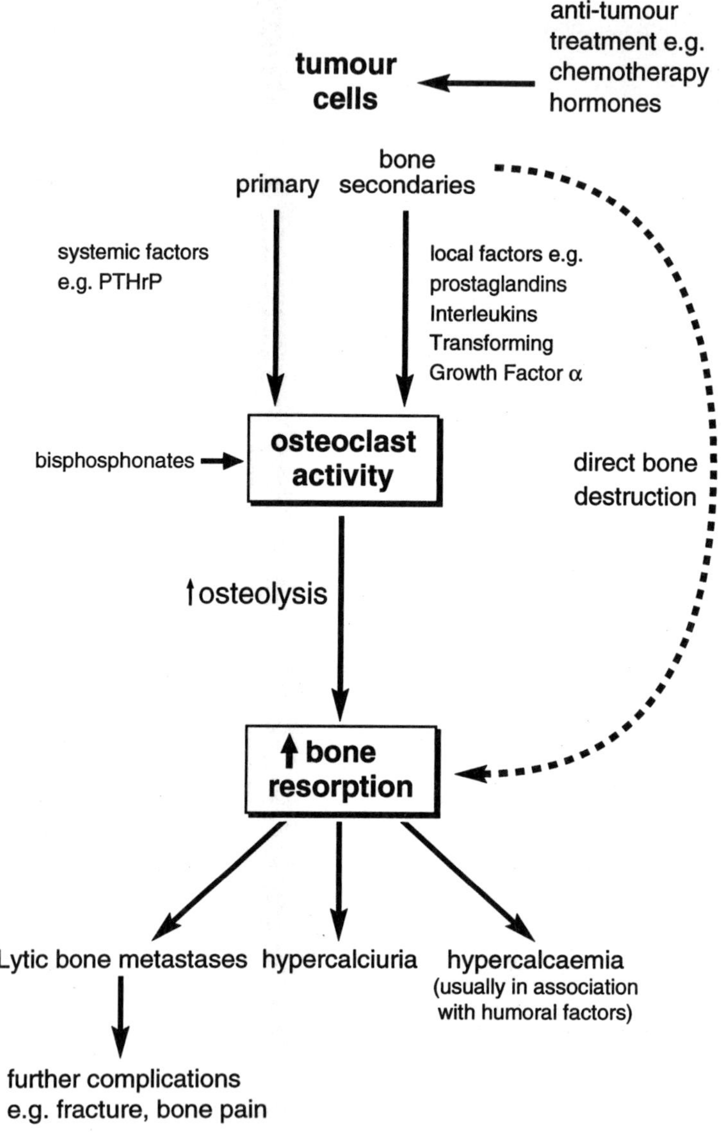

Fig. 7.2 Role of osteoclasts in bone pathology. Primary tumours can affect bone resorption by release of humoral factors into the circulation. Bone metastases have a direct effect on normal bone but their main influence is mediated through the osteoclast. Bisphosphonates act by inhibiting osteoclasts.

than 1.5 cm in diameter with loss of 50% of bone mineral content. Plain radiographs have a low sensitivity and in some sites, such as the thoracic spine, a low specificity.

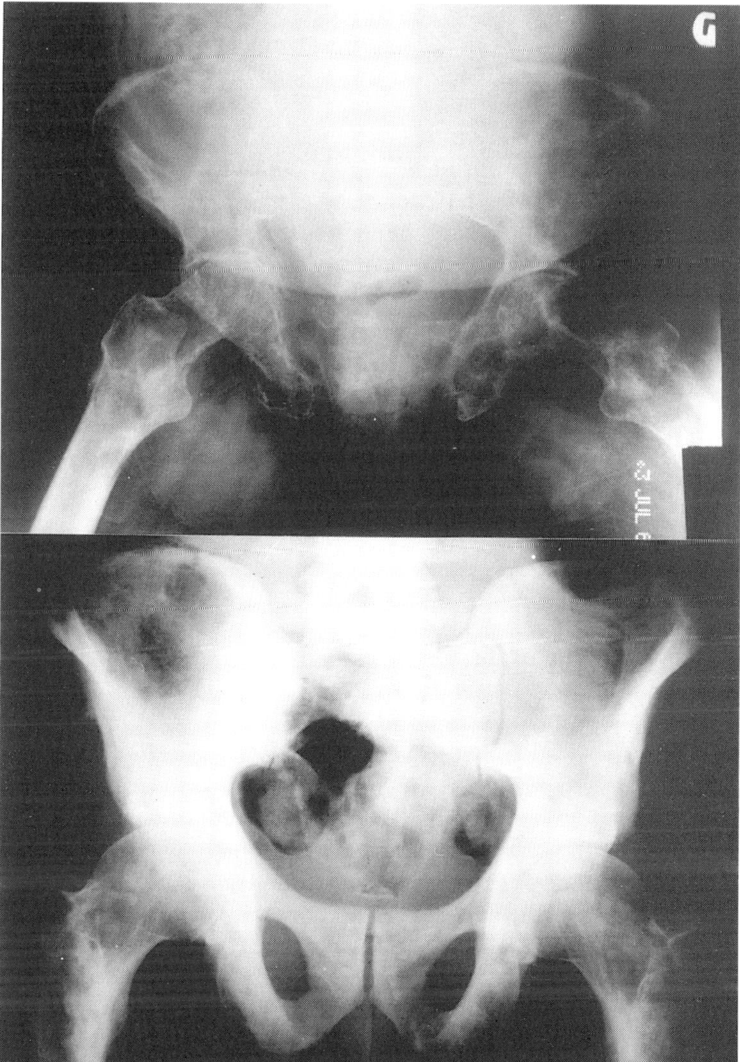

Fig. 7.3 (Top) Osteolytic metastases are common and occur in breast, lung and thyroid cancer. This X-ray shows multiple osteolytic metastases from breast cancer. (Bottom) Sclerotic metastases occur in prostate, lung and bladder cancer, but also rarely from breast cancer. This X-ray shows multiple sclerotic metastases from prostate cancer.

Osteolytic metastases are the most common, appearing as lesions with thinned bone cortex, loss of trabeculae and ill-defined margins, while sclerotic metastases show as areas of thickening (Fig. 7.3).

Bone scintigraphy is the optimal investigation for bone pain. This requires the injection of a technetium-labelled bisphosphonate radioisotope. The major factors influencing adsorption of isotope are osteoblastic activity and skeletal vascularity, with preferential uptake at sites of active bone formation (Fogelman & McKillop 1991). The scan thus reflects the metabolic reaction of the bone to any nonspecific disease process, giving the isotope scan a higher sensitivity of 82% but a specificity of only 79%. Cancer patients with normal radiographs have abnormal isotope scans in 15–35% of cases (Charkes 1973).

In practice, when a lesion is identified on bone scan, plain radiographs are required as they are generally better at assessing the response of osteolytic lesions to treatment than repeated bone scans. Solitary lesions occur in up to 20% of breast cancer patients and cause diagnostic difficulty, occasionally requiring a bone biopsy. Metastases tend to be multiple irregularly distributed foci affecting the axial skeleton. Cancer patients with 5 or more new bone scan abnormalities always have metastatic disease whereas only 11% of single new scan abnormalities prove to be malignant (Jacobson et al 1990). False negative scans occur if the lesion induces no osteoblastic reaction, for example in multiple myeloma where lesions may be purely osteolytic.

Computerised tomography (CT) and magnetic resonance imaging (MRI)

CT is more sensitive than plain radiography, with good soft tissue resolution and excellent definition of soft tissue masses associated with bone metastases and nerve root compression. CT can clarify areas where an isotope scan is positive but plain radiographs are normal. Breast cancer patients with normal plain films and abnormal bone scans have obvious bony metastases on CT in half the cases, while half of the remainder have benign disease and half have no abnormality. None of those with normal or benign CT findings subsequently develop metastases (Muindi et al 1983).

MRI of normal bone marrow gives a high intensity signal due to its high fat content (75% total weight) whilst cortical bone gives no signal on MRI, thus appearing black. Tumour infiltration of the fatty marrow causes a focal decrease in signal intensity, giving an image of the tumour itself, rather than indirect changes in cell activity or cortical reactions (Fig. 7.4). Abnormal signal may be diffuse or focal and changes are usually best seen on T1 weighted images. The advantages of MRI are that it produces multiplanar images with good soft tissue contrast without exposing the patient to ionising radiation. The drawbacks are cost and the time taken for each scan but MRI can be particularly useful in differentiating between the causes of vertebral compression fractures such as osteoporosis and metastatic involvement (Jones et al 1990), allowing accurate diagnosis in 94% of cases (Yuh et al 1989). MRI is the investigation of choice for imaging presymptomatic spinal cord compression (Williams et al 1989) as it can image extradural tissues and the entire cord, defining the upper limit of any block and identifying the 10% of patients who have multiple levels of cord impingement (Bonner & Lichter 1990, Carmody et al 1989). MRI is currently the most sensitive radiological method of detecting bone marrow metastases (Frank et al 1990).

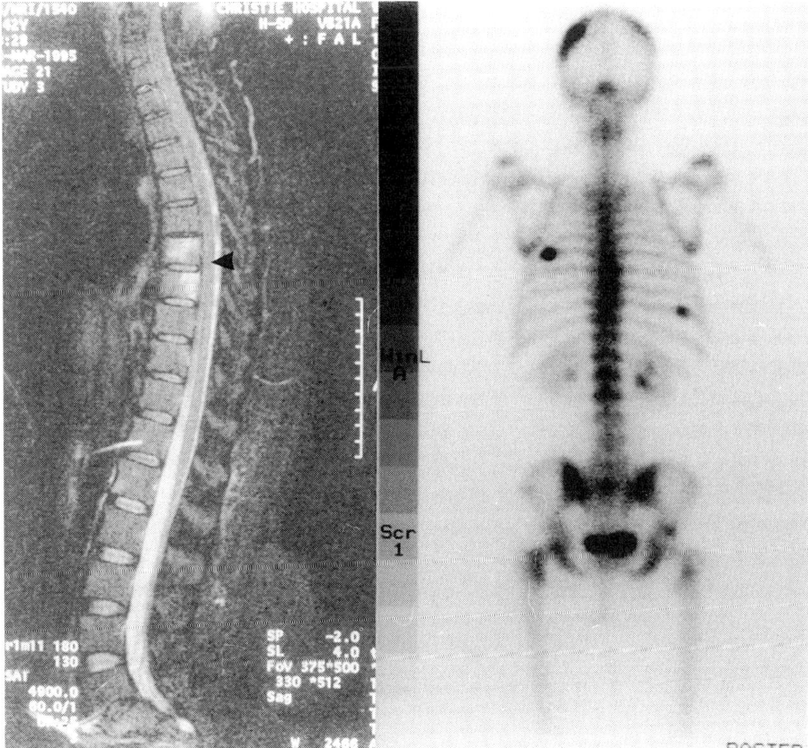

Fig. 7.4 (i) Bone scan showing multiple metastases (right) and (ii) MRI in the same patient (left). On the bone scan, multiple areas of increased activity are seen in the vertebrae, ribs, pelvis and skull. On the MRI, areas of high signal can be seen in T7 and T8 (arrow), showing the extent of vertebral involvement. The spinal cord is clearly visualised.

ASSESSMENT OF THE RESPONSE TO TREATMENT OF BONE METASTASES

Radiological

The treatment of uncomplicated bone metastases depends on the primary tumour. For endocrine sensitive tumours, such as breast and prostate, systemic hormone therapy is used, whilst for unresponsive tumours, radiotherapy, chemotherapy, or radioisotope therapy may be necessary. The treatment of bone metastases complicated by hypercalcaemia, fracture or spinal cord compression is more urgent and will be considered separately.

The objective assessment of response to systemic therapy by skeletal radiography, as defined by the Union Internationale Contre le Cancer (UICC), requires recalcification of lesions to indicate a response. Reported response rates of bone metastases to systemic treatment using these criteria are lower than those at other metastastic sites (Whitehouse 1985). Sclerotic bone metastases are considered non-assessable, as are single metastases which have been irradiated. Recalcification may not be evident for up to 6 months and since the mean response duration for extra-skeletal disease is 7–18 months, there may not be time for sclerosis to occur. When more subjective measures such as pain relief are used, response rates in bone are equivalent to those in visceral or loco-regional sites (Stoll 1985). Patients whose disease remains static for at least 6 months during systemic therapy for breast cancer have a similar overall survival to patients showing objective evidence of remission (Coleman et al 1987). Repeated plain radiographs remain the gold standard method of assessment of response to therapy for bone metastases. Serial isotope scans are difficult to interpret in the first 3–4 months due to the 'flare phenomenon' of increased uptake which can be a sign of healing but also of disease progression. Nevertheless, new lesions appearing on bone scan after 4 months of therapy represent definite disease progression.

Biochemical

In view of the length of time it takes to assess response to therapy in bone radiologically, attempts have been made to predict response earlier by biochemical assessment. Changes in the serum or urine products of bone formation (e.g. alkaline phosphatase), bone resorption (e.g. urinary calcium), or specific tumour markers (e.g. CA 15-3 or prostate specific antigen) have been used to monitor response. Although no specific marker of bone metastatic activity exists, a number of biochemical parameters are disturbed by tumour invasion of bone (Table 7.2). Patients with breast cancer metastases responding to treatment show a transient rise in serum alkaline phosphatase and osteocalcin, both markers of bone formation, within 2 months of starting treatment whereas those with progressing disease do not (Coleman 1991). Myeloma metastases likewise show a transient increase in osteocalcin.

Markers of bone resorption have been more extensively studied. Fasting urinary calcium excretion is a sensitive indicator of net calcium loss from bone and is easily measured. However, urine calcium excretion does not indicate

Table 7.2 Biochemical parameters of bone formation and breakdown that can be used to monitor disease activity in bone

Markers of bone metabolism	Activity involved	Comments
Osteocalcin	Bone formation	Transient rise in response to treatment
Alkaline phosphatase (bone isoenzyme)	Bone formation	
Hydroxyproline	Bone breakdown	Too dependent on diet
Calcium excretion	Bone breakdown	Simple; useful, but altered by bisphosphonate therapy
Pyridinolines	Bone breakdown	Sensitive and specific
Galactosyl hydroxylysine	Bone breakdown	

the amount of bone resorption and formation in the presence of humorally mediated changes in renal reabsorption (e.g. PTHrP secreting tumours) and is often within normal limits in patients with sclerotic metastases.

Type 1 collagen which is produced initially as procollagen constitutes 90% of the bone matrix. This molecule (procollagen) is cleaved to liberate peptides from the C terminal (PICP) and amino terminal ends (PINP), before the collagen chains are bound together in the bone matrix by the cross-linking molecules hydroxyproline and deoxypyridinoline. The procollagen fragments PICP and PINP are potential measures of collagen synthesis (bone formation) while the pyridinoline cross-links and their joining regions with collagen reflect bone resorption. Urinary hydroxyproline was previously used to monitor osteolysis but its excretion is markedly influenced by diet, complement activation, and soft tissue breakdown (e.g. soft tissue metastases), and it has now been superseded.

The amino acids pyridinoline and deoxypyridinoline are released form bone matrix during osteolysis and have proved sensitive urinary biochemical markers in bone disease (e.g. menopause induced osteoporosis). Both cross-links increase in progressing bone metastases at an early stage and levels of both are raised in the urine in 80% of women with bone metastases from breast cancer (Walls et al 1994). These cross-links have the advantage of being completely excreted during collagen breakdown and are unaffected by diet.

In patients with prostate cancer, the alkaline phosphatase levels correlate significantly with urinary cross-link levels and all three are significantly raised in men who develop bone metastases, indicating that cross-links are useful markers, even in sclerotic bone metastases (Sano et al 1994).

Combinations of markers of formation (alkaline phosphatase bone isoenzyme, osteocalcin) and of breakdown (urinary calcium excretion) have been claimed to be the best monitors of disease response (Coleman 1991).

Tumour markers

A number of tumour produced proteins have been used to monitor systemic therapy in breast cancer (CEA, CA15-3) and prostate cancer (prostate specific antigen, acid phosphatase). Although 50–80% of women with metastatic breast cancer have elevated serum levels of carcinoembryonic antigen (CEA), changes in levels are insufficient to provide clinical differentiation between progressing and stable disease.

CA15-3 is a human breast tumour associated antigen, defined and assayed using two monoclonal antibodies, which appears to be a more sensitive predictor of bone metastasis (Kerin et al 1989). CA15-3 is elevated in 70% of women with new bone metastases and changes in CA15-3 are clinically useful in predicting disease response. Some workers have claimed that a combination of CEA, CA15-3 and the erythrocyte sedimentation rate gives a sensitivity of 92% and a specificity of 82% for predicting disease response in breast cancer and suggested that tumour markers can be used to replace the UICC criteria, but this is not universally accepted (Robertson et al 1990).

Prostatic acid phosphatase and prostate specific antigen (PSA) have both been used to monitor disease in prostate cancer; PSA has proven to be more reliable. Metastatic prostate cancer is associated with PSA levels twice the normal reference range and serial measurements are valuable in monitoring response to therapy. Up to 75% of men with responding disease show a fall in PSA levels during the first 6 months of therapy. Bone lesions due to multiple myeloma can be monitored using measurement of serum or urinary myeloma protein.

SYSTEMIC TREATMENT OF BONE METASTASES

Current management of patients with skeletal metastases is aimed at symptom palliation and involves either local or systemic therapy. Although external beam radiotherapy is the treatment of choice for localised bone pain and metastases, the majority of patients have multiple sites of disease and systemic therapy is used to prevent complications and to improve quality of life.

Endocrine therapy

Breast cancer

Breast cancer patients with bone metastases have a median survival of 2 years compared to a median survival of 3 months if liver metastases occur. The concurrent or subsequent development of metastases in extraskeletal sites (e.g. lung or liver) is associated with a much poorer prognosis. Hormonal therapy is used initially in women who develop bone metastases. In postmenopausal women the treatment of choice is the anti-oestrogen tamoxifen, and in premenopausal patients, oophorectomy either medical, surgical, or by irradiation. Response rates to hormonal treatment are better if the primary tumour was well-differentiated, contained oestrogen receptors, or when relapse has occurred a long time after primary surgery (Coleman & Rubens 1987). If the tumour responds to hormone therapy for 6 months or longer, then relapse is usually treated by further endocrine therapy.

Chemotherapy is used in preference to hormone therapy if the bone metastases are associated with life-threatening visceral disease, are rapidly progressive or are known to be oestrogen receptor poor. The rapid relief of bone pain which occurs with hormone therapy is rarely seen during initial chemotherapy.

Complications such as bone pain, pathological fractures or spinal cord compression may occur even in stable responding bone metastases because of loss of integrity of bone structure. However, these complications are, by definition, deemed evidence of progressive disease and usually lead to changes of systemic treatment.

Prostate cancer

Prostate cancer produces osteoblastic metastases (sclerotic lesions on plain radiographs) (Fig. 7.3). Tumour markers such as acid phosphatase and prostate specific antigen are the best disease monitors. At the time of presentation, 30% of patients have skeletal spread and each year 10% of the remainder will develop bone metastases. Pathological fractures and hypercalcaemia occur infrequently and fractures tend to heal well.

Response to endocrine treatment occurs in 80% of cases. The commonest form of endocrine therapy in advanced disease is surgical orchidectomy. Luteinising hormone regulating hormone (LHRH) agonists and flutamide show response rates similar to surgery (Sogani et al 1984, Mauriac 1988) and may be more acceptable to some patients. The use of oestrogens or Megace is becoming less common because of the associated feminisation sometimes seen and the increased risk of cardiovascular events. Combination hormone therapy with an LHRH agonist plus a pure anti-oestrogen (flutamide) produces a 90% response rate with a median duration of 12 months (Neri et al 1992) but the combination is expensive compared to orchidectomy.

Cytotoxic chemotherapy produces pain relief in 11–54% of prostate cancer patients (Eagen et al 1978, Scott et al 1975). Single agent chemotherapy is as good as combination therapy but there is no evidence that either improves survival rates. Moreover, elderly patients with advanced prostate cancer tolerate chemotherapy poorly. Radioactive strontium (^{89}Sr) is concentrated and retained in areas of osteoblastic activity, delivering high doses of radiation locally, with a long half-life (Robinson 1986). It provides effective palliation in prostate cancer but marrow suppression occurs in a number of patients.

Lung cancer

Lung cancer is still the commonest single malignancy in the UK. Untreated, the mean survival from the time of primary diagnosis is less than 3 months. In small cell lung cancer, bone marrow involvement can be found by immunohistochemical means in up to 80% of patients at the time of diagnosis (Trillet et al 1989) and is close to 100% at death. The main role of bone scans in the management of skeletal metastases from lung cancer is in identifying whether local pain is due to metastatic involvement and hence whether it may be amenable to radiotherapy as a means of analgesia.

Systemic inhibition of osteolysis

Tumours produce a number of potent growth factors or cytokines which activate osteoclasts and stimulate bone resorption and recently, therapy directed at inhibiting the osteoclast itself has been developed. Bisphosphonates are synthetic analogues of endogenous pyrophosphate which are adsorbed onto bone mineral, are resistant to enzymatic hydrolysis and are potent inhibitors of bone resorption. They prevent osteoclast attachment to bone matrix as well as recruitment and differentiation. Two main bisphosphonates are currently used; pamidronate and clodronate. About 30% of metastases produce fractures or hypercalcaemia and long term bisphosphonate therapy has been used prophylactically to prevent these complications. Bisphosphonate treatment significantly reduces bone pain in both breast and prostate cancer patients (Van Holten 1991, Clarke et al 1991). A randomised trial of oral pamidronate in breast cancer women showed a highly significant reduction in the cumulative number of complications. The requirement for radiotherapy, and the number of episodes of hypercalcaemia were reduced (Van Holten 1991). Pamidronate-treated women had better mobility, suffered less bone pain and required fewer changes of systemic therapy. In another randomised trial, treatment of patients with multiple myeloma with clodronate delayed bone lesions, decreased pain and reduced the frequency of hypercalcaemic episodes (Lahtinen et al 1992).

Recently, a double-blind controlled study of long-term oral clodronate therapy in breast cancer patients demonstrated a significant reduction in bone pain, pathological fractures, and hypercalcaemic events in the treated group, demonstrating the value of inhibition of osteolysis (Patterson et al 1993). Pamidronate has also been given intravenously as the sole systemic therapy for progressing bone metastases from breast cancer. Intravenous pamidronate significantly reduced urinary calcium excretion and produced falls in tumour markers (CA15-3/CEA) along with a 28% objective response rate (Morton et al 1988). Currently, trials are underway in women at high risk of developing bone metastases who have either large primary breast tumours or advanced disease in other sites to determine whether prophylactic bisphosphonate therapy can prevent the development of bone metastases.

HYPERCALCAEMIA

Hypercalcaemia is the commonest metabolic complication of malignant disease, occurring in 10% of cancer patients overall. Multiple myeloma, lung, breast and ovarian cancers most commonly produce this complication. Two main mechanisms underlie the hypercalcaemia of malignancy. The tumour may release factors which cause increased bone breakdown by osteoclasts, leading to excessive release of calcium and collagen fragments from bone. Secondly, tumours secrete factors into the bloodstream which, as well as activating osteoclasts locally, circulate and increase renal tubular reabsorption of calcium, preventing calcium excretion. All primary tumours which produce hypercalcaemia without metastasizing (e.g. lung cancer) do so via such a humoral mechanism. The extent of bone metastases does not correlate with serum calcium levels in hypercalcaemic cancer patients, and biochemical evaluation suggests a humoral aetiology in the majority of cases, even when bone disease is present.

Parathyroid hormone related protein (PTHrP) has aminoterminus sequence homology to parathyroid hormone (PTH) and a similar ability to increase renal reabsorption of calcium, decrease phosphate reabsorption and increase nephrogenous cyclic AMP production. Like PTH, it stimulates osteoclastic activity in bone, increasing bone resorption. PTHrP can be identified in tumour cell cytoplasm (Bundred et al 1992) and immunoradiometric assays for PTHrP have shown that PTHrP is undetectable in the plasma of normocalcaemic patients, but is detectable in the plasma of 80–90% of hypercalcaemic patients with malignancy (Ratcliffe et al 1992). Evidence to date supports PTHrP as the major mediator of malignant hypercalcaemia. Correspondingly, the highest serum PTHrP levels and detectability occurs in tumours which produce hypercalcaemia by a humoral mechanism, but patients with bone metastases from breast cancer who become hypercalcaemic have detectable plasma PTHrP in 70–80% of cases and 50% have raised urinary cyclic AMP, emphasising the important humoral role of PTHrP even when bone metastases are present. However, PTHrP alone is unlikely to explain all the features of hypercalcaemia of malignancy because, unlike hyperparathyroidism, osteoclastic bone resorption is much more prominent and bone formation is reduced. Moreover, 1,25 vitamin D_3, which is raised in parathyroid disease, is often suppressed in hypercalcaemia of malignancy because of a reduction in renal 1α-hydroxylase activity. This appears to be due to negative feedback from the high circulating serum levels of calcium combined with PTH suppression (Mundy 1988). Since bisphosphonates, by inhibiting osteoclasts, are effective in restoring normocalcaemia in malignancy, the relative importance of osteoclast-mediated bone resorption as a mechanism of hypercalcaemia is clear. However, humoral hypercalcaemia of malignancy does not respond as well to bisphosphonate therapy as hypercalcaemia associated with bone metastases. This is in keeping with evidence that the main action of PTHrP on serum calcium is mediated through the renal tubules, rather than the osteoclast, effects which are uninfluenced by bisphosphonate therapy (Walls et al 1994).

In haematological cancers (myeloma and lymphoma), approximately half of the patients have raised plasma PTHrP but in the remainder, immune-related cytokines such as TNF-β, IL-1 and colony stimulating factors appear to be the main osteoclastic activating factors.

Excessive production of 1,25 vitamin D by lymphoma cells occurs and represents the only example where hypercalcaemia of malignancy is mediated partly by increased intestinal calcium absorption. The majority of hypercalcaemic patients with solid tumours have suppressed Vitamin D levels and some solid tumours may produce a humoral factor which inhibits renal 1α-hydroxylase.

Management

Around 10% of hypercalcaemic patients with concurrent or previous malignancy, but with no evidence of distant disease or recurrence, will have primary hyperparathyroidism as the underlying cause (Walls et al 1994, Ratcliffe et al 1992). The serum PTH should always be measured at presentation and a high normal or elevated value will prove the diagnosis. The majority of patients who have hypercalcaemia of malignancy will have low normal or undetectable serum PTH. Patients with parathyroid disease have often had high or borderline raised serum calcium for some years with minimal symptoms, whereas hypercalcaemia due to malignancy is usually associated with a sudden onset. In patients with underlying parathyroid disease, parathyroidectomy is the treatment of choice. Symptoms of hypercalcaemia range from polydipsia, polyuria, nausea and vomiting to drowsiness, confusion and coma in severe hypercalcaemia which may be life-threatening if not treated promptly. The clinician needs a high index of suspicion as many patients have nonspecific complaints.

Consideration should be given as to whether there will be systemic treatment available to control tumour growth after the hypercalcaemia has been controlled. In the presence of widespread metastatic disease, which has exhausted therapeutic options, further treatment of malignant hypercalcaemia may be inappropriate. Breast cancer metastases and myeloma are usually treatable whereas non-small cell lung cancer or renal cancer are relatively refractory. Nevertheless, the median survival time for any tumour type after an initial episode of hypercalcaemia is only 3 months (Walls et al 1994).

Initial management is by rehydration with 3–4 l of intravenous normal saline to stimulate a calcium diuresis. Rehydration does not affect bone resorption and lowers the calcium by at most 0.5 mmol/l. The poor gastrointestinal absorption of the bisphosphonates, together with the need for rapid reduction in serum calcium has led to their intravenous use in established hypercalcaemia. Intravenous pamidronate (given as a single dose of 60 mg over 2 h) should be given once the diagnosis is confirmed. Normocalcaemia is achieved in 90% of cases within 5 days, an effect which lasts 14–28 days. Bisphosphonates do not affect renal reabsorption of calcium and patients with a marked humoral component to their hypercalcaemia may not achieve normocalcaemia, but symptomatic relief is usually complete.

Glucocorticoids are effective in up to 70% of patients with myeloma or lymphoma but in only 30% of patients with solid tumours. They work mainly by decreasing gastrointestinal absorption of calcium and hence are particularly useful in hypercalcaemia associated with lymphoma.

Calcitonin is a hypocalcaemic hormone which acts mainly on renal reabsorption of calcium. It is effective in combination with glucocorticoids and produces a short-lived rapid reduction in serum calcium but is too expensive for routine management.

LOCAL MANAGEMENT OF BONE METASTASES

Radiotherapy

Irradiation of bone containing metastases leads to degeneration of the tumour and formation of a fibrous stroma which is then replaced by woven bone and finally by lamellar bone and bone marrow. Recalcification of lytic areas reaches a maximum 2 months after treatment. The overall biological effect depends on the total dose of radiation delivered. Radiotherapy is necessary for patients whose bone metastases are causing spinal cord compression, pathological fracture and localised bone pain. Improvement of bone pain after radiotherapy occurs in 85% of patients with complete relief in 50%. Analgesia occurs regardless of tumour type. External beam ionising radiation may be used in the form of either gamma rays or X-rays. Treatment can be localised to single sites or hemibody irradiation may be used for multiple sites of involvement.

When orthovoltage beams are used, bone receives a higher dose of irradiation relative to soft tissue as it has a high atomic weight, but the dose depends on the distance from the source. High energy megavoltage X-ray beams have no differential effect on bone but have better penetration. Superficial bones such as the ribs, sternum and scapula are suitable for orthovoltage treatment but for deeper structures, such as the pelvis and spine, megavoltage beams are required. Tangential beams of megavoltage are employed to attain an even dose over the treatment area. Simulators reproduce treatment beams and can take radiographs, giving an accurate view of the target area.

Where multiple sites of painful metastases are the problem, hemibody irradiation reduces pain in 75% of patients but is more toxic than localised treatment, causing nausea and diarrhoea for 24 h and occasionally alopecia and bone marrow depression (Needham & Hoskin 1994).

Bone metastases selectively take up certain radioisotopes to allow ionising radiation to be targeted to multiple sites. Radioactive iodine (^{123}I) is selectively absorbed by 50–80% of bone metastases from thyroid cancer and if uptake occurs, ablative iodine ^{131}I therapy can be used to knock out the metastases. Patients whose metastases concentrate ^{131}I have a 50% 5-year survival rate. Thus patients presenting with lytic metastases due to thyroid carcinoma require total thyroidectomy and administration of ^{131}I.

Radiotherapy is the treatment of choice for painful bone metastases which are localised. With more widespread disease, hemibody radiation treatment has significant side effects which must be balanced against the limited survival expectations of patients with bone metastases from primaries other than breast cancer.

Orthopaedic management

Of patients with bone metastases, 10% will develop a pathological fracture which may require surgical fixation. They occur twice as frequently in the vertebrae as in the long bones; over 86% of all fractures are caused by four tumour types: lung, prostate, myeloma and breast cancer.

Radiographic features which suggest impending fractures are lytic lesions > 2.5 cm in diameter and involvement of > 50% of the diameter with erosion of the cortex (Beals et al 1971). The risk of fracture correlates with the degree of cortical destruction (Fidler 1981) and if > 50% of the cortex is destroyed, the incidence of fracture is 80%. Prophylactic fixation of these lesions and those either in vulnerable regions (e.g. subtrochanteric region of femur), or causing persistent pain, avoids the morbidity associated with overt fractures. Radiotherapy relieves the pain of bone metastases but temporarily weakens the bone, thus initially increasing the risk of fracture in a painful metastasis.

The treatment of choice for pathological (or impending) fracture of a long bone is internal fixation followed by postoperative irradiation, as pre-operative irradiation delays healing. The type of fixation depends on the site of the lesion but where possible, closed intramedullary nailing is used to spread the load over the remaining normal bone. Isotope scans and radiographs of the entire bone are required as an implant must stabilise all metastases in the affected bone as well as the site of fracture. Large osteolytic lesions should be removed and the defect in the bone filled with bone cement. The implant does not affect subsequent radiation therapy providing that megavoltage (not orthovoltage) irradiation is used. If there is any doubt about the origin of the primary, a biopsy of the lesion is essential.The rate of fracture healing is dependent on the site of the primary tumour and the site of fracture. Transcervical femoral fractures do not unite, due to the additional effect of irradiation on an area where fractures are known to critically reduce vascularity. Replacement arthroplasty gives the best results in this situation with hemiarthroplasty if there is no involvement of the acetabulum by metastatic disease or a more extensive reconstruction if there is widespread pelvic involvement (Harrington 1981).

Humoral fractures are treated by internal fixation, functional cast brace, or replacement arthroplasty. In patients with a reasonable life expectancy (> 3 months), internal fixation produces greater mobility, earlier limb usage, and better pain relief. Arthroplasty is only required for those patients where the site of the fracture, or the degree of bone destruction prevent stabilisation.

Isolated skeletal metastases, with no other evidence of tumour dissemination, are rare, except from renal carcinomas. Resection of the lesion should be considered, especially if fracture has not occurred, as the haematoma resulting from a fracture may prevent excision with adequate margins.

Spinal instability and cord compression

Around 10% of patients with disseminated carcinoma who develop back pain will have spinal instability. The radiographic features are bone destruction with a variable degree of vertebral collapse. Several methods of spinal stabilisation are available but the commonest approach is posteriorly using either Banks' rods or the Hartshill rectangle. Implants must be fixed 2 or 3 vertebrae above and below the unstable segments. If posterior stabilisation is not adequate, as at the level of L5, it may be combined with anterior stabilisation. If anterior decompression for neurological symptoms is required, anterior stabilisation may be the method of choice. Routine investigation to exclude any signs of cord compression must be carried out before surgery.

Spinal cord compression occurs in 5–10% of autopsy series of patients with a variety of primary tumours. The majority of patients have established bone metastases. Soft tissue epidural disease is the main cause of the compression (75%), rather than bone collapse (24%) (Pigott et al 1994). Symptoms include, in order of frequency, motor weakness (96%); pain (94%); sensory disturbance (79%); and sphincter disturbance (61%) (Hill et al 1993). Magnetic resonance imaging is necessary to determine if the block is due to extradural disease, in which case radiotherapy is the treatment of choice, or vertebral collapse, in which case decompressive surgery is necessary.

Occasionally both modalities of treatment are required. Those patients who were ambulant before therapy usually remain so (96%) whilst those who are not ambulant have only a 7% chance of regaining their ability to walk after treatment. Median survival following spinal cord compression is only 4-7 months.

Patients who receive spinal radiotherapy for pain control and who are particularly at risk of developing spinal cord compression should be alerted to the warning symptoms and told to seek attention at the earliest opportunity if they occur.

KEY POINTS FOR CLINICAL PRACTICE

- Involvement of the skeleton is a common manifestation of metastatic malignancy. The management of patients with bone metastases requires skilful multidisciplinary palliative and supportive therapy to minimise morbidity and maximise the patients quality of life.

- Of patients with breast and prostate cancer 70% will develop bone metastases and one-third of these will develop complications such as hypercalcaemia, pathological fracture or spinal cord compression.

- Bone scintigraphy is the optimal investigation of bone pain; metastases tend to be multiple irregularly distributed lesions affecting the axial skeleton.

- Radiographic features which suggest impending fracture are lytic lesions > 2.5 cm in diameter and involvement of > 50% of the diameter with erosion of the cortex. Plain radiographs are better at assessing the response of osteolytic lesions to treatment than repeated bone scans.

- CT and MRI are excellent for defining soft tissue masses associated with bone metastases and nerve root compression. Both are useful to clarify an area where bone scans are positive but plain films are not diagnostic (e.g. the cause of vertebral collapse). MRI is the investigation of choice in spinal cord compression.

- Management of patients with skeletal metastases aims for symptom palliation and prevention of complications using local or systemic therapy. External beam radiotherapy is the treatment of choice for localised bone pain but patients with multiple sites of disease require systemic therapy, such as hormonal treatment or bisphosphonates.

- Hypercalcaemia of malignancy requires rehydration and intravenous bisphosphonate therapy to inhibit osteolysis, return the patient to normocalcaemia and allow time to initiate systemic anti-cancer treatment.

- In spinal cord compression, if constriction is due to extradural disease, early radiotherapy is the treatment of choice, but if vertebral collapse is the cause, orthopaedic decompression is necessary.

- Even in the presence of bone metastases, thyroid cancer requires total thyroidectomy to allow ablation of metastases with radioactive iodine.

REFERENCES

Asdourian PZ, Weidenbaum M, DeWald RL et al 1990 The pattern of vertebral involvement in metastatic breast cancer. Clin Orthop 250: 164-170
Batson OV 1940 The function of the vertebral veins and their role in the spread of metastases. Ann Surg 112: 138-149
Beals RK, Lawton GD, Swell WE 1971 Prophylactic internal fixation of the femur in metastatic breast cancer. Cancer 28: 1350-1354
Bonner JA, Lichter AS 1990 A caution about the use of MRI to diagnose spinal cord compression. New Engl J Med 322: 556-557
Boyce BF 1991 Normal bone remodelling and its disruption in metastatic bone disease. In: Rubens RD, Fogelman I eds. Bone metastases: diagnosis and treatment. Springer-Verlag, London, pp 11-30
Bundred NJ, Walker RA, Ratcliffe WA et al 1992 Parathyroid hormone related protein and skeletal morbidity in breast cancer. Eur J Cancer 28: 690-692
Carmody RF, Yang PJ, Seeley GW et al 1989 Spinal cord compression due to metastatic disease: diagnosis with MR imaging versus myelography. Radiology 173: 225-229
Chackal-Roy M, Niemayer C, Moore M, Zetter BR 1989 Stimulation of human prostatic carcinoma cell growth by the factors present in human bone marrow. J Clin Invest 84: 43-50
Charkes ND 1973 Bone and soft tissue sarcomas; current status of radioisotopes in the diagnosis of bone cancer. In: Proceedings of the Seventh National Cancer Conference. JB Lippincott, Philadelphia, pp 915-919
Clarke NW, Holbrook IB, McClure J, George NJ 1991 Osteoclast inhibition by pamidronate in metastatic prostate cancer: a preliminary study. Br J Cancer 63: 420-423
Coleman RE, Rubens RD 1987 The clinical course of bone metastases from breast cancer. Br J Cancer 55: 61-66
Coleman RE 1991 Assessment of response to treatment. In: Rubens RD, Fogelman I (eds) Bone metastases: diagnosis and treatment. Springer-Verlag, London
Coombes RC, Dady P, Parson C et al 1983 Assessment of response of bone metastases to systemic treatment in patients with breast cancer. Cancer 52: 610-614
Eagen RT, Hahn RG, Myers RP 1978 Adriamycin versus 5-fluorouracil and cyclophosphamide in the treatment of metastatic prostate cancer. Cancer Treat Rep 60: 115-117
Elston CW, Blamey RW, Johnson J 1980 The relationship of estradiol receptor (ER) and histological tumor differentiation with prognosis in human primary breast carcinoma. In: Mouridsen HT, Palshof T (eds) Breast cancer; experimental and clinical aspects. Pergamon, Oxford, p 59
Fidler IJ 1970 Metastasis: quantitative analysis of distribution and fate of tumour emboli labelled with ^{125}I-5-iodo-2′-deoxyuridine. J Natl Cancer Inst 45: 773-782.
Fidler M 1981 Incidence of fracture through metastases in long bones. Acta Orthop Scand 52: 623-627
Fogelman I, McKillop JH 1991 The bone scan in metastatic disease. In: Rubens RD, Fogelman I (eds) Bone metastases: diagnosis and treatment. Springer-Verlag, London, pp 11-30
Frank J, Ling A, Patronas NJ et al 1990 Detection of malignant bone tumours by MR imaging versus scintigraphy. Am J Roentgenol 155: 1043-1048
Galasko CSB 1976 Mechanisms of bone destruction in the development of skeletal metastases. Nature 263: 507
Galasko CSB 1981 The anatomy and pathways of skeletal metastases. In: Weiss L, Gilbert AH (eds) Bone metastases. GK Hall, Boston, pp 49-63
Harbeck N, Untch M, Pache L, Eirmann W 1994 Tumour cell detection in the bone marrow of breast cancer patients at primary therapy: results of a 3-year follow-up. Br J Cancer 69: 566-571
Harrington KD 1981 The management of acetabular insufficiency secondary to metastatic malignant disease. J Bone J Surg (Am) 63: 653-684

Hill ME, Richards MA, Gregory WM et al 1993 Spinal cord compression in breast cancer: a review of 70 cases. Br J Cancer 68: 969-973

Hoskin PJ 1991 Radiotherapy in the management of bone metastases. In: Rubens RD, Fogelman I (eds) Bone metastases; diagnosis and treatment. Springer-Verlag, London pp 171-185

Jacobson AF, Stomper PC, Jochelson MS et al 1990 Association between number and sites of new bone scan abnormalities and presence of skeletal metastases in patients with breast cancer. J Nucl Med 31: 387-392

Jones AL, Williams MP, Powles TJ et al 1990 Magnetic resonance imaging in the detection of skeletal metastases in patients with breast cancer. Br J Cancer 62: 296-298

Kerin MJ, McAnena OJ, O'Malley VP et al 1989 CA15-3: its relationship to clinical stage and progression to metastatic disease in breast cancer. Br J Surg 76: 838-839

Lahtinen R, Laakso M, Palva I et al 1992 Randomised, placebo-controlled multicentre trial of clodronate in multiple-myeloma. Lancet 340: 1049-1052

Mansi JL, Easton D, Berger U et al 1991 Bone marrow micrometastases in primary breast cancer; prognostic significance after 6 years follow up. Eur J Cancer 27: 1552-1555

Mauriac L, Cote P, Richard P et al 1988 Clinical study of an LHRH agonist (ICI 118.630, Zoladex) in the treatment of prostate cancer. Am J Clin Oncol 11(suppl 2): 117-119

Morton AR, Cantrill JA, Pillai GV, McMahon A, Anderson DC, Howell A 1988 Sclerosis of lytic bone metastasis after di sodium aminohydroxypropylidene bisphosphonate (APD) in patients with breast carcinoma. BMJ 297: 772–773

Muindi J, Coombes RC, Golding S et al 1983 The role of computed tomography in the detection of bone metastases in breast cancer patients. Br J Radiol 56: 223-236

Mundy GR 1988 Hypercalcaemia of malignancy revisited. J Clin Invest 82: 1-6

Nagy KP 1965 A study of normal, atypical and neoplastic cells in the white cell concentrate of peripheral blood. Acta Cytol 9: 61

Needham PK, Hoskin PJ 1994 Radiotherapy for painful bone metastases. Palliative Med 8: 92-104

Neri B, Gemelli MT, Sambataro S et al 1992 Subjective and metabolic effects of clodronate in patients with advanced breast cancer and symptomatic bone metastases. Anticancer Drugs 3: 87-90

Patterson AHG, Powles TJ, Kanis JA et al 1993 Double-blind controlled trial of clodronate in patients with bone metastases from breast cancer. J Clin Oncol 11: 59-65

Pigott KH, Baddeley H, Maher EJ 1994 Pattern of disease in spinal cord compression on MRI scan and implications for treatment. Clin Oncol 6: 7-10

Powell GJ, Southby J, Danks JA et al 1991 Localisation of parathyroid hormone related protein in breast cancer metastases; increased incidence in bone compared with other sites. Cancer Res 51: 3059-3061

Ratcliffe WA, Hutcheson ACJ, Bundred NJ, Ratcliffe JG 1992 Role of assays for parathyroid hormone related protein in investigation of hypercalcaemia. Lancet 339: 164-167

Robertson JFR, Ellis IO, Price M et al 1990 Objective serum measurement of response to endocrine therapy in breast cancer. Br J Cancer 62 (suppl XII): 18

Robinson RG 1986 Radionuclides for the alleviation of bone pain in advanced malignancy. Clinic Oncol 5: 39-49

Sano M, Kushida K, Takahashi M et al 1994 Urinary pyridinoline and deoxypyridinoline in prostate carcinoma patients with bone metastasis. Br J Cancer 70: 701-703

Scott WW, Johnson DE, Schmidt JE, et al 1975 Chemotherapy of advanced prostatic carcinoma with cyclophosphamide or 5-fluorouracil: results of the first national randomised study. J Urol 114: 909-911

Sogani PC, Vagaiwala MR, Whitmore Jr WF 1984 Experience with flutamide in patients with advanced prostatic cancer without prior endocrine therapy. Cancer 54: 744-750

Stoll BA 1985 Mechanisms in endocrine therapy of bone metastases. J R Soc Med 78 (suppl 9); 11-14

Trillet V, Revel D, Combaret V et al 1989 Bone marrow metastases in small cell lung cancer: detection with magnetic resonance imaging. Br J Cancer 60: 83-88

Van Holten-Verzantvoort AT, Zwinderman AH, Aaronson NK 1991 The effect of supportive pamidronate treatment on aspects of quality of life of patients with advanced breast cancer. Eur J Cancer 27: 544-549

Walls J, Ratcliffe WA, Assiri A et al 1994 Urinary cross-links: mechanisms of hypercalcaemia in women with breast cancer (abstract). Br J Surg 81: 755

Whitehouse JM 1985 Site-dependent response to chemotherapy for carcinoma of the breast. J R Soc Med 78 (suppl 9); 18-22

Williams MP, Cherryman GR, Husband JE 1989 Magnetic resonance imaging in suspected spinal cord compression. Clin Radiol 40: 286-290
Yoneda T, Sasaki A, Mundy GR 1994 Osteolytic bone metastasis in breast cancer. Breast Cancer Res Treat 32: 73-84
Yuh WT, Zachar CK, Barloon TJ 1989 Vertebral compression fractures; distinction between benign and malignant causes with magnetic resonance imaging. Radiology 172: 215-218

8

CT and MRI in general surgery

R.M. Blaquière

Conventional computed tomography (CT) also known as computerised tomography and computerised axial tomography has an established role in the management of a wide range of conditions which present to the general surgeon. It was thought that a plateau in terms of application was achieved in the late 1980s but technical advances in the design of CT scanners over the last few years have changed this attitude. The advent of spiral CT, also termed helical or volume CT, has significantly extended the capabilities of CT and this chapter discusses this recent advance.

Magnetic resonance imaging (MRI), formerly termed nuclear magnetic resonance (NMR) imaging, but frequently abbreviated to MR, now occupies a pivotal place in the management of many central nervous system and orthopaedic disorders. Its use in the abdomen is less well established but the technique is developing rapidly and it is likely that by the time of publication this will have changed. The present role of MRI and its likely evolution is also discussed in this chapter.

A comprehensive discussion of the role of CT and MRI in the myriad of conditions a general surgeon encounters is beyond the scope of this chapter. Instead, attention is focused on a number of diseases in which the recent developments in CT and MR are likely to have most impact. Similarly a detailed exposition of the physics underlying either CT (Boyd et al 1992) or MR (Stark & Bradley 1992, Horowitz 1992) is inappropriate here, but it is important that the reader has some understanding of the principles so that the potential of the techniques can be appreciated.

PRINCIPLES OF CT

Most CT machines consist of an X-ray tube mounted on a gantry opposite a bank of solid state or inert gas filled detectors which rotate around the subject. One manufacturer uses an alternative arrangement consisting of a fixed ring of detectors within which the X-ray tube rotates. All the machines have X-ray tubes which emit a narrow fan shaped X-ray beam and irradiate the subject from different angles. The detectors pick up the X-ray photons which have traversed the subject and by a comparison of the number of photons which have been stopped, or attenuated, by the subject at different incident angles, the X-ray density or attenuation value of the elements within the subject, as well as their relative positions can be computed. From this information, an image is generated of a slice of the subject corresponding to the width of the X-ray beam.

In conventional CT, the table on which the subject is placed is moved by a predetermined amount varying between 1–10 mm. Separate scans are obtained after each separate table movement. The width of the slice of tissue scanned can also be varied between 1–10 mm. Depending on the requirements of the examination, the slice width may be the same as the table movement or the table movement may be greater than the width of each slice, which leaves an area between each slice which is not examined. The time taken for each cycle of table movement, scanning and image reconstruction varies but a typical time on a fast scanner examining the abdomen would be 10 s. Thus to cover 20 cm in the upper abdomen taking contiguous slices would require 3 min 20 s. Many patients are unable to keep still for this length of time and, furthermore, are unable to take a constant inspiration or breath hold on successive scans. This leads to movement artefact or blurring of the image and also misregistration of slices, i.e. failing to scan some areas of the patient while rescanning others.

The direction of rotation of the X-ray tube in conventional CT alternates between clockwise and anticlockwise on successive scans because of the constraints applied by the cables which supply the electricity and transmit the data obtained to the computers. In spiral CT scanners, the X-ray tube and detectors are mounted on conducting metal rings (slip rings) which replace the cables and allow the system to rotate continuously in the same direction. If the table and the subject is moved at a steady rate through the machine while the tube is rotating in this fashion, a helix or spiral is described around the subject (hence the terms spiral, helical and volume scanning). Instead of only one slice being irradiated at a time, a much larger volume of tissue is examined. The scanning time required to examine a given area is significantly reduced compared to conventional CT. Thus the 200 s required to examine a length of 20 cm using conventional methods can be reduced to about 30 s in total. This has a number of obvious advantages. In restless patients there is better image quality since less movement artefact occurs. Since the examination can be obtained during a single breath hold there is no misregistration of slices. Sick patients have to spend less time on the scanner. Overall there is potentially a higher throughput of patients.

Apart from the speed of the technique there are other advantages. In all forms of CT, the slice width is determined before the examination, but in spiral CT, data from a large volume of tissue have been obtained, so the width of the slice to be reconstructed as an image can be varied. Thus, while the X-ray beam may be collimated to say 8 mm (the slice width) the image can be reconstructed using an effective slice width of only 4 mm. This not only increases the detection of small lesions, but also allows a more detailed retrospective examination of the suspicious abnormalities visualised on the initial series of images. This avoids any need for rescanning and thus re-irradiating the patient. Reformatting of image data in planes other than axial, using computer software, has been available for some time. This enables the investigator to depict an area of interest coronally, sagittally or in three dimensions. However, these reformatted images have suffered from significant image degradation. The ability of spiral CT to overlap the effective slices greatly improves the quality of the reformatted images. In addition to this, the speed of acquisition of the data means that the passage of intravenous contrast through various organs and systems can be demonstrated in great detail. When this is allied to three dimensional reformatting the vascular anatomy can be demonstrated with an accuracy which is approaching that of angiography.

Although it might be thought that the radiation dose to the patient would have to increase to allow this sort of information to be obtained, this is not the case. Generally, tube currents in spiral CT are lower, to allow long continuous scans and this reduces the radiation dose. The need to rescan areas either because of patient movement or to allow more detailed examination of problem areas is reduced. Thus dosage is comparable to and possibly lower than that from conventional CT.

PRINCIPLES OF MRI

Human tissues contain, with a number of notable exceptions, large numbers of hydrogen nuclei. These are charged particles which have an odd number of protons, so they exhibit nuclear spin, or angular momentum, that is they rotate around their axes. It is the properties of these particles that are exploited in MR imaging of the human body, although magnetic resonance is a property common to many other less common nuclei within the body.

When charged nuclei spin, they create a small magnetic field, that is they behave like small bar magnets. When they are then placed in a strong magnetic field they will align themselves parallel to that field and we can think of the sum of all the fields of the individual bar magnets as a vector pointing in the direction of the strong magnetic field. The individual vectors of the small bar magnets are not stationary however but rather spin or precess around their long axes in a movement analogous to a spinning top.

A magnetic resonance scanner consists of a tunnel in which the patient lies. The main field is along the long, or Z axis of the tunnel. It is in this direction that the magnetic vector within the patient is pointing. The axes which define a cross-section of the patient are termed X and Y, X being from right to left and Y being from anterior to posterior. If we apply briefly an alternating electric current or radio frequency (RF) pulse in such a way that its magnetic field component is at right angles to the Z axis, it causes the magnetic vector within the patient to tip over towards the X–Y plane. It also causes the main magnetic vector along the Z axis to precess in the same way that the individual nuclei or small bar magnets have been precessing like tiny spinning tops. The frequency of the RF pulse is selected to equal the precession frequency of the hydrogen nuclei and it is this phenomenon of magnetic 'resonance' which allows imaging to be performed and gives rise to the name of the process.

When the RF pulse stops, the nuclei begin to return to their base line position, or to relax. As they do so, they emit a signal which can be detected and it is this signal which is used to construct the image. The two major components of relaxation are termed T1 and T2. The reader will recall that the magnetic vector within the patient was tipped into the X–Y plane by the RF pulse. The return of the vector to the Z axis is the T1 relaxation process and the decay of the vector in the X–Y plane is the T2 relaxation process. The times that these two processes take vary for different tissues and this forms the basis for the contrast within the image.

In order that an image can be produced, the whole process has to be repeated many times with relaxation and signal measurement after each RF application (typically 128 or 256 signal samples are performed). This multiple repetition of RF pulses is necessary not only for spatial orientation of the signal but also for maximising the differences (contrast) in the signal emanating, or echoing, from different tissues. By changing the sequence of RF pulses the signal will vary depending on the T1 and T2 times of the tissues being imaged. This gives rise to T1 (T1W) or T2 (T2W) weighted scans. Since neither T1 nor T2 effects can be completely eliminated from an MR image the term weighting is used to reflect the way the image is biased.

The T1 and T2 times of tissues are dependent not just upon the number of 'free' or non-bonded hydrogen nuclei but also the atomic lattice in which they lie, as well as the magnetic effect that neighbouring atoms exert. Thus the image produced by MRI is dependent upon far more factors than those involved in the interaction of X-rays or ultrasound with tissue. This means that a whole new series of tissue characteristics have to be understood. For example the presence of a large number of free protons in inflammatory or neoplastic tissue will result in a lot of signal being returned from these tissues providing the correct T2W pulse sequence is used. On a T1W sequence the same tissue will return less signal and may be indistinguishable from adjacent normal tissue. While these factors may be initially confusing they hold out the promise of contrast resolution, and therefore disease detection, far in excess of previous imaging techniques.

A major drawback to MR has been the time required to acquire the information to generate the image. Unlike CT where scans of individual slices are acquired sequentially, in MR information about all the slices is being acquired throughout the scanning period. This means that if the patient moves during the MR acquisition all the slices will be degraded. To a certain extent this can be overcome in parts of the body where there is physiological motion such as the abdomen because the average position of a lesion in a moving part such as the liver will remain the same over the 5 or 6 min taken to acquire a conventional T1W image. However numerous ingenious pulse sequences have been devised to shorten the time taken to acquire the necessary information. These images often suffer from reduction in 'quality' but when taken in conjunction with a conventionally acquired image produce useful new information. As a result imaging of the abdomen, pelvis, mediastinum and lungs is now routinely performed.

In addition, it is likely that ultra fast MR will become a reality in the near future. Echo planar sequences use a different technique for producing an image and are very much quicker than 'conventional' MR. Although these sequences have been known for many years, it is only recently that technological advances have allowed them to be developed for clinical practice. The speed of this type of MRI opens up the vista of near 'real time' imaging with all the benefits that this entails for examination of the abdomen and chest (Edelman et al 1994).

Intravenous contrast agents have been devised based on salts of gadolinium. These have similar enhancement characteristics to those found in iodinated intravenous contrast media as used in X-ray based studies. They can often provide additional information in the same way that contrast can in CT. Interventional techniques in MR have been hampered partly by the need for non-ferromagnetic instruments and partly by the time needed to produce an image. However, these obstacles now appear surmountable and MR guided biopsy as well as therapeutic intervention is likely to become a reality in the near future.

APPLICATIONS

The liver

CT

The assessment of primary and secondary hepatic malignancy is one of the most important aspects of abdominal CT. The success of surgical techniques such as partial hepatic resection, liver transplantation and portal catheter placement for chemotherapy in managing patients with hepatic malignancy has given added impetus to the need for accurate radiological staging. Dynamic contrast enhanced CT remains a highly accurate method for detecting liver tumours, as intravenous contrast increases the attenuation difference between a tumour and the normal liver parenchyma. However this attenuation difference can be transient since with time contrast will leak into the tumour and raise its attenuation while at the same time the adjacent normal liver excretes the contrast and, therefore, lowers its attenuation. Thus, there will be a point at which the densities of both the tumour and the normal liver are the same; indeed, after a few hours, the attenuation of some tumours is higher than that of the normal liver.

Over the last few years an enormous effort has been made to determine the best method of delivering contrast, the optimum volume and the ideal timing for the commencement of the scan sequence (Foley et al 1994, Small et al 1994). The consensus has emerged that approximately 150 ml of contrast delivered rapidly (2–5 ml/s) via a power injector in either a uniphasic or biphasic fashion with scanning commencing at about 40–50 s, and covering the liver in 2 min, will detect the vast majority of abnormalities.

CT with arterial portography (CTAP)

CTAP involves placing a catheter in the superior mesenteric or splenic artery, injecting contrast and then scanning rapidly through the liver as the contrast bolus returns through the portal venous circulation. This more invasive method will detect more tumours than conventional dynamic CT and has become an important procedure in planning surgery for patients with hepatic metastases (Soyer et al 1991, Soyer et al 1994b) (Fig. 8.1).

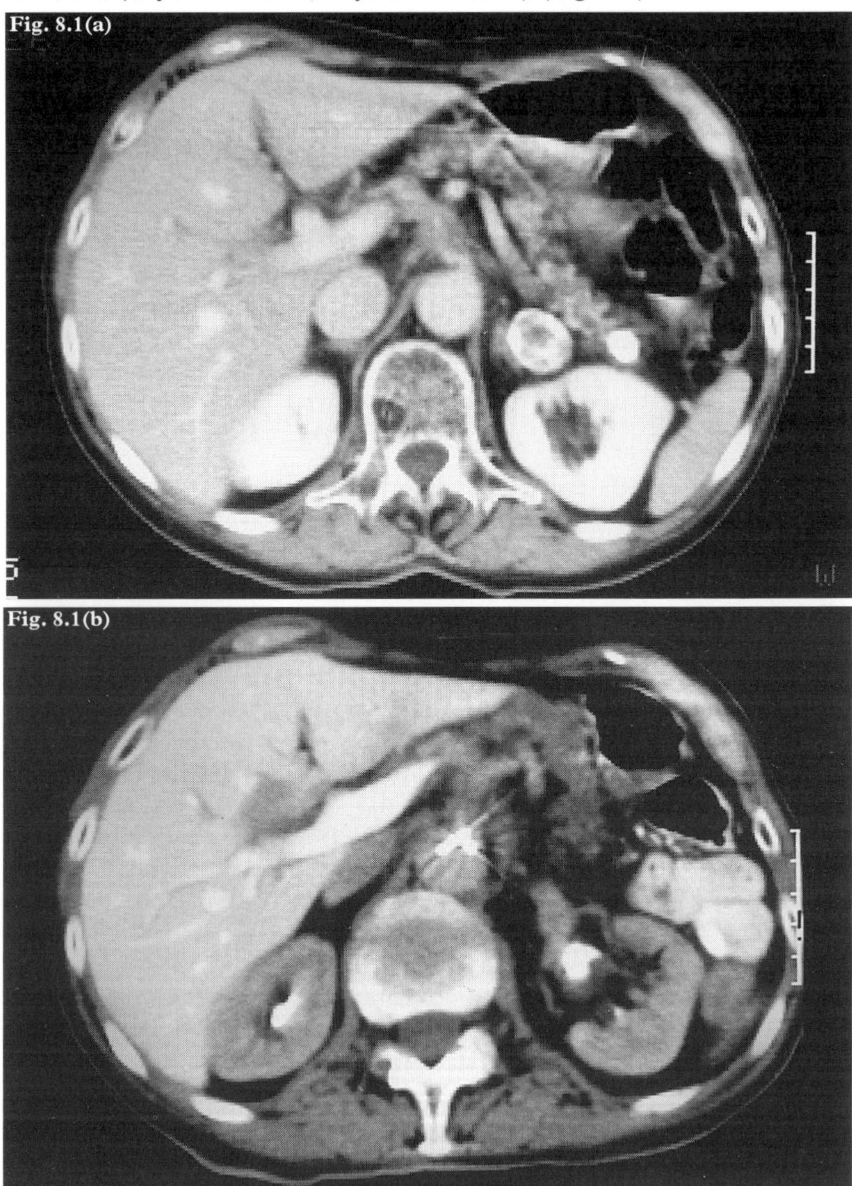

Fig. 8.1 Conventional dynamic CT (a) and CTAP (b) of the liver in a patient with carcinoma of the pancreas. The conventional study (a) shows soft tissue infiltration around the root of the superior mesenteric artery but no evidence of liver metastases. The CTAP section at the same level made within 14 days (b) clearly shows hepatic defects due to metastases.

All these techniques rely upon the whole of the liver being imaged while the differences in attenuation between the tumour and the liver parenchyma are at their maximum. Heiken et al (1993) suggest that the window of opportunity during which liver enhancement is raised by 40 Hounsfield units only lasts for 31 ± 13 s. Conventional CT cannot cover the liver in such a short time. Furthermore, it is not uncommon for patients to breathe slightly differently between each scan which means that some areas of the liver are not scanned at all while others are scanned twice. Spiral CT can examine the whole liver in one breath hold in approximately 30 s and this can overcome both problems. The speed of spiral CT also means that the liver can be scanned initially to look at the hepatic arterial phase and then again during the portal venous phase (Fig. 8.2).

Some hypervascular metastases, such as those from carcinoid and islet cell tumours, enhance very rapidly and in up to 39% of patients they will be isodense compared to the normal liver on conventional CT (Bressler et al 1987). If such tumours are scanned in the arterial phase as well as the portal venous phase they are less likely to be missed. While large studies examining the accuracy of spiral CT versus conventional CT have yet to be published, it is likely that spiral CT and CTAP will improve the detection of metastases. The overall accuracy of conventional CT in detecting liver metastases is approximately 80–85% (Bluemke et al 1994) while for lesions greater than 1 cm, accuracies as high as 99% have been reported (Chezmar et al 1988). CTAP appears to be as accurate for even smaller lesions (Moran et al 1994). Using MR, accuracies similar to conventional CT have been possible for some time (Reinig et al 1989). As experience increases and the relative values of the different MR techniques are analysed (Steinberg et al 1990), the published papers are tending to show that MR is more sensitive than conventional CT (Larson et al 1994, Rummeney et al 1992). Whether spiral CT will reverse this trend remains to be seen.

The CT appearances of many metastases are relatively non-specific, being similar to those found in benign lesions such as cysts and haemangiomas. Greater specificity can be achieved by studying the way in which the lesion handles intravenous contrast. Thus while many metastases show slight early peripheral enhancement and moderate patchy late enhancement, cysts show no enhancement at all. Haemangiomas show a typical pattern of early nodules of peripheral enhancement with centripetal 'filling in' of the mass (Quinn & Benjamin 1992).

While this section has concentrated on CT of the liver, it must be remembered that the technique also provides superb demonstration of the rest of the abdomen (Chezmar et al 1988). Thus malignant enlargement of nodes in the mesentery, retroperitoneum and porta are routinely shown as are occult masses within other solid organs. The imaging of peritoneal cavity disease by CT remains unsurpassed.

MR

The T1 value of the liver is shorter than that of the spleen, and this means

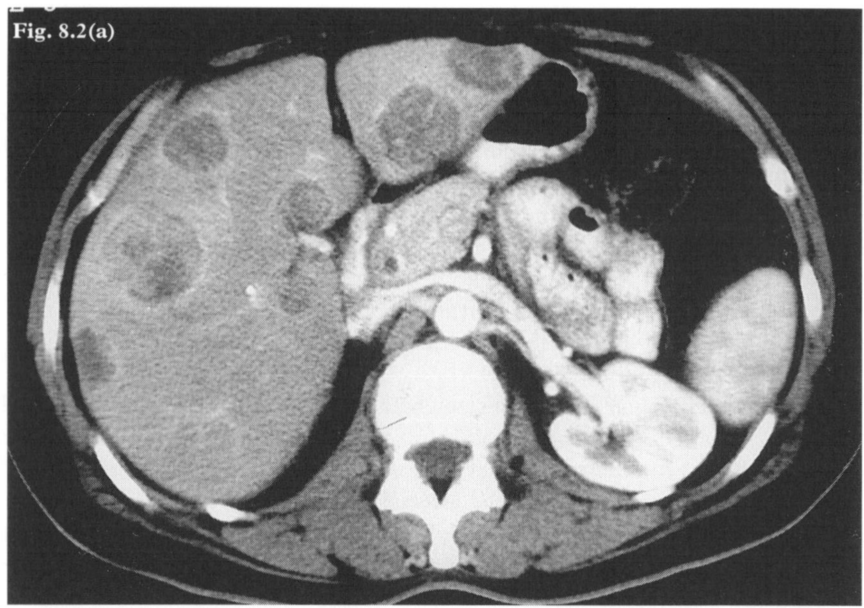

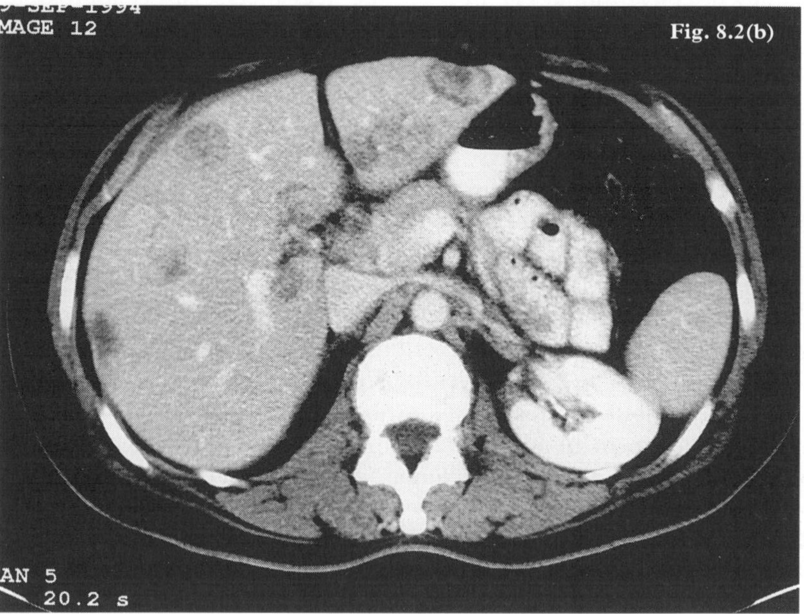

Fig. 8.2 Spiral CT scans in a patient with liver metastases. (a) Arterial phase (b) portal venous phase. Note how a number of the lesions are less clearly seen in the venous phase compared to the arterial phase.

that the liver has a higher signal intensity on T1 weighted sequences. The T2 value is also relatively short and conversely this means that it is lower in signal intensity than the spleen. The T1 and T2 values of metastases are variable but are typically prolonged. Thus they are usually of low signal on T1W and high signal on T2W. A major drawback to MR of the liver has been the time required to acquire the images. This has been a particular problem with T2W sequences because of their susceptibility to respiratory blurring. However fast T2W multiple section acquisition during a breath hold is now possible (Rydberg et al 1995, Taupitz et al 1995).

MR has even greater contrast resolution than CT and is, therefore, more sensitive to the delineation of the varied composition of metastases. Various forms of signal alteration are characteristic of metastases (Fig. 8.3) and doughnut, halo and light bulb signs have all entered the radiological lexicon (Wittenberg et al 1988, Outwater et al 1991). One of the main challenges is the differentiation of metastases from cysts and haemangiomas. The homogenous fluid content of cysts and the very long T2 relaxation times of haemangiomas can be emphasised by manipulation of the various sequences, and sensitivities of 100% in the distinction between haemangiomas and malignant tumours have been reported (McFarland et al 1994).

The use of gadolinium as an intravenous contrast agent adds further specificity to the differentiation of benign from malignant lesions (Hamm et al 1994, Mahfouz et al 1994, Yamashita et al 1994). Haemangiomas have characteristic enhancement features (Semelka et al 1994) which are similar to those found in CT and if present provide an accuracy of 100% (Mitchell et al 1994).

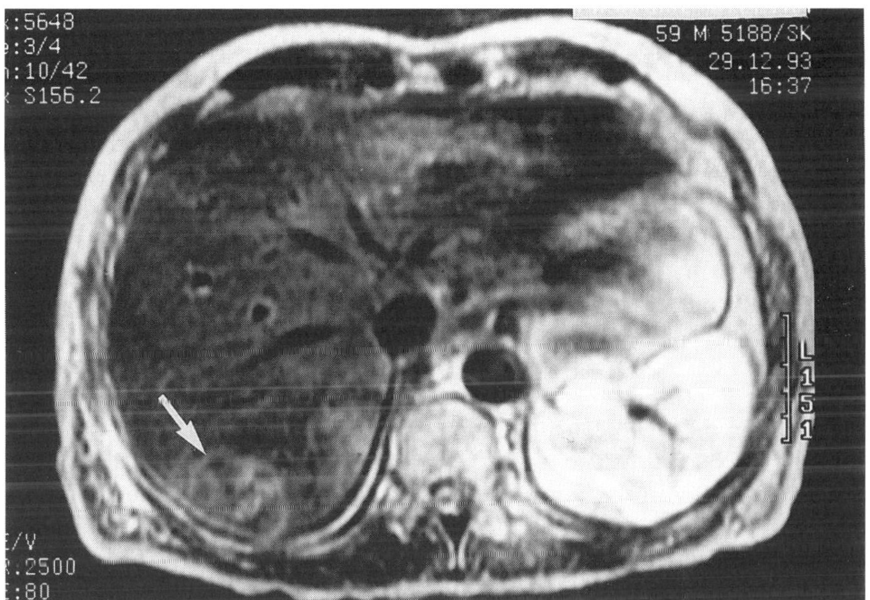

Fig. 8.3 T2 weighted section of the liver showing a metastasis (arrow) with a typical halo of high intensity around a lower intensity centre.

Furthermore, new sequences which allow much faster acquisition of data with reduced artefact are being developed and are likely further to improve the role of MR. Arterial portography can also be applied to MR in the same way that it is applied to CT, but it seems that this has no greater accuracy than CTAP (Soyer et al 1994a).

Summary

In summary it appears that short of intra-operative assessment with ultrasound, CTAP is still the most sensitive method for detection of liver lesions. MR allows more specificity in the characterisation of these lesions while CT gives more information than either about extra-hepatic manifestations of disease.

Pancreas and biliary tree

CT

CT is the established non-invasive method for assessing the pancreas and biliary tree, particularly in suspected neoplasia (Zeman & Silverman 1995a). However, MR and endoscopic ultrasound are making strong challenges to this primacy (Muller et al 1994), while the advent of spiral CT has added an important new element to the equation.

Neoplasia

Using CT, pancreatic adenocarcinoma is recognisable partly as a result of the enlargement or distortion of the pancreatic contour it produces, and partly because of the difference in attenuation between the tumour and the adjacent pancreatic parenchyma. This density difference is frequently accentuated by intravenous contrast enhancement. Spiral CT can provide narrow sections of the pancreas with simultaneous delivery of large volumes of contrast in both the arterial and venous phases, while avoiding respiratory misregistration. It is hoped that this will improve the delineation of pancreatic pathology and enable earlier detection of small tumours before they have caused morphological changes. It is likely that spiral CT will be particularly useful in the detection of small islet cell tumours which tend to be hypervascular and are often difficult to see on conventional CT. However, no studies detailing the effect of spiral CT on management or outcome have yet been published.

There has been considerable interest in the ability of radiological techniques to detect vascular invasion in patients with adenocarcinoma since this affects resectability (Fig. 8.1a). Obliteration of the fat plane around a vessel leading to encasement and invasion is a sign of vascular involvement but conventional CT shows such changes inconsistently (Warshaw et al 1990). Spiral CT enables a rather better assessment of vessels partly because of the technical factors mentioned above but partly because of the ability to overlap the slices.

Not only does this mean that areas of potential invasion are not missed but also that high quality 3D renditions of the peri-pancreatic vessels can be obtained. This in turn can improve the assessment of the tumour's resectability (Zeman et al 1994a).

Obstructive jaundice

Ultrasonography and conventional CT are sensitive in demonstrating biliary duct dilatation and accurate in determining the level of obstruction. However, unless a mass is present, both techniques often have difficulty in demonstrating the cause, whether this is a stricture, a small bile duct tumour, or a stone. Early experience suggests that spiral CT improves the delineation of these pathologies, partly because the transient enhancement of small cholangiocarcinomas is demonstrable (Zeman & Silverman 1995a) and partly because thin overlapping slices are less likely to miss small lesions.

3D reconstruction of the obstructed biliary tree can also be obtained using spiral CT. The relationship of a tumour to the confluence of the hepatic ducts, or the length of the common hepatic duct above a tumour are perhaps more easily appreciated using this method and this can be of value if surgery is being planned. In the non-obstructed system, an intravenous cholangiogram combined with spiral CT and 3D reconstruction provides an excellent demonstration of the anatomy (Stockburger et al 1994, Van Beers et al 1994). Although it is claimed that this will be of value in planning laparoscopic surgery, this potential benefit may be outweighed by the known toxicity of intravenous cholangiographic contrast.

MR

On T1W images, the signal from the normal pancreas is higher than that from the liver whereas adenocarcinoma typically returns a low signal similar to that from the spleen; thus a tumour lying within a normal pancreas stands out as a low signal area (Vellet et al 1992) (Fig. 8.4). The contrast of the tumour is increased if the signal from the fat is suppressed (Mitchell et al 1991), a technique which is available on the majority of newer machines. Scanning in the early (arterial) phase after intravenous injection of gadolinium also makes the tumours more prominent but timing is crucial since, after 1 min or more, many tumours enhance (Semelka et al 1991).

Many carcinomas are associated with atrophy or pancreatitis of the non-neoplastic gland which reduces the signal. This makes differentiation from tumours more difficult, although again intravenous gadolinium helps in the diagnosis since chronic pancreatitis enhances more than adenocarcinoma (Semelka & Ascher 1993). Conventional T2W images are relatively unhelpful (Steiner et al 1989) partly because the signal intensity of normal pancreas is variable. However the ducts and any associated fluid collections stand out clearly on T2 weighting particularly when the newer faster spin echo sequences are used. This is particularly useful in the display of the biliary tree and pancreatic ducts. MR cholangiopancreatography has been described recently and this seems to compare favourably with ERCP (Takehara et al 1994).

MR has been compared to CT in the assessments of patients with severe acute pancreatitis (Saifuddin et al 1993). Scanning using rapid sequences after

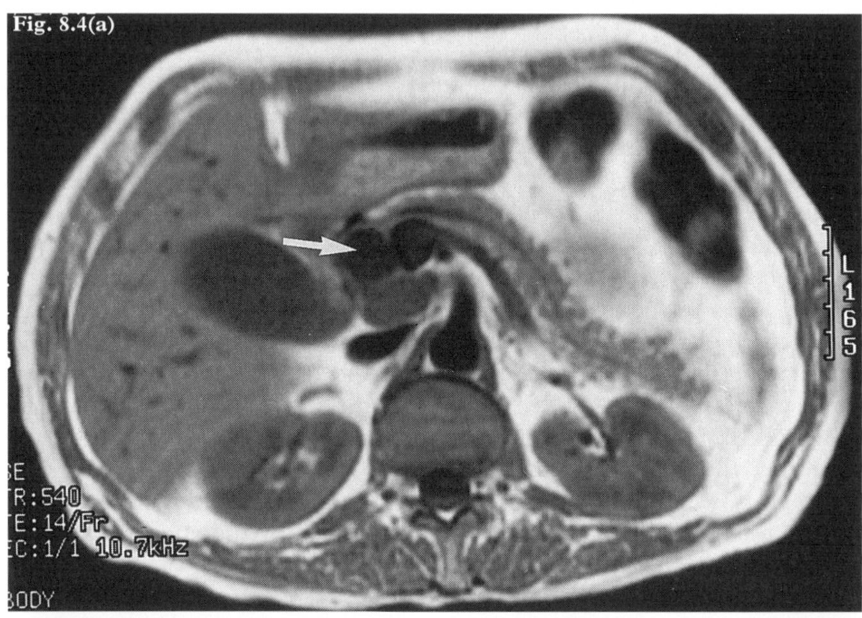

Fig. 8.4(a)

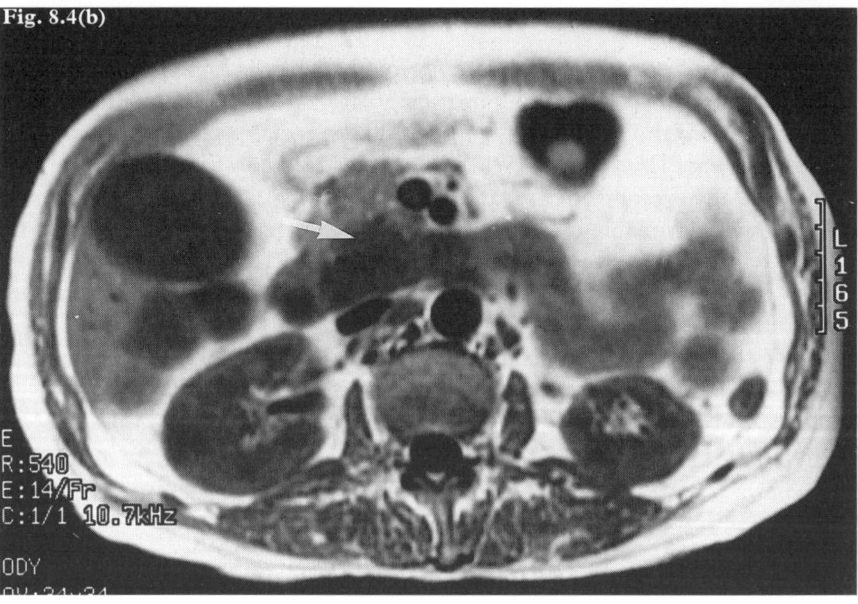

Fig. 8.4(b)

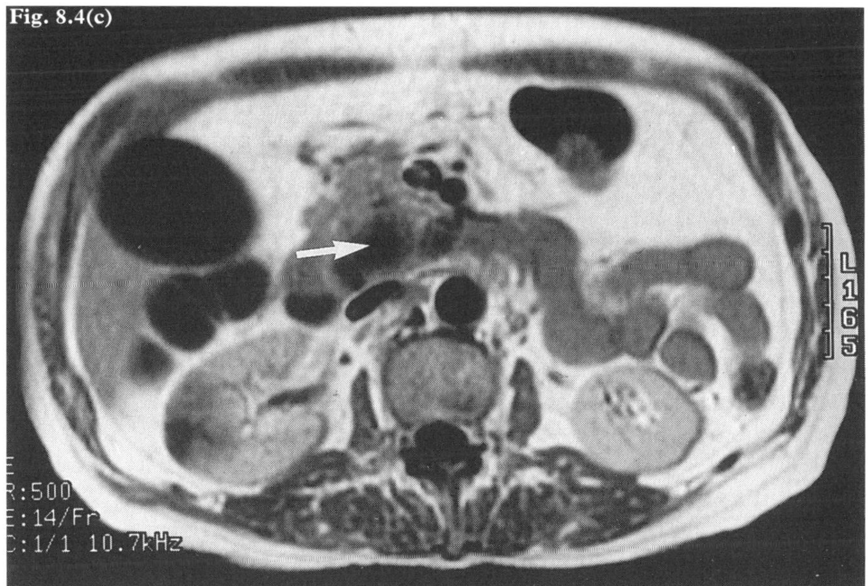

Fig. 8.4 (a) The normal pancreatic signal and morphology is well shown on T1 weighted unenhanced sequences. Note the dilated low signal common bile duct (arrow) and also the low signal from the prominent pancreatic duct, both the result of an obstructing tumour inferiorly. (b) T1W section at a level inferior to (a) showing a low signal area within the head of the pancreas caused by a carcinoma (arrow). (c) T1W section after intravenous gadolinium at the same level as (b). The definition of the tumour is improved as a result of the enhanced signal from the normal pancreatic parenchyma compared to the poorly enhancing carcinoma (arrow).

intravenous gadolinium demonstrates 'viable' pancreatic tissue with an accuracy identical to that of contrast enhanced CT. The sensitivity of MR to fluid makes the technique potentially very useful in patients with extensive disease and a mixture of necrosis with peri-pancreatic collections. The difficulties in scanning acutely unwell patients are well known and a clinically useful superiority of MR over good quality CT has yet to be established. Nonetheless, as in other areas, the lack of ionising radiation in MR is an important consideration in patients having multiple follow-up examinations.

One of the great advantages of MRI is its ability to depict flowing blood without the need for intravenous injection. Using gradient echo techniques flowing blood is of high signal intensity and processing of the images enables their demonstration as an MR angiogram. As with spiral CT, vascular involvement can be assessed on both the individual images and on the reconstructed angiogram.

Islet cell tumours have longer relaxation times than adenocarcinomas and are therefore more conspicuous (Tjon et al 1989). This makes MR theoretically preferable to CT but the technical requirements are stringent for optimisation of the signal differences. Nonetheless, the studies published show a significant advantage for MR over other techniques (Moore et al 1995).

The most recent comparisons between MR and CT show that MR is more sensitive in the detection of pancreatic tumours, although endoscopic ultrasonography maybe better than either (Muller et al 1994). However, it is not clear whether MR is better than CT in the detection of peripancreatic tumour spread (Gabata et al 1994). Comparisons of MR with spiral CT have not yet been published and while the present snapshot of the literature favours MR the leap-frogging of the different modalities as a result of the rapid technical advances means that the bias may well change over the next few years.

Abdominal vascular pathology

Spiral CT and MR have the potential to revolutionise vascular radiology. Both techniques enable highly accurate mapping of the vascular tree in the abdomen and elsewhere using relatively noninvasive methods (Fig. 8.5). The value of these techniques in the assessment of tumour encasement has been alluded to above in the section on the pancreas and the potential of MR in the detection of renal artery stenosis has been recognised for some time (Galanski et al 1993, Kim et al 1990). However, the techniques are likely to have most impact for the general surgeon in the assessment of abdominal aortic aneurysm (AAA). Ultrasonography is the standard screening technique for AAA (LaRoy et al 1989) but pre-operative assessment usually requires CT or angiography. MR

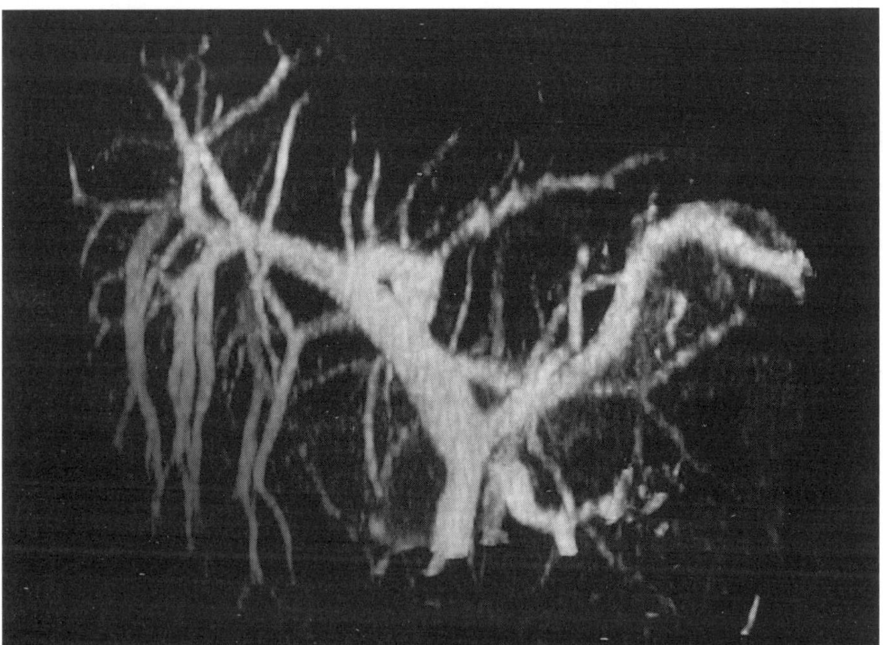

Fig. 8.5 Following an intravenous contrast injection the portal vein and its branches can be demonstrated by performing a spiral CT series, taking the maximum intensity points from the data and reformatting the information.

angiography can successfully and accurately demonstrate a range of thoracic aortic diseases (Hartnell et al 1994) and, although the technique is not yet widespread for assessing the abdominal aorta, the indications are not only that it is accurate (Kaufman et al 1994) but that in many patients it can replace conventional arteriography (Ecklund et al 1994). However, artefact from surgical clips reduces its value in the post-operative patient (Rubin & Jeffrey 1995).

CT

Conventional axial CT using IV contrast shows accurately the size of an aneurysm, any intramural thrombus and also extra aortic changes (Siegel & Cohan 1994). However, in up to 16% of patients, the extent of the aneurysm is incorrectly estimated and it is easy to miss accessory renal arteries as well as renal artery stenosis (Papanicolaou et al 1986). The advantages of spiral CT can be fully exploited in evaluating AAA and significantly improve the accuracy of CT in this disease (Zeman et al 1994b) (Fig. 8.6). While on the axial images it often remains difficult to identify the extent of an aneurysm, the 3D reformats are invaluable in clarifying the anatomy (Rubin et al 1993) in a way which surgeons often find useful. The reformatted images rely on computer software to strip away other structures within the image and then render the high attenuation contrast within the vessel in various visually acceptable formats (Fig. 8.7). Depending on the type of format chosen, calcification may be obscured or enhanced and the vessels may appear opaque or relatively translucent (Zeman 1995b). This, however, is a time consuming and labour

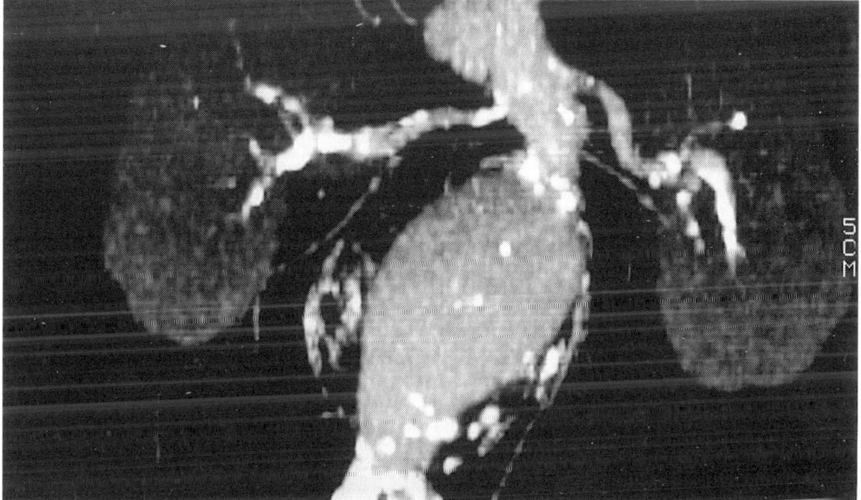

Fig. 8.6 Spiral CT demonstration of an abdominal aortic aneurysm and its relationship to the renal arteries using a maximum intensity profile technique following intravenous contrast injection.

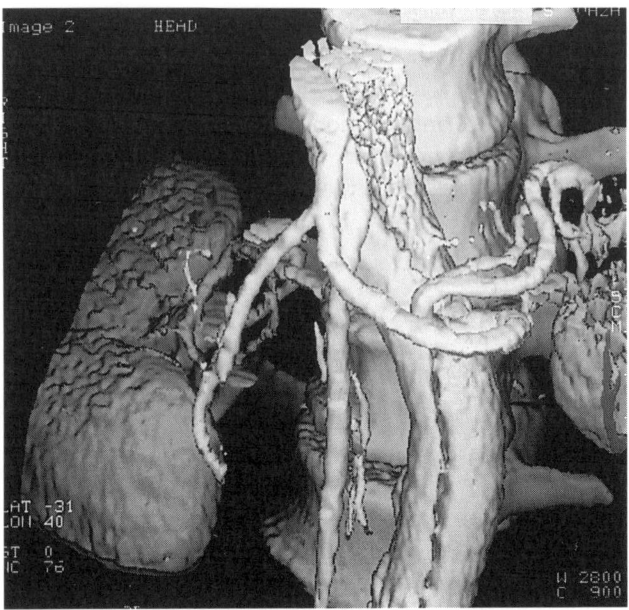

Fig. 8.7 Spiral CT 3D reconstruction of an abdominal aortic dissection manipulated to 'look down' on the lesion. The image has been reconstructed to show the aorta, spine and kidneys while stripping away the other structures.

intensive operation and makes the technique less suitable for emergency situations.

MR

The sensitivity of MR angiography in detecting renal stenosis extends to pathology in the other major abdominal vessels, including occlusion of the portal vein (Rodgers et al 1994). The ability of MR to image directly in any plane is a major advantage over other techniques, and this ability extends to MR angiography (Miyazaki et al 1995). However, in addition to this, recent work has shown that differences in superior mesenteric arterial blood flow in the fasting and post prandial states can be detected using MR (Li et al 1994). The same group has work in progress assessing superior mesenteric arterial and venous blood flow simultaneously as well as measuring the oxygen saturation of venous blood using MR (Li et al 1995a, Li et al 1995b). If these findings are confirmed then there are clear implications for improving our understanding of mesenteric ischaemia.

Bowel disease

Although CT and MR are not usually thought of as primary tools in the investigation of bowel disorders, it is becoming increasingly clear that they have a useful role to play in certain circumstances. Suspected small bowel obstruction is usually confirmed by plain film radiography but non-obstructed small bowel dilatation can look identical radiologically. Conventional CT has been used with success to differentiate these two entities (Gazelle et al 1994) and also to determine the cause and location of any obstruction (Frager et al 1994). While CT is obviously not necessary in all patients, it should be considered when clinical and plain film findings are inconclusive.

CT is also being used more widely in the assessment of patients with large bowel pathology and, in particular, those with colitis. In these patients, mural thickening and mesenteric infiltration are common findings on CT which can also show the distribution of the changes. While such findings are highly suggestive of inflammatory bowel disease, there is not consistent differentiation between Crohn's disease and ulcerative colitis (Philpotts et al 1994). Unfortunately the CT changes do not necessarily correlate with clinical severity (Boland et al 1995). MR of large and small bowel pathology has been hindered by technical difficulties and the absence of a suitable oral contrast agent. However, some of the technical problems have been resolved and work using MR in association with intravenous gadolinium in the investigation of inflammatory bowel disease is particularly promising. Active Crohn's disease shows enhancement of the thickened bowel wall and the degree of thickening and enhancement have been correlated with activity (Kettritz et al 1995).

Perianal fistula is a particularly distressing complication of Crohn's disease and often difficult to treat. CT can be used to show the abscesses and fluid collections associated with these fistulae but it is often difficult to demonstrate the fistulas themselves and their extent. The sensitivity of MR to free fluid and its ability to image directly in any plane is well suited to the demonstration of such complications. Saline can be used as a contrast agent (Myhr et al 1994) but is not always required. Direct coronal imaging enables the classification of fistulae with respect to the levator ani and musculocutaneous junction of the anus. This enables the correct surgical procedure to be selected and is likely to become the investigation of choice in assessing these patients (Barker et al 1994).

KEY POINTS FOR CLINICAL PRACTICE

- Spiral CT is becoming more widely available. Its speed will increase the utility of CT in restless and acutely unwell patients, while other technical improvements are likely to expand its application and accuracy.

- The speed of acquisition of MR sequences is likely to increase dramatically, making MR a routine procedure for the examination of the abdomen.

- MR appears to be the best non-invasive technique for assessing focal hepatic lesions but CTAP remains the most sensitive for their detection.

- MR is good at detecting pancreatic tumours and probably better than CT for small lesions. However MR is no better than CT in assessing peri-pancreatic spread of tumour.

- Both MR and spiral CT cholangiopancreatography may develop and become a useful noninvasive adjunct to diagnostic ERCP.
- Both MR and spiral CT angiography have enormous potential to improve the assessment of vascular pathology.
- Both MR and CT can be useful in patients with inflammatory bowel disease particularly when complicated by fistulas.

REFERENCES

Barker PG, Lunniss PJ, Armstrong P, Reznek RH, Cottam K, Phillips RK 1994 Magnetic resonance imaging of fistula-in-ano: technique, interpretation and accuracy. Clin Radiol 49: 7-13

Bluemke DA, Urban D, Fishman EK 1994 Spiral CT of the liver: current applications. Semin Ultrasound CT MRI 15: 107-121

Boland GW, Lee MJ, Cats AM, Ferraro MJ, Matthia AR, Mueller PR 1995 *Clostridium difficile* colitis: correlation of CT findings with severity of clinical disease. Clin Radiol 50: 153-156

Boyd DP, Parker DL, Goodsitt MM 1992 Principles of computed tomography. In: Computed tomography of the body. W.B. Saunders, Philadelphia, pp 1355-1383

Bressler EL, Alpern MB, Glazer GM, Francis IR, Ensminger WD 1987 Hypervascular hepatic metastases: CT evaluation. Radiology 162: 49-51

Chezmar JL, Rumancik WM, Megibow AJ, Hulnick DH, Nelson RC, Bernardino ME 1988 Liver and abdominal screening in patients with cancer: CT versus MR imaging. Radiology 168: 43-47

Ecklund K, Hartnell GG, Hughes LA, Stokes KR, Finn JP 1994 MR angiography as the sole method in evaluating abdominal aortic aneurysms: correlation with conventional techniques and surgery. Radiology 192: 345-350

Edelman RR, Wielopolski P, Schmitt F 1994 Echo-planar MR imaging. Radiology 192: 600-612

Foley WD, Hoffmann RG, Quiroz FA, Kahn CE, Perret RS 1994 Hepatic helical CT: contrast material injection protocol. Radiology 192: 367-371

Frager D, Medwid SW, Baer JW, Mollinelli B, Friedman M 1994 CT of small-bowel obstruction: value in establishing the diagnosis and determining the degree and cause. Am J Roentgenol 162: 37-41

Gabata T, Matsui O, Kadoya M et al 1994 Small pancreatic adenocarcinomas: efficacy of MR imaging with fat suppression and gadolinium enhancement. Radiology 193: 683-688

Galanski M, Prokop M, Chavan A, Schaefer CM, Jandeleit K, Nischelsky JE 1993 Renal arterial stenoses: spiral CT angiography. Radiology 189: 185-192

Gazelle GS, Goldberg MA, Wittenberg J, Halpern EF, Pinkney L, Mueller P R 1994 Efficacy of CT in distinguishing small-bowel obstruction from other causes of small-bowel dilatation. Am J Roentgenol 162: 43-47

Hamm B, Thoeni RF, Gould RG et al 1994 Focal liver lesions: characterization with nonenhanced and dynamic contrast material-enhanced MR imaging. Radiology 190: 417-423

Hartnell GG, Finn JP, Zenni M et al 1994 MR imaging of the thoracic aorta: comparison of spin-echo, angiographic, and breath-hold techniques. Radiology 191: 697-704

Heiken JP, Brink JA, McClennan BL, Sagel SS , Forman HP, DiCroce J 1993 Dynamic contrast-enhanced CT of the liver: comparison of contrast medium injection rates and uniphasic and biphasic injection protocols. Radiology 187: 327-331

Horowitz AL 1992 MRI physics for radiologists, 2nd edn. Springer Verlag, New York

Kaufman JA, Geller SC, Petersen MJ, Cambria RP, Prince MR, Waltman AC 1994 MR imaging (including MR angiography) of abdominal aortic aneurysms: comparison with conventional angiography. Am J Roentgenol 163: 203-210

Kettritz U, Shoenut JP, Semelka RC 1995 MR imaging of the gastrointestinal tract. Magn Reson Im Clin North Am 3: 87-98

Kim D, Edelman RR, Kent KC, Porter DH, Skillman JJ 1990 Abdominal aorta and renal artery stenosis: evaluation with MR angiography. Radiology 174: 727-731

LaRoy LL, Cormier P, Matalon TAS, Patel SK, Turner DA, Silver B 1989 Imaging of abdominal aortic aneurysms. Am J Roentgenol 152: 875-792

Larson RE, Semelka RC, Bagley AS, Molina PL, Brown ED, Lee JKT 1994 Hypervascular malignant liver lesions: comparison of various MR imaging pulse sequences and dynamic CT. Radiology 92: 393-399

Li KCP, Wright GA, Pelc LR et al 1995a Oxygen saturation of blood in the superior mesenteric vein: in vivo verification of MR imaging measurements in a canine model. Radiology 194: 32-325

Li KCP, Hopkins KL, Dalman RL, Song CK 1995b Simultaneous measurement of flow in the superior mesenteric vein and artery with cine phase-contrast MR imaging: value in diagnosis of chronic mesenteric ischemia. Radiology 194: 327-330

Li KCP, Whitney WS, McDonnell CH et al 1994 Chronic mesenteric ischemia: evaluation with phase-contrast cine MR imaging. Radiology 190: 175-179

McFarland EG, Mayo-Smith WW, Saini S, Hahn PF, Goldberg MA, Lee MJ 1994 Hepatic hemangiomas and malignant tumours: improved differentiation with heavily T2-weighted conventional spin-echo MR imaging. Radiology 193: 43-47

Mahfouz AE, Hamm B, Wolf KJ 1994 Peripheral washout: a sign of malignancy on dynamic gadolinium-enhanced MR images of focal liver lesions. Radiology 190: 49-52

Mitchell DG, Saini S, Weinreb J et al 1994 Hepatic metastases and cavernous hemangiomas: distinction with standard-and triple-dose gadoteridol-enhanced MR imaging. Radiology 193: 49-57

Mitchell DG, Vinitski S, Saponaro S, Tasciyan T, Burk DL, Rifkin MD 1991 Liver and pancreas: improved spin-echo T1 contrast by shorter echo time and fat suppression at 1.5 T. Radiology 178: 67-71

Miyazaki T, Yamashita Y, Shinzato J, Kojima A, Takahashi M 1995 Two-dimensional time-of-flight magnetic resonance angiography in the coronal plane for abdominal disease: its usefulness and comparison with conventional angiography Br J Radiol 68: 351-357

Moore NR, Rogers CE, Britton BJ 1995 Magnetic resonance imaging of endocrine tumours of the pancreas. Br J Radiol 68: 341-347

Muller MF, Meyenberger C, Bertschinger P, Schaer R, Marincek B 1994 Pancreatic tumors: evaluation with endoscopic US, CT, and MR imaging. Radiology 190: 745-751

Myhr GE, Myrvold HE, Nilsen G, Thoresen JE, Rinck PA 1994 Perianal fistulas: use of MR imaging for diagnosis. Radiology 191: 545-549

Outwater E, Tomaszewski JE, Daly JM, Kressel HY 1991 Hepatic colorectal metastases: correlation of MR imaging and pathologic appearance. Radiology 180: 327-332

Papanicolaou N, Wittenberg J, Ferrucci JT et al 1986 Preoperative evaluation of abdominal aortic aneurysms by computed tomography. Am J Roentgenol 146: 711-715

Philpotts LE, Heiken JP, Westcott MA, Gore RM 1994 Colitis: use of CT findings in differential diagnosis. Radiology 190: 445-449

Quinn SF, Benjamin GG 1992 Hepatic cavernous hemangiomas: simple diagnostic sign with dynamic bolus CT. Radiology 182: 545-548

Reinig JW, Dwyer AJ, Miller DL, Frank JA, Adams GW, Chang AE 1989 Liver metastases: detection with MR imaging at 0.5 and 1.5 T. Radiology 170: 149-153

Rodgers PM, Ward J, Baudouin CJ, Ridgway JP, Robinson PJ 1994 Dynamic contrast-enhanced MR imaging of the portal venous system: comparison with X-ray angiography. Radiology 191: 741-745

Rubin GD, Jeffrey RB 1995 3D spiral CT angiography of the abdomen and thorax. In: Spiral CT principles, techniques and clinical applications. Raven Press, New York, p 187

Rubin GD, Walker PJ, Dake MD et al 1993 Three-dimensional spiral compute tomographic angiography: an alternative imaging modality for the abdominal aorta and its branches. J Vasc Surg 18: 656-665

Rummeny EJ, Wernecke K, Saini S et al 1992 Comparison between high-field-strength MR imaging and CT for screening of hepatic metastases: a receiver operating characteristic analysis. Radiology 182: 879-886

Rydberg JN, Lomas DJ, Coakley KJ, Hough DM, Ehman RL, Riederer SJ 1995 Comparison of breath-hold fast spin-echo and conventional spin-echo pulse sequences for T2-weighted MR imaging of liver lesions. Radiology 194: 431-437

Saifuddin A, Ward J, Ridgeway J, Chalmers AG 1993 Comparison of MR and CT scanning in severe acute pancreatitis: initial experiences. Clin Rad 48: 111-116

Semelka RC, Brown ED, Ascher SM et al 1994 Hepatic hemangiomas: a multi-institutional study of appearance on T2-weighted and serial gadolinium-enhanced gradient-echo MR images. Radiology 192: 401-406

Semelka RC, Ascher SM 1993 MR imaging of the pancreas. Radiology 188: 593-602

Semelka RC, Kroeker MA, Shoenut JP, Kroeker R, Yaffe CS, Micflikier AB 1991 Pancreatic disease: prospective comparison of CT, ERCP, and 1.5-T MR imaging with dynamic gadolinium enhancement and fat suppression. Radiology 181: 785-791

Siegel CL, Cohan RH 1994 CT of abdominal aortic aneurysms. Am J Roentgenol 163: 17-29

Small WC, Nelson RC, Bernardino ME, Brummer LT 1994 Contrast-enhanced spiral CT of the liver: effect of different amounts and injection rates of contrast material on early contrast enhancement. Am J Roentgenol 163: 87-92

Soyer P, Roche A, Gad M et al 1991 Preoperative segmental localization of hepatic metastases: utility of three-dimensional CT during arterial portography. Radiology 180: 653-658

Soyer P, Laissy JP, Sibert A et al 1994a Focal hepatic masses: comparison of detection during arterial portography with MR imaging and CT. Radiology 190: 737-740

Soyer P, Bluemke DA, Hruban RH, Sitzmann JV, Fishman EK 1994b Hepatic metastases from colorectal cancer: detection and false-positive findings with helical CT during arterial portography. Radiology 193: 71-74

Stark DD, Bradley WJ 1992 Unit 1. In: Magnetic resonance imaging, 2nd edn, vol 1. Mosby Yearbook, St Louis

Steinberg HV, Alarcon JJ, Bernardino ME 1990 Focal hepatic lesions: comparative MR imaging at 0.5 and 1.5 T. Radiology 174: 153-156

Steiner E, Stark DD, Hahn PF et al 1989 Imaging of pancreatic neoplasms: comparison of MR and CT. Am J Roentgenol 152: 487-491

Stockberger SM, Wass JL, Sherman S, Lehman GA, Kopecky KK 1994 Intravenous cholangiography with helical CT: comparison with endoscopic retrograde cholangiography. Radiology 192: 675-680

Takehara Y, Ichijo K, Tooyama N et al 1994 Breath-hold MR cholangiopancreatography with a long-echo-train fast spin-echo sequence and a surface coil in chronic pancreatitis. Radiology 192: 73-78

Taupitz M, Speidel A, Hamm B et al 1995 T2-weighted breath-hold MR imaging of the liver at 1.5 T: results with a three-dimensional steady-state free precession sequence in 87 patients. Radiology 194: 439-446

Tjon A, Tham RTO, Falke THM, Jansen JBMJ, Lamers CBHW 1989 CT and MR imaging of advanced Zollinger-Ellison syndrome. J Comput Assist Tomogr 13: 821-828

Van Beers BE, Lacrosse M, Trigaux JP, de Canniere L, De Ronde T, Pringot J 1994 Noninvasive imaging of the biliary tree before or after laparoscopic cholecystectomy: use of three-dimensional spiral CT cholangiography. Am J Roentgenol 162: 1331-1335

Vellet AD, Romano W, Bach DB, Passi RB, Taves DH, Munk PL 1992 Adenocarcinoma of the pancreatic ducts: comparative evaluation with CT and MR imaging at 1.5 T. Radiology 183: 87-95

Warshaw AL, Gu ZY, Wittenberg J, Waltman AC 1990 Preoperative staging and assessment of resectability of pancreatic cancer. Arch Surg 125: 230-233

Wittenberg J, Stark DD, Forman BH et al 1988 Differentiation of hepatic metastases from hepatic hemangiomas and cysts by using MR imaging. Am J Roentgenol 151: 79-84

Yamashita Y, Hatanaka Y, Yamamoto H et al 1994 Differential diagnosis of focal liver lesions: role of spin-echo and contrast-enhanced dynamic MR imaging. Radiology 193: 59-65

Zeman RK, Silverman PM 1995a Abdomen and pelvis. In: Helical/spiral CT: a practical approach. McGraw-Hill, New York, p 187, 203

Zeman RK 1995b Vascular system and three-dimensional CT angiography. In: Helical/spiral CT: a practical approach. McGraw-Hill, New York, p 269

Zeman RK, Davros WJ, Berman P et al 1994a Three-dimensional models of the abdominal vasculature based on helical CT: usefulness in patients with pancreatic neoplasms. Am J Roentgenol 162: 1425-1429

Zeman RK, Silverman PM, Berman PM, Weltman DI, Davros WJ, Gomes MN 1994b Abdominal aortic aneurysms: evaluation with variable-collimation helical CT and overlapping reconstruction. Radiology 193: 555-560

9

Recent advances in nutritional support of surgical patients

B. J. Moran

Surgeons have been at the forefront in practically all the major developments in nutritional support down through the ages. In 1790, John Hunter first described the use of a tube to feed a patient enterally and, almost a century later, the first successfully performed surgical gastrostomy was reported in 1876 (Gauderer & Stellato 1986). Another century elapsed before the concept of 'nutritional support' was popularized. Nutritional support, as we know it today, has really emanated from the demonstration of the first successful use of total parenteral nutrition (TPN) by Dudrick and colleagues in 1968.

In broad terms, modern nutritional support involves a range of activities, extending from prescribing the oral intake of specialized (usually liquid) enteral feeds, and providing access to the available functioning gut (in the form of enteral tubes and stomas) to bypassing the intestinal tract in patients with intestinal failure (in the form of TPN). In this context, the concept of 'intestinal failure' is useful. Intestinal failure is defined as a 'reduction in functioning gut mass below the minimum necessary for the adequate digestion and absorption of nutrients' (Fleming & Remington 1981). The only absolute indication for TPN is intestinal failure and the surgeon should aim to feed all other patients enterally, though this may require ingenious methods to gain access to the gut.

The fundamental aspects of nutritional support may be broadly categorized into three specific areas (Table 9.1).

SELECTION OF PATIENTS IN NEED OF NUTRITIONAL SUPPORT

The selection of patients for intervention has, in many ways, been the most

Table 9.1 Three main considerations in the provision of nutritional support

- Determine which patients require nutritional support and whether they have a functioning gastrointestinal tract
- Select the appropriate substrate
- Obtain and maintain access for delivery of the substrate to the patient

Table 9.2 Methods to assess malnutrition

1. Methods to assess body composition, or anthropometric measurements
   - Body weight
     — compared with usual (for individual) or ideal
   - Muscle stores
     — mid arm muscle circumference (MAMC)
   - Fat stores
     — skinfold thickness, triceps skinfold thickness (TSF)
     — bioelectrical impedance analysis
   - Research methods (expensive and impractical)
     — in vivo neutron activation analysis
     — isotopic labelling studies
2. Methods which attempt to measure body function
   - Muscle function
     — grip strength
   - Immune function
     — lymphocyte count
     — delayed skin hypersensitivity
   - Biochemical markers
     — albumin
     — transferrin
     — retinol binding protein
     — thyroxine binding prealbumin
3. Clinical assessment techniques
   - Dietary history
     — dietary recall/prospective
   - History and examination by an experienced clinician
     — 'End-Of-The-Bedogram'

contentious aspect of nutritional support. Indeed, little progress has been made in refining the selection criteria. At the centre of the controversy lies the search for the optimal method, or methods, for nutritional assessment. The methods used to measure malnutrition fall into three broad groups (Table 9.2).

Whilst many of these methods can serve as indices of malnutrition, they may not necessarily indicate the necessity for adjuvant nutritional support, nor do they permit ready appraisal of the efficacy of any nutritional therapy. Despite some recent enthusiastic, though unsubstantiated, claims for individual techniques, such as bioelectrical impedance analysis for example, the selection of patients for nutritional support and the assessment of nutritional status remain largely a clinical decision. This decision-making process has been called 'subjective global assessment' by Detsky and colleagues (1987). A more simplistic term which we have coined in Southampton is the 'End-

Of-The-Bedogram'. However, all clinical techniques entail the clinician being aware of

- the symptoms and signs of malnutrition
- the prevailing disease and the likely effects of treatment
- the available methods and techniques for nutritional therapy.

Thus, when conclusions are drawn that clinical methods are best for nutritional assessment, it should be appreciated that these conclusions have been drawn by clinicians with an awareness and interest in nutritional support.

Any mechanism which helps to identify patients in need of nutritional support is to be encouraged, provided the limitations of the technique are taken into consideration. Simple nutritional assessment of all patients (by measuring body weight and height and obtaining a history of weight loss and current food intake), together with serial monitoring on a weekly basis, provide valuable information on the presence or likely development of serious undernutrition.

PERIOPERATIVE NUTRITIONAL SUPPORT

Another major unresolved issue has been the concept of perioperative nutritional support. Grossly malnourished patients have an increased incidence of postoperative complications, and this has been noted in several studies since Studley observed in 1936 that patients with greater than 20% weight loss had a 33% mortality following gastrectomy for peptic ulcer compared with 3% in those with less than 20% weight loss. Improving nutritional status in malnourished individuals ought to improve outcome following major surgery, but scientific evidence has been lacking.

Perioperative TPN

A recent major study tried to address the issue of the benefits of perioperative nutrition by a randomized prospective study of 7–10 days preoperative TPN in malnourished patients undergoing major abdominal or non-cardiac thoracic surgery (Buzby et al 1991). The initial entry criteria excluded 3% of the patients who had an absolute requirement for TPN (that is, they had prolonged intestinal failure). Following randomization of 395 patients, approximately 5% were classified as severely malnourished and appeared to derive benefit from TPN. In the remaining 95% who were less severely malnourished, TPN resulted in an increase in major complications, mainly infectious in nature, compared with controls. These data have been presented as suggesting that perioperative TPN has an unproven role and may be detrimental (Detsky 1991). However, this is misleading, as patients with intestinal failure in whom TPN was essential were excluded. Furthermore, those with an intact functioning gastrointestinal tract (presumably practically all those randomized) could have been more appropriately nourished with enteral nutrition.

A realistic analysis of this study suggests that TPN is life-saving in patients with intestinal failure and, in addition, improves the outcome in those who are severely malnourished. In borderline-to-severe malnutrition however, the risks of TPN outweigh the benefits. As it was the risks of TPN that altered the risk-benefit equation, the results suggest that preoperative and perioperative enteral nutrition (which is cheaper, safer and metabolically superior to TPN) may well prove beneficial but evaluation is awaited.

Postoperative enteral nutrition to improve outcome

Enteral supplementation postoperatively has been shown to improve outcome in orthopaedic patients. Bastow et al (1983) looked at the effects of a liquid feed (1000 ml, 1000 kcal/day) given postoperatively via a fine bore nasogastric tube in elderly malnourished women following surgical treatment of fractured neck of femur. In this randomized prospective study, there were significant improvements in the time to rehabilitation and the time to discharge from hospital in the group which received nutritional supplements.

A similar study by Delmi et al (1990) simplified the method of nutrient administration. These authors used an oral nutritional supplement (250 ml, 20 g protein, 254 kcal) for a mean of 32 days in a randomized prospective study of 59 elderly patients with femoral neck fractures. The median duration of hospital stay was significantly shorter in the supplemented group (24 versus 40 days). Clinical outcome during the stay in the convalescent hospital was also significantly better in the supplemented group (59% favourable course versus 13% in the controls). The rates of deaths and complications were also significantly lower in the supplemented patients (44% versus 87%) and these differences in morbidity and mortality were maintained at 6 months (40% versus 74%).

Enteral supplementation of general surgical patients

A recent study (Rana et al 1992) looked at the effects of supplementing patients recovering from abdominal operations. A total of 54 patients who were scheduled to undergo predetermined moderate to major gastrointestinal surgical procedures entered the study. They were randomly assigned to receive a normal ward diet postoperatively or the same diet supplemented *ad libitum* by an oral nutritional sip feed. The study period commenced when the surgical team indicated that the patient could have 'clear fluids'. Supplemented patients maintained their preoperative weight, whereas control patients had lost a significant amount of their preoperative weight at the time of discharge (4.7 ± 1.2 kg, $P \pm 0.02$). Preoperative muscle function, as evidenced by grip strength dynamometry decreased to a greater extent in the control than in the treatment group. There was a tendency towards fewer complications in the supplemented group but the small numbers did not allow definitive conclusions. This study has been repeated with 100 patients randomized and there is a significant reduction in postoperative complications in the supplemented group (Silk 1995, personal communication).

These recent studies suggest that it is possible to improve outcome following surgery by nutritional support. However, there are several other factors which influence outcome following surgery, for example the skill of the surgeon, the age of the patient, the severity of the disease and the presence of malignancy. It is difficult to evaluate nutritional intervention in isolation from these confounding variables. The fact that there is a paucity of scientific evidence to support perioperative nutritional intervention more likely reflects methodological problems rather than the absence of genuine benefit in selected patients.

SELECTION OF THE APPROPRIATE SUBSTRATE

The appropriate substrate for nutritional support depends primarily on the function of the gastrointestinal tract. Patients with prolonged intestinal failure require intravenous nutrients and it is now possible, for instance, to maintain individuals indefinitely on parenteral nutrition in the form of home-based TPN. The past decade has seen an explosion of interest in the formulation of nutritional substrates, and we are in the era of 'disease specific nutrients' with, in general, excessive and unsubstantiated claims for their efficacy in clinical practice. The concept of 'disease specific nutrients' extends to both enteral and parenteral feeds and much research has been channelled into this area.

Enteral nutrients

All companies in the enteral nutrition market now produce a range of liquid enteral feeds. Enteral feeds can be used to nourish a patient completely (often via an enteral feeding tube), or may be used to supplement an inadequate oral intake (often by oral voluntary intake or what is commonly referred to as 'sip-feeding'). Enteral feeds may be broadly categorized by their composition (Table 9.3).

The polymeric, elemental and disease specific feeds are 'complete' feeds containing a reasonable balance of macronutrients (protein, carbohydrate and fat) and micronutrients (vitamins and trace elements). In sufficient

Table 9.3 Categories of enteral feeds

- Polymeric or 'whole protein feeds'
- Elemental (also called predigested or 'chemically defined')
- Disease specific
- Modular or supplemental

quantities, these feeds can be used as the sole nutrient intake for indefinite periods. Modular, or supplemental, feeds are incomplete and often are composed of one macronutrient, such as carbohydrate, and may only be used to supplement, not to replace normal dietary intake.

Polymeric feeds

These feeds are made from whole protein (approximately 5 g nitrogen/l), usually contain 1 kcal/ml and are almost all lactose- and gluten-free. Thus 2.5 l of a polymeric feed contains 2500 kcal and 12.5 g nitrogen and is a suitable daily intake. Recent variations contain 1.5–2 kcal/ml which allow adequate nutrient intake in a smaller volume, which is often better tolerated and allows adequate nutritional support in patients whose oral fluid intake is restricted.

Another recent advance is the introduction of polymeric feeds containing fibre. These fibre-containing feeds have paradoxically been found to be useful in patients with either constipation or diarrhoea. The beneficial effect on constipated patients is to be expected. It is likely that fibre-containing feeds improve diarrhoea by altering colonic flora and thus colonic fluid and electrolyte metabolism (Moran and Jackson 1992). Polymeric feeds are cheaper and relatively palatable (by comparison with the other feeds), are available in various flavours and are the most acceptable for oral consumption.

Elemental feeds

Elemental, or chemically defined feeds contain predigested protein in the form of oligopeptides or amino acids. These feeds are vigorously promoted by nutritional companies for use in patients with reduced absorptive capacity, such as patients with short bowel syndrome, and patients with pancreatic or small bowel mucosal disease. However, research studies have shown that the majority of patients will absorb whole protein feeds (Payne-James & Silk 1988). There is some evidence to support the use of elemental feeds in a small number of patients with severe pancreatic insufficiency or severe Crohn's disease. The disadvantages of these feeds are their expense, their unpalatability (which almost invariably limits their use to tube feeding) and their increased osmolarity due to an increase in the number of particles per unit volume.

Disease specific feeds

The production of disease specific feeds stems from theoretical principles of nutrient metabolism and requirements in specific diseases or specific organ dysfunctional states. The majority of these feeds contain (with some notable exceptions, such as the respiratory specific feed) variations in the type and amount of the amino acid content. Thus branched chain amino acid (BCAA) enriched solutions have been used in liver disease and in trauma because of the reduced plasma levels of BCAA noted in individuals with these conditions. Theoretical advantages have not been confirmed in clinical practice (Morgan 1990).

Glutamine. Current enthusiasm in disease specific amino acid solutions relates predominantly to the use of glutamine, and, to a lesser extent, arginine. Glutamine is considered a non-essential amino acid but is the most abundant amino acid in the free amino acid pool of the body. Glutamine plays an important role in the transport of nitrogen between tissues and is essential for renal ammoniagenesis. It is also the essential energy substrate for enterocytes, lymphocytes and other rapidly dividing cells (Dudrick & Souba 1991). Thus, glutamine enriched solutions may be theoretically beneficial in almost every seriously ill patient. Indeed it has been hypothesized that glutamine-enriched solutions might reduce the incidence of multiple organ failure which may be related to bacterial translocation from the intestinal lumen in patients whose immune system is compromised by severe illness. Glutamine was not, until recently, included in TPN formulations due to its instability in solution. Research continues into both enteral and parenteral supplementation with glutamine-enriched solutions, but early enthusiasm, mainly from animal experimentation, has not been substantiated by subsequent clinical studies.

Other modifications of the amino acid solutions, by arginine supplementation or by utilization of essential amino acid solutions (in particular in patients with renal disease), continue to generate interest. However, clinical trials to date have not demonstrated major advantages for these nutrients, either individually or in combination.

Parenteral nutrients

The use of parenteral nutrients to completely feed an individual is relatively new, and continues to undergo modification. The main constraints in intravenous nutritional support remain the hypertonicity of the nutrient solutions which result in injury to the vein wall, and the chemical interactions involved when nutrients are mixed prior to infusion. Chemical and pharmaceutical constraints continue to limit the supply of intravenous nutrients. A typical example is the amino acid glutamine, which is unstable in solution, and therefore has not been added to intravenous solutions. Recent studies suggest that ill patients may have very large glutamine requirements which are vastly in excess of the patient's ability to synthesize glutamine endogenously. For this reason, attempts are currently being made to supply glutamine for TPN either as free glutamine added just prior to infusion, or as glutamine dipeptides. Further research continues in this area and results are awaited, though initial enthusiastic claims should be viewed with caution.

Other areas of current interest include the use of medium chain triglycerides (MCT) which have theoretical advantages over currently used long chain triglyceride solutions in that MCT hydrolysis is not dependent upon lipoprotein lipase, and MCT metabolism is independent of carnitine. Here again, no clear clinical benefits have been shown to date.

METABOLIC MANIPULATION

It is now well established that nutrient provision in the severely ill, metabolically stressed patient may reduce, but does not prevent, body protein breakdown and nitrogen loss. The metabolic response to injury and illness can be modified through cytokine manipulation and by hormonal therapy. Indeed, nutrients (such as alternative fat solutions) can alter both the cytokine and hormonal response and such nutrients have been termed 'nutraceuticals', that is nutrients functioning in a pharmaceutical fashion. To date, however, no readily available nutrient manipulations have been shown to have obvious benefits in clinical practice.

A further recent area of interest has been the use of growth hormone to promote protein synthesis and considerable research is in progress.

CURRENT STATUS OF NUTRITIONAL SUPPORT

The theoretical advantages and anecdotal reports of benefits of alterations in nutrient manipulations have not been confirmed in clinical practice. The majority of individuals who require nutritional support are adequately treated with readily available standard enteral and parenteral substrates. Although selected patients may require specialized substrates, indications for many of these expensive compounds are often poorly defined. It is useful to consider nutritional support in severe illness as a 'damage limitation' therapy whilst disease is being treated with drugs, surgery and other interventions. The concept of 'disease specific nutrients' in severe illness is, as yet, a research tool and of little clinical significance in modern clinical practice.

ACCESS TECHNIQUES

The limiting factor in nutritional support of the vast majority of patients is the attainment and maintenance of safe access, whether it be to the venous system for TPN, or to the gut for enteral nutrition. Surgeons are commonly the most appropriately trained personnel available in a hospital with the various technical skills of enteral and parenteral access.

Access routes for enteral nutrition

Three important developments in enteral access techniques during the past 20 years have been:

- fine bore naso-enteral feeding tubes
- needle catheter jejunostomy
- percutaneous endoscopic gastrostomy (and jejunostomy).

Fine bore naso-enteral feeding tubes

Although the term 'enteral feeding' usually refers to nasogastric feeding, feeding tubes can be passed nasally into the duodenum and jejunum. There is little justification for using a Ryle's nasogastric tube for prolonged nutritional support, though if already in place, a Ryle's tube may be used for a short time (approximately 1 week).

Fine bore polyurethane tubes are superior to Ryle's tubes, as they are better tolerated by the patient, less likely to cause gastro-oesophageal reflux or ulceration and are easier to pass. These tubes can be inserted by patients themselves for supplemental overnight feeding. In addition, they can be positioned accurately by being passed over a guidewire, under fluoroscopic or endoscopic control, into the stomach, duodenum or upper jejunum.

Nasojejunal feeding may be successful in some cases where nasogastric feeding has failed, because of gastric statis or severe gastro-oesophageal reflux.

Despite the advantages of fine-bore tubes, they are still subject to most of the general complications of any feeding tube, namely failure to obtain access, misplacement, displacement, tube blockage or fracture.

There is a variety of tube designs. The tip of the tube may be modified by altering the shape of the opening or by adding weights, though manufacturers' claims for several of these design modifications have not been substantiated in clinical practice (Payne-James & Silk 1988).

Due to some recent evidence that gastric stasis often prevents enteral feeding, particularly in the postoperative period, double lumen tubes are now available whereby one lumen is positioned in the stomach for nasogastric decompression and the distal lumen is positioned in the upper jejunum for feeding (Fig. 9.1).

Needle catheter jejunostomy

In 1973, Delaney and colleagues described a technique to obtain access to the jejunum via a catheter inserted at operation into the proximal jejunum. The catheter is tunnelled subserosally for several centimetres (using techniques similar to that for tunnelling a central venous catheter) prior to entering the lumen. A needle catheter jejunostomy is recommended for patients who are undergoing major upper gastrointestinal surgery such as oesophagectomy, gastrectomy or pancreatic surgery as these may be complicated postoperatively by a leaking gastrointestinal anastomosis.

A second laparotomy for complications of a primary procedure is another indication for jejunostomy as postoperative nutritional support is essential.

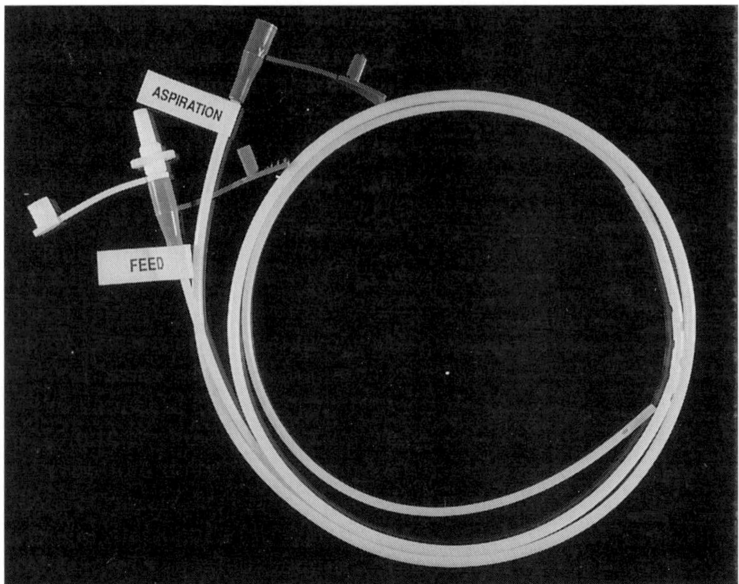

Fig. 9.1 A double lumen naso-enteral tube. The aspiration ports are sited in the stomach for nasogastric decompression. The tip of the tube is positioned at operation or placed over a guidewire (radiologically or endoscopically) into the duodenum or upper jejunun for infusion of feed.

The main complications of these catheters are tube displacement, intraperitoneal leakage and small bowel perforation but these complications are minimal with modern catheter kits. Jejunostomy tubes can, however, only be inserted at laparotomy and their use, therefore, is limited.

Percutaneous endoscopic gastrostomy (PEG)

Surgical gastrostomy has been one of the most common methods of providing long-term enteral support, but the surgical techniques have recently been superseded. In 1980, Gauderer and Ponsky described the technique of percutaneous endoscopic gastrostomy (PEG) for placing a gastrostomy tube without a laparotomy. The technique is relatively simple and is partly illustrated in Figure 9.2. All current PEG kits contain detailed instructions which should be studied before the procedure. Several variations of the original technique have been reported, including a radiological technique, and all are described in detail elsewhere (Moran et al 1990).

Percutaneous endoscopic jejunostomy (PEJ)

It is possible to pass a tube through a previously placed PEG and guide the tube into the upper jejunum, a technique referred to as percutaneous endoscopic jejunostomy. Jejunostomy is indicated for patients who suffer reflux

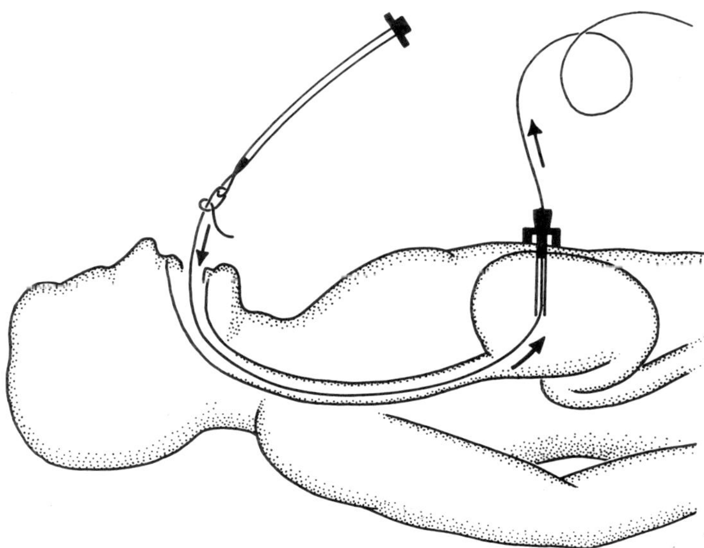

Fig. 9.2 Percutaneous endoscopic gastrostomy. The gastroscope is passed into the stomach, the stomach is inflated and a cannula is introduced into the stomach through the anterior abdominal wall under local anaesthetic. A wire, or thread, is passed through the cannula, grasped with a biopsy forceps and retrieved out of the mouth. The wire, or thread, is tied to the gastrostomy tube and the tube is pulled down through the oesophagus and out through the anterior abdominal wall until the internal retainer apposes the stomach wall to the anterior abdominal wall.

resulting in aspiration pneumonia, which occurs in approximately 5% of patients with a PEG.

The main indications for PEG (or PEJ) are summarised in Table 9.4. There are few complications of PEG. A failure rate of 5% has been reported due to an inability to transilluminate the stomach, but this is usually in patients with previous extensive upper gastrointestinal surgery or patients with extreme obesity (Moran et al 1990).

It is often impossible to predict survival of the patient, but, as a general rule, a PEG should only be used if it is anticipated that enteral feeding will be required for at least 3 weeks. Other patients may best be treated with a fine

Table 9.4 Indications for PEG or PEJ

- Acute neurological events (e.g. stroke or severe head injury) which necessitate supplemental feeding for prolonged periods
- Chronic neurological diseases (e.g. multiple sclerosis and motor neurone disease) which affect swallowing
- Patients with head and neck cancer (to facilitate surgery or radiotherapy)
- Patients with growth failure or anorexia (e.g. cystic fibrosis and scleroderma)

bore nasogastric tube, but the option of a PEG for even short term palliation should not be completely ruled out. There have been recent reports of the use of skin level gastrostomies or gastrostomy buttons in patients who require long-term gastrostomy feeding and already have an established gastrostomy tract. They are cosmetically more acceptable but are more difficult to use and require more expensive giving sets.

ADVANCES IN PARENTERAL ACCESS

Parenteral nutrition, by definition, involves intravenous feeding and, therefore, requires venous access. Indeed, the historic breakthrough in the successful use of TPN resulted from the realisation by Dudrick and colleagues in 1968 that central venous access was required to infuse the hypertonic nutrients. More recently, however, there has been a shift in emphasis away from central access with renewed interest in peripheral vein parenteral nutrition.

Peripheral venous access

Novel solutions, with a lower osmolality, continue to be developed to allow peripheral TPN which is certainly now feasible for at least 7–10 days and much longer in some institutions. However, some patients will be unsuitable for any form of peripheral vein feeding due to the unavailability of suitable peripheral veins. In patients with suitable veins, the main limitation is still the hypertonicity of the solutions, caused in particular by the amino acid solutions, but also, the glucose required to provide a cost effective energy supply. Recent changes in TPN practice, such as the recognition of lower calorie requirements than were previously considered necessary, together with the availability of lipid emulsions and the use of all-in-one mixtures contained in a 3-l bag, have all facilitated peripheral vein feeding. There have also been several recent reports of techniques to prolong the life of the peripheral vein. In order of clinical significance these are:

Catheters

The use of very fine paediatric venous catheters which are threaded into a peripheral vein has been very successful when used by experts, but serious complications of TPN infusion (e.g. thrombophlebitis and infection) may still occur. Modern fine catheters are usually manufactured from polyurethane or silicone, but polyurethane is the preferred material (Everitt et al 1993). An infusion pump is required to reduce the risk of blockage.

Vasodilators

The application of glyceryl trinitrate (GTN) patches distal to the infusion site has been shown to prolong significantly the peripheral catheter infusion time. Side effects from the GTN, such as dizziness and nausea, occasionally occur.

Infusion site

Rotation of the site of the infusion every 24–48 h is effective, but costly in terms of consumables, patient discomfort, and medical and nursing time.

Anticoagulants and anti-inflammatory agents

The addition of low dose heparin to the infusion at a concentration of 1000 units/l may help prolong infusion site use.

The use of both local and systemic anti-inflammatory agents, including low dose steroid additions to the infusion, may be helpful.

These techniques can be combined to achieve further prolongation of catheter life. A major continuing problem with peripheral parenteral nutrition is its lack of 'credibility' compared with central venous TPN. Unfortunately, medical and nursing staff do not apply the same degree of attention to detail in the care of a peripheral line. The best results are achieved in units with a multidisciplinary nutrition team where meticulous attention to protocols for TPN lines is applied. This involves insertion of the peripheral cannula under sterile conditions, by an experienced individual, with line care using protocols similar to those used in the care of central venous TPN catheters. The peripheral cannula should be used exclusively for TPN and carefully observed for the early signs of thrombophlebitis with replacement as necessary. Undoubtedly, peripheral venous cannulation is safer than central venous cannulation and peripheral parenteral nutrition is likely to be the method of choice in an increasing number of patients who require intravenous feeding.

Central venous access

Currently, central venous access is the optimal route for prolonged effective TPN. Techniques themselves have varied little, with the main routes being subclavian and internal jugular, by a direct cutdown or increasingly (even in children) by a closed percutaneous technique. The common complications are outlined in Table 9.5. An excellent review of the various techniques, and

Table 9.5 Complications of central venous catheters

1. Insertion
    - Failure (approximately 5–10% but generally under-reported)
    - Malposition
    - Pneumothorax (approximately 5% overall for subclavian lines)
    - Arterial stab (usually of no consequence if it is recognised and pressure is applied)
2. In use
    - Line sepsis (reduce incidence by: experienced insertor; dedicated TPN line; nursing protocols)
    - Line displacement (fallout)
    - Fracture
    - Blockage

their complications, is to be found elsewhere (Grant 1992). It is salutary to note that the cumulative complication rate for insertion of 12 987 catheters, in 14 large recently reported series, was approximately 10% with failure to cannulate, misplacement, pneumothorax and arterial puncture being the most common.

There is controversy as to whether percutaneous subclavian or jugular vein cannulation is the safer or better route. Subclavian catheters are easier to tunnel, more comfortable for the patient and have a lower incidence of catheter tip infection. The incidence of pneumothorax is, however, higher with subclavian catheters than with jugular cannulation.

Catheter sepsis in most institutions is unacceptably high in the absence of a dedicated nutrition team. In the hands of an experienced clinician, the complication rate of subclavian catheters can be reduced significantly and this is, therefore, the preferred route, particularly for prolonged intravenous nutrition.

Techniques for central venous access have also been improved by recent developments, such as new catheter materials, percutaneous catheters which incorporate a dacron cuff and the increasing use of double and triple lumen catheters for TPN.

Catheter material

Silicone and polyurethane are the only two materials suitable for prolonged central venous access. Polyurethane is stronger and has been reported to be less thrombogenic than silicone. Polyurethane catheters with a much larger lumen compared with the external diameter (i.e. thin walled) are available, and, these facilitate percutaneous insertion and also reduce the amount of intravascular foreign material.

Catheters incorporating a dacron cuff

A significant advance in central venous access for chemotherapy or prolonged TPN was the development and use of a catheter which incorporates a dacron cuff by Hickman and colleagues in 1979 (Fig. 9.3). There have been several modifications of the cuffed silicone catheter, including the description of techniques for percutaneous insertion under local anaesthetic (Fig. 9.4), and the family of such catheters is now referred to as the 'Hickman-Broviac' catheters. The dacron cuff is located subcutaneously and becomes incorporated in fibrous tissue which keeps the catheter in place and which may reduce catheter infection.

The difficulty in attaching a dacron cuff to polyurethane has recently been overcome with a report of the first clinical trial of prolonged use of a cuffed polyurethane catheter (Moran et al 1992).

Cuffed catheters are not required in most patients, however, and their use has generally been reserved for patients receiving chemotherapy or home parenteral nutrition.

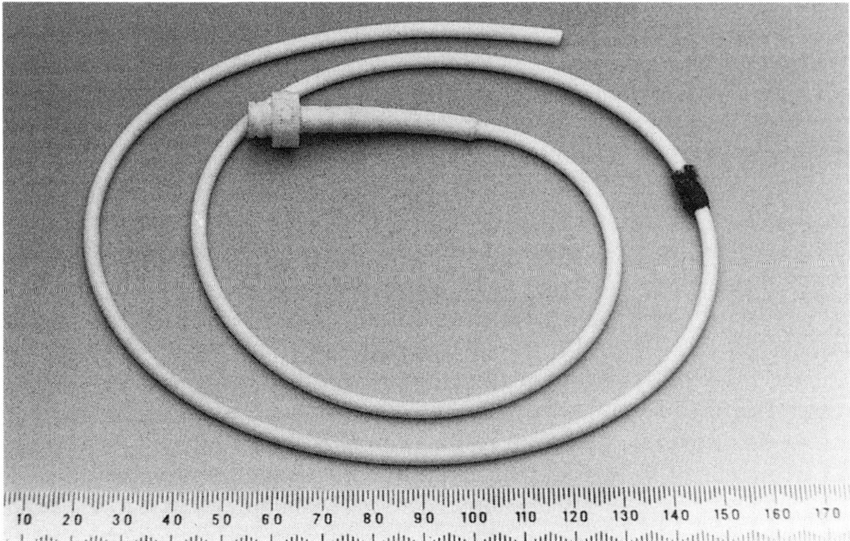

Fig. 9.3 A Hickman catheter composed of silicone and incorporating a dacron cuff.

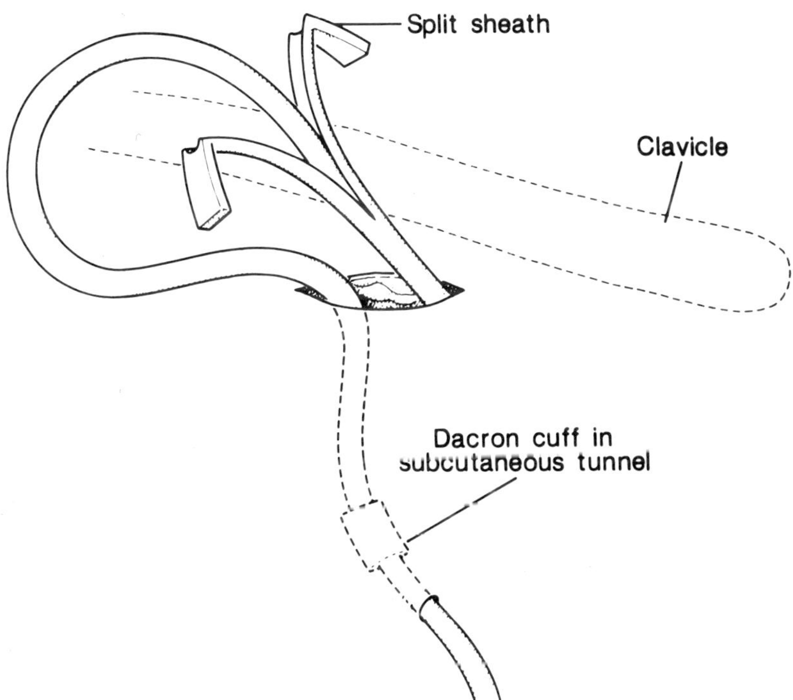

Fig. 9.4 A diagrammatic representation of a percutaneous technique for inserting a cuffed catheter. The technique requires a 'splittable' introducer.

Multilumen catheters for TPN

There is increasing interest in the use of multilumen catheters for TPN. Whilst this may be essential in some patients, such as small children being intensively treated with cytotoxic chemotherapy, and advantageous in many others, our practice has been generally to avoid and discourage the use of multilumen lines for TPN. Recent reports indicate that the incidence of infection may be greater with catheters possessing more than one lumen. Based on recent cumulative evidence in a review of 15 publications, Grant (1992) reported an increased incidence of sepsis in triple lumen lines (168 cases in 1910 triple lumen lines, compared with 56 cases in 1482 single lumen lines ($P < 0.0001$). However, this observation may be because the patients in whom multilumen catheters are generally used are invariably at greater risk of infection due to more active disease and also because of a greater degree of immunosuppression. Furthermore, the requirement for, and frequency of, fine usage is greater in patients with multilumen lines. If these factors are taken into account, there may be no difference in the actual complication rates of single and multilumen lines. In either case, strict adherence to a line-care protocol minimizes the risk of infection.

HOME-BASED TPN

The principles of venous access for home-based TPN are similar to those for short or medium term venous access. In general, catheters which incorporate a dacron cuff (Hickman/Broviac or the novel cuffed polyurethane catheter) are used and some centres advocate the use of subcutaneous implantable systems similar to those used for prolonged chemotherapy (Fig. 9.5). Venous access is crucial in home TPN patients and the complications of venous access are the leading cause of morbidity and mortality in this group of patients.

CONCLUSIONS

Nutritional support is now an essential part of the practice of surgery, particularly surgery of the gastrointestinal tract (Moran & Jackson 1993). Controversy continues as to the cost benefit of nutritional support, particularly TPN. There are difficulties in designing studies to prove the assumed benefits and many of the reported studies suffer from major flaws in study design. An explosion of interest in novel substrates has diverted attention from one of the key issues, which is the precise selection of patients who will benefit from adequate nutritional support.

All techniques for achieving access to the venous system or the gut have complications, and some of these complications are fatal. Operator experience minimizes, but never abolishes, the risks. Undoubtedly a multidisciplinary nutritional support team plays a key role in selecting patients for nutritional support, choosing appropriate substrates, deciding on the route of access and in the safe provision and maintenance of enteral and parenteral access.

KEY POINTS FOR CLINICAL PRACTICE

- Undernutrition is common in surgical patients and can be treated using current nutritional therapies which range from supplemental oral feeding and enteral tube feeding to TPN.
- There are no readily available accurate and reliable tests for measuring malnutrition and any such claims should be viewed with caution.
- Serial measurements of body weight and approximate documentation of daily food intake provide valuable information.
- The concept of 'intestinal failure' (a functioning gut mass below the minimum necessary for the adequate digestion and absorbtion of nutrients) is useful.
- Intestinal failure is the only absolute indication for TPN: all other patients should be fed enterally using modern enteral tubes.

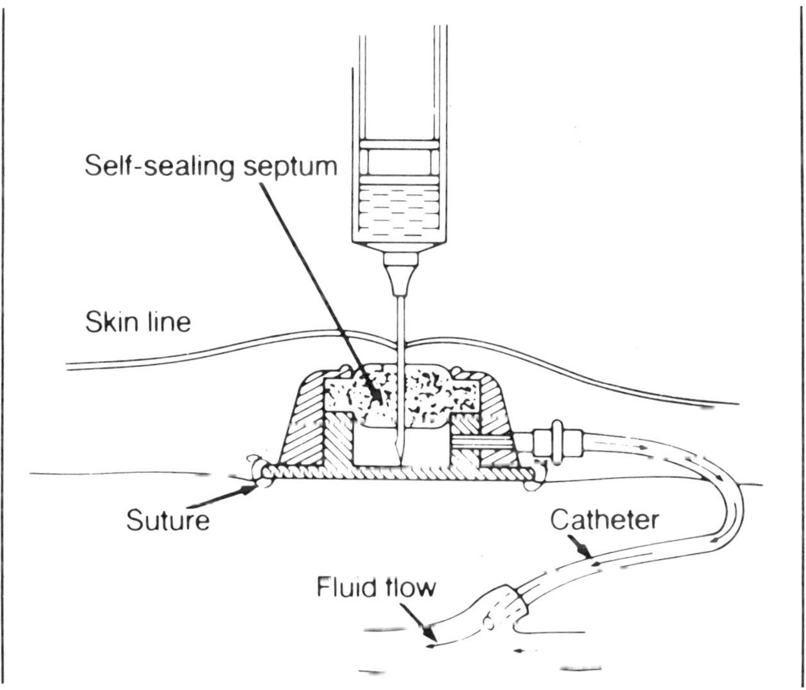

Fig. 9.5 A diagrammatic representation of a subcutaneous implantable port device, commonly used for chemotherapy but increasingly used for 'Home TPN'.

- The limiting factor in the provision of nutritional support in the majority of patients is achieving access to the gut or the venous system: the specific substrate is usually of much less importance.

- Fine bore nasogastric feeding tubes, PEG, needle catheter jejunostomy and double lumen tubes have been significant advances in enteral nutrition.

- Many patients who require TPN can now be fed by a peripheral vein, especially using fine bore peripheral cannulae and 'all-in one' mixtures.

- All techniques for obtaining access to the gut or the venous system have complications: experience minimizes, but never abolishes, the risks.

- Nutritional support of the seriously ill patient is a 'damage limitation' exercise: nutritional support may limit the degree of malnutrition.

REFERENCES

Bastow MD, Rawlimgs J, Allison SP 1983 Benefits of supplementary tube feeding after fractured neck of femur: a randomized controlled trial. BMJ 287: 1589-1592
Buzby GP The Veterans Affairs Total Parenteral Nutrition Co-operative Study Group 1991 Perioperative total parenteral nutrition in surgical patients. N Engl J Med 325: 525-532
Delaney HM, Carnevale NJ, Garvey JW 1973 Jejunostony by a needle catheter technique. Surgery 73: 768-780
Delmi M, Rapin CH, Bengoa JM et al 1990 Dietary supplementation in elderly patients with fractured neck of femur. Lancet 335: 1013-1016
Detsky AS, McLoughlin JR, Baker JP et al 1987 What is subjective global assessment of nutritional status? JPEN 11: 8-13
Detsky AS 1991 Parenteral nutrition: is it helpful? N Engl J Med 325: 573-575
Dudrick SJ, Wilmore DW, Vars HM, Rhoads JR 1968 Long term total parenteral nutrition with growth, development and positive nitrogen balance. Surgery 64: 134-142
Dudrick PS, Souba WW 1991 The role of glutamine in nutrition. Curr Opin Gastroenterol 7: 306-311
Everitt NJ et al 1993 Finebore rubber and polyurethane catheters for the delivery of complete intravenous nutrition. Clin Nutr 12: 261-265
Fleming CR, Remington M 1981 Intestinal failure. In: Hill GL (ed) Nutrition and the surgical patient. Churchill Livingstone, Edinburgh 219-235
Gauderer MWL, Stellato TA 1986 Gastrostomies: evolution, techniques, indications and complications. Curr Probl Surg 13: 661-719
Gauderer MWL, Ponsky JL, Izant RJ 1980 Gastrostomy without a laparotomy: a percutaneous endoscopic technique for feeding gastrostomy. J Pediatr Surg 15: 872-875
Grant JP. 1992 Handbook of total parenteral nutrition 2nd edn. WB Saunders, Philadelphia
Hickman RO, Buckner CD, Clift RA et al 1979 A modified right atrial catheter for access to the venous system in marrow transplant patients. Surg Obstet Gynecol 148: 871-875
Moran BJ, Sutton GLJ, Karran SJ 1992 Clinical evaluation and long-term usage of a new cuffed polyurethane catheter for central venous access. Ann R Coll Surg Engl 74: 426-429
Moran BJ, Taylor MB, Johnson CD 1990 Percutaneous endoscopic gastrostomy: a review. Br J Surg 77: 858-862
Moran BJ, Jackson AA 1992 Function of the human colon. Br J Surg 79: 1132-1137
Moran BJ, Jackson AA 1993 Perioperative nutritional support. Br J Surg 80: 4-5.
Morgan MY 1990 Branched chain amino acids in the management of chronic liver disease. Facts and fantasies. J Hepatol 11: 133-141
Payne-James J, Silk DBA 1988 Enteral nutrition: background, indications and management. Baillieres Clin Gastroenterol 2: 815-847

Rana SK, Bray J, Menzies-Gow et al 1992 Short term benefits of postoperative oral dietary supplements in surgical patients. Clin Nutr 11: 337-344
Studley HO 1936 Percentage of weight loss: a basic indicator of surgical risk in patients with chronic peptic ulcer. JAMA 106: 458-460.

10

Wound healing and the plastic surgeon

A. D. Wilmshurst

The disruption of tissue sets in train a complex series of related and interdependent events which results in wound repair by formation of scar. The completeness of the repair and the speed with which it occurs are dependent on a number of factors present in the organism and in the immediate wound environment. In the past few years, there has been a dramatic increase in the understanding of some of the mechanisms of wound healing, particularly in the biochemistry of collagen and the role of growth factors. The point has been reached where therapeutic manipulation of the healing wound is being considered as a realistic possibility to improve healing time.

Further light is being shed on repair processes by the study of healing in the mammalian fetus. The absence of scar formation in these models has been the pivot for investigation of the differing actions of the variety of growth factors thought to be involved in both adult and fetal wound healing.

The plastic surgeon is concerned with the problems of healing in a number of tissues, including bone, muscle and tendon, but it is skin which assumes the greatest significance in the clinical setting. Our consideration of wound healing will be confined to this tissue, but the basic mechanisms appear to be very similar in all tissues that undergo repair. Certainly, the deleterious effects of repair by scar are seen in a wide variety of clinical situations, including, for example, bile duct stenosis, hepatic cirrhosis, post-traumatic epilepsy, or tendon adhesions.

THE PHASES OF WOUND HEALING

It is traditional to divide the events of wound repair into phases, but this is somewhat artificial as there is marked overlap and interdependence between the phases. The process should be regarded as a continuous stream of interrelated responses. Nevertheless, it is helpful to discuss the subject under distinct headings.

Inflammation

Acute inflammation establishes haemostasis and mobilises components of the immune system as a response to the injury and the breach in the defences.

Vascular response

A brief period of vasoconstriction is accompanied by activation of the coagulation cascade. Platelet adhesion and aggregation lead to formation of a clot and degranulation of the platelets releases several protein growth factors, which are potent chemotactic factors for inflammatory cells.

Vasoconstriction is followed by active vasodilatation and increased permeability of the capillaries, caused by histamine, released from mast cells, and by serotonin. Blood flow slows and protein and white cells leave the circulation and enter the extracellular space adjacent to the wound. Increased vascular permeability continues for about 72 h. This vascular phase gives rise to the clinical appearance of inflammation – heat, redness, swelling and pain.

Cellular response

Within a few hours of the injury, chemotactic factors attract neutrophils to migrate across the vessel walls into the wound, followed by macrophages and lymphocytes. Necrotic cellular material, foreign bodies and bacteria are scavenged. In the absence of infection or contamination, the inflammatory phase is rapidly succeeded by proliferation of collagen and wound repair, but effective healing cannot take place where inflammation continues. The macrophage appears to be the crucial controller cell at this stage of repair (Knighton & Fiegel 1989). Growth factors secreted by macrophages stimulate migration of fibroblasts, epithelial cells and endothelial cells to the wound (Wahl et al 1989).

Proliferation

As fibroblasts and other cells migrate into the injured area, they begin to proliferate and the cellularity of the wound increases. This is the start of the proliferative phase of the repair process, which normally lasts for up to 3 weeks, although in adverse conditions it may continue for much longer.

Epithelialisation

The epithelial barrier prevents the access of bacteria and toxic agents and the loss of water and electrolytes. Restoration of this cell layer involves mobilisation of basal cells at the wound margin, their migration to the area of loss and proliferation by mitosis. Migration of cells continues relentlessly as long as there are denuded areas which remain. Contact inhibition occurs as epithelial cells come into contact with each other. Finally, the cells differentiate and assume keratinocyte function, and the cell layer gradually increases in thickness, in some cases by as much as 1 mm/ day.

Whereas in a wound closed primarily, epithelialisation may be complete by 48 h, in wounds healing by secondary intention, migration of cells does not occur until an adequate bed of granulation exists, usually at 4–5 days.

Partial thickness skin wounds, such as split skin graft donor sites or superficial burns, heal by epithelialisation alone without granulation. Cellular restoration takes place from epidermal appendages in the dermis as well as from the margins.

Contraction

Contraction is the second phenomenon involved in the closure of an open wound, accompanying epithelialisation. It may account for up to 80% of the closure of excised wounds in experimental animals. The process is largely due to the action of the myofibroblast, a cell that has both fibroblast and smooth muscle characteristics (Gabbiani et al 1972). They are distributed throughout the granulation tissue, which thus serves as a contractile organ in which the myofibroblasts shrink the wound, followed by collagen deposition and cross-linking to maintain the contraction.

Fibroplasia

Scar tissue develops from the formation of collagen molecules by fibroblasts. The intracellular protein in the fibroblast is known as procollagen and must be secreted by the cell before being formed, in the appropriate environment of the ground substance, into large stable collagen fibres by intra- and intermolecular bonds. Extracellular transport of procollagen proline requires hydroxylation to the amino acid hydroxyproline which is almost unique to collagen. Fibres and fibrils, formed by intermolecular aldehyde crosslinking, are woven into an ordered pattern and this occurs early in the process of fibroplasia. Capillary ingrowth takes place during this stage and is influenced by tissue oxygen concentration and angiogenic growth factors.

The other components of the extracellular matrix include fibronectin and the glycosaminoglycans. Their roles in wound repair are the subject of considerable study at present, but it is apparent that they are important for the regulation and synthesis of collagen as well as influencing cell motility and differentiation (Grinnell 1984, Nogami et al 1989).

Remodelling

At the end of 20 days, the healed wound can resist moderate stresses placed across it. An excess of collagen has been formed, and wound strength progressively increases over several weeks. However, by the end of 3 weeks, collagen degradation is already proceeding at an equal rate to synthesis. Wound strength reaches its maximum at 3–6 months, but never achieves the tensile strength of normal skin.

Scar maturation takes place by remodelling of the collagen fibres, which have been laid down primarily in a disordered fashion. The fibres are rewoven in response to stress and become lined up along stress lines. This process occurs in the context of a fine balance between the synthesis and degradation of collagen. The degradative system is a function of a whole group of depolymerising collagenase enzymes, made by many cell types and having specific functions under different conditions (Werb 1982).

The scar reaches maturity in a period which varies widely but usually lies between 6–12 months. At this time, the collagen is dense and avascular and the scar is pale and flat.

GROWTH FACTORS

It is becoming clear that the control of wound healing on a molecular level is regulated by a group of peptide growth factors, known as cytokines. An extensive literature has developed in recent years, but a final elucidation of all facets of this complex system is still some way off. Of interest to surgeons involved in the management of difficult repair problems is the potential therapeutic role of these factors. Impressive laboratory studies and reports of clinical trials are beginning to appear in this context. A valuable source of up-to-date information is to be found in the literature reviews of the subject which appear periodically, such as that by Bennett and Schultz (1993).

Production of growth factors

Growth factors are secreted mainly by the cells involved in the phases of wound healing, although some are also released from cell cytoplasm and basement membranes damaged by the initial injury. Platelet degranulation in the early inflammatory phase produces high levels in the coagulum of several cytokines, their role being primarily chemotactic for inflammatory cells at this stage. Platelet derived growth factor (PDGF), insulin-like growth factor-1 (IGF-1), epithelial growth factor (EGF) and transforming growth factor β (TGFβ) are the principal factors released by platelets. However, the much more prolonged actions required for control of the healing wound during repair and remodelling necessitate the continuous synthesis and secretion of these factors by controller or ‘effector’ cells. The most important cell in this respect is the macrophage, but fibroblasts, epithelial cells and vascular endothelial cells all have a role. Each of the growth factors appear to be produced by a number of different cell types.

Actions of growth factors

The actions of growth factors are chemotactic and hormonal. Mitosis of the cells involved in wound healing may be either stimulated or inhibited, as may be the synthesis of extracellular matrix components. There is some selectivity for the cell type that each growth factor attracts or stimulates, but the overlap of actions is very broad. Studies continue to throw light on this complex system.

It is possible, for some of the better understood growth factors, to give an overview of their principal actions. PDGF is initially produced from platelets and is important in an initial phase of strong chemotaxis for inflammatory cells. One of its main roles thereafter becomes the control of fibroplasia, which requires its more prolonged production and this appears to be taken over by macrophages and endothelial cells, which both secrete an almost identical factor to PDGF. There is attraction of fibroblasts and smooth muscle cells and stimulation of their mitosis. IGF-1 is another factor identified as being responsible for the regulation of cell division of these mesodermal cells, and it is also chemotactic for endothelial cells.

Epithelial growth factor is, as its name specifies, important in epithelialisation. It is chemotactic and a mitogen for epithelial cells, but is also responsible for fibroblast proliferation, the synthesis of fibronectin, and has a role in angiogenesis. Basic fibroblast growth factor (bFGF) appears to be a strong inducer of angiogenesis, attracting endothelial cells and stimulating their mitosis. It has similar effects on fibroblasts.

TGFβ is an intriguing cytokine, with at least three isoforms which have differing actions. It is a powerful stimulator of collagen synthesis and thus of scar formation. Attraction of fibroblasts and the laying down of collagen are important effects, but it also decreases the production of collagenase and inhibits epithelial cell mitosis.

It is easy to imagine the uses of growth factors if they could be employed in the clinical situation. Problems in achieving sound wound healing are not confined to the chronic ulcers or irradiated skin fields presented to the reconstructive surgeon: they include challenges as disparate as anastomotic healing in gastrointestinal surgery, the infarcted myocardium, corneal grafts, and injured neural tissue. The healed skin scar itself may be weak, stretched, keloidal, or contracted. Some of the clinical and experimental evidence now available suggests that it might become possible to manipulate the cellular components of healing and eliminate the unfavourable scar by the application of the right combination of growth factors. This could ultimately lead to the elimination of scar formation and the production of scarless healing.

WOUND HEALING IN CLINICAL PRACTICE

One of the preoccupations of the plastic surgeon is with problems in the healing of the skin and integument. It may be of interest to consider the implications on the clinical situation of some of the recent advances in wound and scar research. Only a brief review of this extensive topic is possible here.

Problems in obtaining healing

The chronic wound

Wounds which do not heal and become chronic ulcers represent a heavy burden both to the patient and to the services which provide care.

Underlying conditions causing the ulcer, such as prolonged pressure, diabetes, vasculitis, venous hypertension, or ischaemia, also form an obstacle to successful reconstructive surgery by graft or flap.

Bennett and Schultz (1993) studied wound fluids collected from patients. Their findings suggested that growth factor levels were reduced in chronic wounds and, perhaps more significantly, that levels of protease activity were very high. There may thus be an intrinsic molecular defect in chronic wounds which prevents their healing. Platelet extract from patients' own blood has been used in trials where it has been applied to chronic wounds (Knighton et al 1986, 1990). Impressive healing was obtained in both percentage achieved and time to full epithelialisation.

Platelets contain a number of cytokines which may be implicated in these effects. Studies using purified factors have been possible more recently. In a small trial of EGF on long-standing nonhealing ulcers, Brown et al (1991) obtained healing in 9 of 10 wounds in an average of 34 days. A larger and better controlled trial of PDGF-BB in pressure sores also produced impressive results and gave an indication of effective dose levels (Robson et al 1992). Clearly further carefully designed studies are required to determine which factors, and in what combination, are most effective, and what are the specific chemical abnormalities in a chronic wound which appear to neutralise the healing response.

The hypoxic wound

Numerous factors influence the healing of wounds, and many of these have a well established place in the surgical literature. Important examples are factors such as nutritional status, the role of vitamins, steroid therapy, chemotherapy, and the technical aspects of wound closure. One area in which there has been a resurgence of interest in recent years, however, is the importance of tissue oxygen concentration in wound healing, and how factors which are assumed to have an adverse effect on oxygenation, such as smoking, may influence healing.

It has long been known that healing in the animal model is prejudiced by anaemia, dehydration, and acute haemorrhage, but it has only become possible much more recently to correlate healing rates with direct measurements of oxygen tension in wounds. Hunt and his colleagues (Hunt et al 1978, Knighton et al 1981) particularly stressed that arterial pO_2 does not necessarily reflect tissue pO_2 and that correct blood volume is important. This was confirmed in studies on postoperative patients by Chang et al (1983). The rationale was established for maintenance of a normal circulating volume and cardiac output in surgical patients. In another study of patients with healing surgical wounds, peripheral perfusion, collagen deposition and tissue oxygen tension were monitored and found to be directly proportional to each other. Collagen production was not significantly related to either blood loss or haematocrit (Jonsson et al 1991).

Delayed wound healing is a well recognised entity in smokers, and the potential mechanisms by which the toxic constituents of cigarette smoke may interfere with healing are understood (Silverstein 1992). Experimentally, nicotine has been shown to cause vasoconstriction, increase platelet stickiness, and reduce mitosis of macrophages and fibroblasts. Carbon monoxide dramatically interferes with oxygen carriage by the blood, and hydrogen cyanide, another constituent of cigarette smoke, blocks oxidative metabolism at the cellular level.

Controlled studies on two groups of normal subjects of the short-term effects of cigarette smoking have been carried out, in the context of possible deleterious effects on wound healing. Skin circulation in the thumb was assessed using laser Doppler flowmetry during smoking, and a marked decrease was demonstrated (van Adrichem et al 1992). Subcutaneous tissue oxygen tension measured using a tonometer similarly showed a significant reduction (Jensen et al 1991) and the authors suggested that activation of the adrenergic system was the cause. In a retrospective review of their experience with free microvascular tissue transfer, Reus and colleagues (1992) found that smokers had a significantly higher rate of delayed wound healing and of the number of secondary wound closure procedures required. Interestingly, there was no difference in the flap survival rate. Plastic surgeons are particularly aware of the incidence of healing problems in smokers. Any operation in these patients where there has been extensive undermining or mobilisation of the skin, or where a skin flap has been transferred, carries an increased risk of wound breakdown and delayed healing. Smokers are firmly advised to stop smoking before operation and while recovering.

The skin graft donor site

Routine use of the versatile and widely applicable technique of split skin grafting depends for its success on the principle that the site from which the graft is harvested will heal spontaneously. Failure of healing, as occasionally occurs, may result in a worse defect than that with which the patient started. Epithelial growth factor commences within 24 h of the creation of a partial thickness wound. Most occurs from epithelial remnants in the dermis, such as hair follicles, sebaceous glands and sweat glands, although migration also take place from the wound margins. Very thin grafts will leave a donor site which heals rapidly, often within 7 days. Thicker defects heal more slowly, and may present a difficult problem in patients with very thin skin, such as those receiving steroid therapy.

Another challenge is the control of donor site pain. It is normal for there to be more discomfort from the donor site than from the recipient operative site, and this is due to the exposure of multiple sensory nerve endings in the raw dermal surface. Much effort has been invested in the search for donor site dressings that reduce pain to a minimum, and at the same time provide absorbency and convenient application. A bonus is gained if acceleration of healing can be obtained with the same material.

Calcium alginate has been investigated as a donor site dressing material by Attwood (1989). In a prospective controlled trial comparing alginate with paraffin gauze, there was a significant and marked reduction in mean time to healing from 10.5 days in the conventional group to 7 days using a preparation of alginate in sheets of convenient size. Improvements in patient comfort and in the quality of regenerated skin were also found. Calcium alginate in the presence of moisture and sodium ions forms an hydrophilic gel at the wound surface. Available calcium ions augment the coagulation cascade when applied to the fresh wound and the dressing may be useful in reducing blood loss where extensive cropping of skin is required. The gel provides a close to ideal healing environment and probably makes dressing removal easier. Butler et al (1993) used alginate sheets wetted with a solution of bupivacaine. This significantly reduced early postoperative pain at 24 and 48 h after skin grafting, compared with the same material used dry or moistened with saline.

Employed in this manner, alginate sheets are becoming the standard dressing material among plastic surgeons in the UK for covering donor sites. Clinical experience confirms the published evidence.

Studies of the influence of growth factors on partial thickness wounds have been carried out on animal models and in humans. The rate of epidermal regeneration has been accelerated by the topical application of various factors to wounds produced by a dermatome or a partial thickness burn (Schultz et al 1987, Lynch et al 1987, Nanney 1990). In humans, donor sites have been treated with epidermal growth factor and epithelialisation time was reduced by an average of 1.5 days (Brown et al 1989). These results suggest that it may not be entirely true that it is not possible to persuade a wound in the normal healthy individual to heal in any less time than it would under standard conditions. In other words, existing growth factor concentrations may not be optimal for the maximal healing rate. In the clinical context, although moderate improvements in healing rates may be of little consequence in small wounds, in the extensive burn or in the compromised patient, a significant reduction in time to healing may be of great benefit. The management of large burns frequently requires recropping of the same donor areas, and rapid healing of these sites is clearly advantageous.

Problems with the scar

Creation of a normal scar is of crucial interest to the surgeon. The concept implies not only quality of appearance, but the functional aspects of tensile strength and absence of contracture. The natural process of fibrous tissue repair by deposition of collagen may in itself result in serious defects in appearance and function, if 'overhealing' occurs by excessive collagen formation or aggravated contraction. Fetal wound healing research has given glimpses of a return down the phylogenetic scale to regeneration rather than repair by scar. Means of manipulating adult wound healing in an attempt to approach this same goal are beginning to be reported. Meanwhile, ugly scars remain as a challenge to conventional management.

The stretched scar

A wide scar may result from disruption of a repaired wound with subsequent healing by secondary intention and the laying down of a broad band of collagen. More commonly, however, the phenomenon is seen in a healed wound closed under apparent tension or in one orientated in a direction running across lines of relaxed skin tension. In an attempt to relate scar appearances to the pattern of local skin tension, Meyer and McGrouther (1991) repeated one of Langer's original studies on cadavers but confined their attention to the presternal area, a site notorious for the incidence of problem scars. Circular incisions were made with a trephine. It was observed that the holes assumed a transverse elliptical orientation in the epigastrium but over the sternum itself they remained circular. They correlated these findings with the earlier observations of Elliot et al (1985) who had studied a group of patients with median sternotomy wounds. In general, the part of the scar that extended below the xiphisternum was liable to stretch while that over the sternum would often undergo hypertrophy but not stretch. Stretching is more likely to occur where skin tension is strong and in one direction; where tension is more uniformly distributed hypertrophy may result. In either case the explanation on a cellular level might be that tension across the healing wound stimulates the active fibroblasts to respond by producing an excess of collagen (McGraw 1986).

Conventionally, the argument is made that to avoid stretching of scars not only should wounds be securely closed but good deep dermal support must be provided to eradicate tension in the epidermal closure. This is clearly a simplistic view, which fails to take into account the very active remodelling phase of wound repair, when collagen is constantly being synthesised, degraded and deposited, responding as it does so to existing tensions across the wound. Any deep sutures in place will remain intact but will become progressively irrelevant as the scar remodels, and widens, around them.

However there is good evidence to show that scar stretching can be modified to some degree by supplying long-term support to the dermal closure. Several studies have compared subcuticular techniques with each other and with conventional interrupted sutures. Sommerlad and Creasey (1978) found that a subcuticular nylon suture retained for 3 weeks significantly reduced scar stretching in comparison with interrupted sutures. They also demonstrated that 80–90% of the increase in width took place over 6 months, regardless of suture technique. Attempts to support the wound over a time span approaching this duration require either non-absorbable sutures left in place, or one of the newer synthetic absorbables which have a relatively prolonged and predictable absorption rate. Polyglycolic acid (Dexon®), in most respects a very satisfactory subcuticular suture, has been shown to perform poorly in terms of scar stretching, being significantly less effective than buried polypropylene (Prolene®) (Nordstrom & Nordstrom 1986) or subcuticular polydioxanone (PDS®) (Chantarasak & Milner 1989). In another prospective trial in patients with excision wounds, Elliot and Mahaffey (1989) showed that subcuticular Prolene allowed significantly less stretching when left in for 6 months than when in place for only 3 weeks. They suggested that the inconvenience of using long-term nonabsorbables might be circumvented by the new monofilament absorbables such as polyglyconate (Maxon®) or PDS, and this was demonstrated with the latter material by Chantarasak and Milner (1989). Prolonged dermal support clearly has a role to play where there is tension across the closed wound.

The proliferative scar

Hypertrophic and keloid scars are forms of abnormal healing characterised by overabundant deposition of collagen. Keloid differs from hypertrophic scar in that it extends beyond the boundaries of the original scar and invades normal tissue, behaving as a neoplasm in this respect. It does not resolve or involute with the passage of time. Both types are associated with broadening of the scar, are very likely to recur after excision and they have a similar histological appearance. They may occur anywhere on the body surface but both are commoner on the trunk, shoulder, neck and 'beard area'. They differ in their genetic, familial and racial incidence.

It is known that the various components of the extracellular matrix, including fibronectin, the glycosaminoglycans and the subtypes of collagen have important roles in the regulation of wound healing. There have been many studies on the production, concentration and distribution of these molecules in healing wounds and mature scars. The formation of hypertrophic and keloid scars is included among these studies, but there has been a notable lack of clinical benefit derived thus far, in terms of control or prevention of abnormal scarring.

Of greater relevance to the practising surgeon are reports of trials of two of the more promising lines of treatment of proliferative scars. Intralesional injection of steroid, commonly triamcinolone, has been used for over 30 years for the treatment of hypertrophic and keloid scars (Maguire 1965). It is not fully understood how steroids inhibit scar formation, but is likely to be by the combined effects of increased collagen degradation and reduced synthesis. Steroids may be utilised in combination with excisional surgery and are given at the time of surgery and serially afterwards, or they may be injected as a course without excising the scar. The aims are the same as other treatments of these scars; namely to reduce the symptoms of pain and pruritis and to produce softening and flattening of the scar. Tang (1992) reported excellent results in a small series of scars which were mostly keloids, in which excision was combined with triamcinolone injection into the wound and was followed by an intensive regimen of further weekly injections into the scar. Some wide scars with atrophic surrounding skin resulted, but these may be regarded as an acceptable price to pay for permanent control of keloid.

Other approaches to the management of proliferative scars include superficial radiotherapy, of limited popularity due to its potential for inducing neoplasia, and pressure, applied in the form of elasticated garments worn over the offending scar for a prolonged period. Initially it was considered that pressure was the principal mechanism by which silicone gel sheeting produced its effects when applied to these scars. This has been used with considerable effect on hypertrophic burn scars (Perkins et al 1982) and its use has been extended to hypertrophic scars in general. However, its mode of action has been the subject of debate. Sawada and Sone (1990) eliminated the pressure component by using a hydrated silicone oil cream applied under an occlusive dressing. Significant improvement was obtained in comparison with their control group which employed the same cream without occlusion. They suggested that a combination of hydration and occlusion was the mode of action of silicone on hypertrophic scars. The same authors (Sawada & Sone 1992) later obtained good results with a cream that provided hydration but did not contain silicone, under occlusion. It appears that silicone gel sheet is simply a convenient vehicle for conveying both occlusion and hydration to the scar.

SCARLESS HEALING

The demonstration that fetal wounds, including those in the human, heal without visible scar has excited interest in the development of human fetal surgery. Due to the considerable inherent risks involved in such surgery, it is, at present, restricted to a few life-threatening conditions such as diaphragmatic hernia and hydronephrosis. However, investigation of the biology of scarless healing with the aim of modifying surgical scarring in the adult is of much wider interest to surgeons. The goal envisaged would be to reduce or even eliminate the scar with its accompanying unwelcome features: potential impairment of growth and function and the unpleasant appearance of broad, hypertrophic or contracted scars.

Fetal wound healing exhibits a virtual absence of the inflammatory response. Fibroplasia in the wound approximates to regeneration with the laying down of a normal collagen pattern without scar, and there is a lack of wound contracture (Krummel et al 1986). Healing also occurs remarkably rapidly, and this may be a result of the composition of the extracellular matrix in the fetus. Tenascin and fibronectin are deposited early in the wound and are important for the migration of epithelial cells. Hyaluronic acid is present for much longer in the fetal than in the adult wound, allowing a more organised deposition of collagen fibrils and more rapid remodelling (Longaker & Adzick 1991). Collagen itself is present in the same types as in the adult wound but in different proportions, with the production of more type III and V, thus approximating to the pattern in normal fetal tissue. The lack of a typical inflammatory response is associated with an absence of neutrophils. Macrophages appear to play a much more dominant role, and may be important in remodelling of the extracellular matrix as well as in the production of factors.

Growth factors are present in the healing fetal wound but their actions appear to be modified in comparison with their role in the adult. Intense fibroplasia can be induced experimentally in the fetal wound by the addition of PDGF or TGF-β, suggesting that these factors are by some mechanism suppressed or inhibited *in utero*. Extension of these studies with TGFβ to the adult animal has produced fascinating results. Neutralising antibody to TGF-β injected into healing wounds in the adult rat resulted in virtually scarless healing (Shah et al 1992). Following the isolation of the three isoforms of TGF-β, the same workers have shown an identical effect with neutralising antibody to TGF-β1 and TGF-β2. Application of the third isoform, TGF-β3, produces the same marked reduction of scarring as the neutralising antibodies, demonstrating that the actions of the isoforms differ fundamentally and suggesting a modulatory role for TGF-β in wound healing (Shah et al 1994, Shah & Ferguson 1993). Of further interest is that healing in these models proceeded at a normal rate, that histological appearances approximated to normal, and that tensile strength across the healed wounds was also normal, in spite of the reduced collagen deposition. Radical pharmacological control of scar formation in the human appears to be a realistic possibility.

KEY POINTS FOR CLINICAL PRACTICE

- Wound healing is as dependent on normal circulating blood volume as on haemoglobin level. Arterial pO_2 may not reflect tissue pO_2.
- Smoking adversely affects the healing of complicated wounds.
- Alginate sheets soaked in bupivacaine solution are the dressing of choice for skin graft donor sites.
- Scars should whenever possible be placed in lines of relaxed skin tension, to reduce the risk of stretching.
- Prolonged dermal support with subcuticular sutures may reduce the incidence of scar stretching.
- Judicious injection of hypertrophic or keloid scars with triamoinolone is an effective treatment but may require to be repeated as a course. Re-excision of these scars without adjunctive measures is likely to result in recurrence with exacerbation.
- Silicone gel sheet is a convenient vehicle for conveying hydration and occlusion treatment to hypertrophic scars.

REFERENCES

Attwood AI 1989 Calcium alginate dressing accelerates split skin graft donor site healing. Br J Plast Surg 42: 373-379

Bennett NT, Schultz GS 1993 Growth factors and wound healing: Part II. Role in normal and chronic wound healing. Am J Surg 166: 74-81

Brown GL, Nanney LB, Griffen J et al 1989 Enhancement of wound healing by topical treatment with epidermal growth factor. N Engl J Med 321: 76-79

Brown GL, Curtsinger L, Jurkiewicz MJ et al 1991 Stimulation of healing of chronic wounds by epidermal growth factor. Plast Reconstr Surg 88: 189-194

Butler PEM, Eadle PA, Lawlor D et al 1993 Bupivacaine and Kaltostat reduces post-operative donor site pain. Br J Plast Surg 46: 523-524

Chang N, Goodson WH, Gottrup F et al 1983 Direct measurement of wound and tissue oxygen tension: in postoperative patients. Ann Surg 197: 470

Chantarasak ND, Milner RH 1989 A comparison of scar quality in wounds closed under tension with PGA (Dexon) and Polydioxanone (PDS). Br J Plast Surg 42: 687-691

Elliot D, Mahaffey PJ 1989 The stretched scar: the benefit of prolonged dermal support. Br J Plast Surg 42: 74-78

Elliot D, Cory-Pearce R, Rees GM 1985 The behaviour of presternal scars in a fair-skinned population. Ann R Coll Surg Engl 67: 238-240

Gabbiani G, Hirschel BJ, Ryan GB et al 1972 Granulation tissue as a contractile organ: a study of structure and function. J Exp Med 135: 719

Grinnell F 1984 Fibronectin and wound healing. J Cell Biochem 26: 107-116

Hunt TK, Conolly WB, Aronson SB et al 1978 Anaerobic metabolism and wound healing: an hypothesis for the initiation and cessation of collagen synthesis in wounds. Am J Surg 135: 328

Jensen JA, Goodson WH, Hopf HW et al 1991 Cigarette smoking decreases tissue oxygen. Arch Surg 126: 1131-1134

Jonsson K, Jensen JA, Goodson III WH et al 1991 Tissue oxygenation, anaemia, and perfusion in relation to wound healing in surgical patients. Ann Surg 214: 605-613

Knighton DR, Fiegel VD 1989 The macrophages: effector cells in wound repair. Prog Clin Biol Res 299: 217-226

Knighton DR, Silver IA, Hunt TK 1981 Regulation of wound-healing angiogenesis – effect of oxygen gradients and inspired oxygen concentration. Surgery 90: 262

Knighton DR, Fiegel VD, Austin LL et al 1986 Classification and treatment of chronic nonhealing wounds. Ann Surg 204: 322-330

Knighton DR, Ciresi K, Fiegel VD et al 1990 Stimulation of repair in chronic, nonhealing, cutaneous ulcers using platelet-derived wound healing formula. Surg Gynecol Obstet 170: 56-60

Krummel TM, Nelson JM, Diegelmann RF et al 1986 Wound healing in the foetal and neonatal rabbit. Surg Forum 37: 595

Longaker MT, Adzick NS 1991 The biology of foetal wound healing: a review. Plast Reconstr Surg 87: 788

Lynch SE, Nixon JC, Colvin PB et al 1987 Pole of platelet-derived growth factor in wound healing: synergistic effects with other growth factors. Proc Natl Acad Sci USA 84: 7696-7700

McGraw WT 1986 The effect of tension on collagen remodelling by fibroblasts; a stereological ultrastructural study. J Conn Tiss Res 14: 229

Maguire HC 1965 Treatment of keloids with triamoinolone acetonide injected intralesionally. JAMA 192: 325

Meyer M, McGrouther DA 1991 A study relating wound tension to scar morphology in the pre-sternal scar using Langers technique. Br J Plast Surg 44: 291-294

Nanney LB 1990 Epidermal and dermal effects of epidermal growth factor during wound repair. J Invest Dermatol 94: 624-629

Nogami R, Maekawa Y, Kudo S 1989 Glycosaminoglycan content in the media of cultured fibroblasts derived from burn scar and normal skin. J Dermatol 16: 42-46

Nordstrom REA, Nordstrom RM 1986 Absorbable versus nonabsorbable sutures to prevent postoperative stretching of wound area. Plast Reconstr Surg 78: 186

Perkins K, Davey RB, Wallis KA 1982 Silicone gel: a new treatment for burn scars and contractures, Burns 9: 201

Reus III WF, Colen LB, Straker DJ 1992 Tobacco smoking and complications in elective microsurgery. Plast Reconstr Surg 89: 490-494
Robson MC, Phillips LG, Thomason A et al 1992 Platelet-derived growth factor BB for the treatment of chronic pressure ulcers. Lancet 339: 23-25
Sawada Y, Sone K 1990 Treatment of scars and keloids with a cream containing silicone oil. Br J Plast Surg 43: 683-688
Sawada Y, Sone K 1992 Hydration and occlusion treatment for hypertrophic scars and keloids. Br J Plast Surg 45: 599-603
Schultz GS, White M, Mitchell R et al 1987 Epithelial wound healing enhanced by transforming growth factor -α and vaccinia growth factor. Science 235: 350-352
Shah M, Ferguson MWJ 1993 Transforming growth factor-beta 3 reduces scarring in adult rodent wounds. Presented at the British Association of Plastic Surgeons, Oxford, UK
Shah M, Foreman DM, Ferguson MWJ 1992 Control of scarring in adult wounds by neutralising antibody to transforming growth factor β. Lancet 339: 213-214
Shah M, Foreman DM, Ferguson MWJ 1994 Neutralising antibody to TGF-beta 1, 2 reduces cutaneous scarring in adult rodents. J Cell Sci 107: 1137-1157
Silverstein P 1992 Smoking and wound healing. Am J Med 93: 22S-24S
Sommerlad BC, Creasey JM 1978 The stretched scar: a clinical and histological study. Br J Plast Surg 31: 34
Tang YW 1992 Intra- and postoperative steroid injections for keloids and hypertrophic scars. Br J Plast Surg 45: 371-373
van Adrichem LNA, Hovius SER, van Strik R et al 1992 Acute effects of cigarette smoking on microcirculation of the thumb. Br J Plast Surg 45: 9-11
Wahl SM, Wong H, McCartney-Francis N 1989 Role of growth factors in inflammation and repair. J Cell Biochem 40: 193-199
Werb Z 1982 Degradation of collagen. In: Weiss JB, Jayson MIV (eds) Collagen in health and disease. Churchill Livingstone, Edinburgh, 121

11

Peptide receptors and gastrointestinal cancers

S. A. M. Laws   H. S. Chave

Cancer of the gastrointestinal tract is a common cause of cancer related mortality and morbidity. It often presents to the clinician at an advanced stage of development when cure by surgical resection is no longer possible. Adjuvant therapies are available but improvement in survival and quality of life associated with their use appears limited. There is clearly a need for the development of more effective palliative strategies. Carcinomas are disorders of control of proliferation within an epithelial cell population. Hormones and growth factors play an important part in the control of normal cell growth and differentiation and there is evidence for functional conservation of certain hormone receptors after malignant transformation. In this review, we discuss the need for non-toxic, palliative, systemic therapy for gastrointestinal malignancies and the rationale for developing treatments based on hormone manipulation.

THE SCALE OF THE PROBLEM

Malignancy of the gastrointestinal tract is a major cause of cancer related death in the Western world. Colon cancer causes 12% of all cancer deaths in the UK and there has been no significant fall in mortality in the last 40 years. Stomach cancer causes 7% of cancer deaths although its incidence is declining. The incidence of squamous carcinoma of the oesophagus is falling while adenocarcinoma of the lower third of the oesophagus and cardia is increasing. The incidence of carcinoma of the pancreas is also increasing and, unfortunately, the age at presentation is falling (CRC factsheet 1.1.1991). Although cancer of the gastrointestinal tract tends to afflict the elderly, the percentage of the population over 65 years of age is rising and hence gastrointestinal malignancy can be expected to require a significant proportion of the health care budget. The aetiology of these cancers remains to be elucidated but the role of preventative intervention should not be underestimated. Dietary manipulation and increasing colonic transit times may reduce the incidence of colonic cancer in a population. The eradication of *Helicobacter pylori*, which has been implicated in the aetiology of gastric cancer, may also reduce the incidence of this disease in future generations (Callam 1994). However, at present the prognosis for patients with advanced

Table 11.1 Incidence and outcome of gastrointestinal malignancies in the UK

Type of cancer	Incidence M:F	5-year survival	% cancer mortality
Oesophagus	100:71/million	7.7%	3.5%
Stomach	270:167/million	10.5%	7%
Pancreas	115:112/million	4.3%	4.5%
Colorectal	486:478/million	36.8%	12%

gastrointestinal malignancy remains dismal even when treated by radical surgery (Table 11.1).

CONVENTIONAL TREATMENT

Surgery

The vast majority of gastrointestinal cancers are too advanced at presentation for curative surgery. Less than 10% of pancreatic and 20% of oesophageal cancers are amenable to any form of 'curative' surgery and although the operative mortality is declining it still remains in the region of 4–10%. The 5-year survival rate after oesophagectomy for stage I disease is 60–80% but only 10% of patients present at this stage. The 5-year survival rate for stage II and III disease after operation is only 15%. Treatment regimes using pre-operative chemotherapy and radiotherapy have increased the number of cases coming to operation but without decreasing the overall mortality (Saltz & Kelsen 1992). Radical gastrectomy for early gastric cancer has been associated with a reduction in the mortality of this disease in Japan but it remains to be seen whether this can be extrapolated to Western populations. The surgical treatment of colonic and rectal cancers is more satisfactory but more than half of all patients still die of recurrent disease (Abulafi & Williams 1994). Because of the vague nature of symptoms from gastrointestinal cancers, presentation is frequently at an advanced stage when the cancer has already metastasised. Resection is often undertaken in order to provide effective palliation.

Radiotherapy

There is no evidence to support the use of radiotherapy in gastric cancer. Although the definitive treatment of cancer of the colon and rectum is surgical resection, local recurrence may be reduced by either pre- or postoperative radiotherapy but the combination does not significantly improve survival rates. The combination of radiotherapy and chemotherapy has been shown to improve moderately the survival of patients with rectal cancer. Pancreatic and oesophageal adenocarcinomas cannot be cured by radiotherapy but there is some evidence to support its use both as an adjunct to surgery and as palliation (Jeekel & Treurniet-Donker 1991, Gastrointestinal Tumour Study Group 1987). Long-term survival appears unaffected (Kalser & Ellenberg 1985, Gastrointestinal Tumour Study Group 1988).

Chemotherapy

Chemotherapy can be used either as an adjunct to surgery either pre- or post-operatively or as palliative treatment for advanced disease. In combination with radiotherapy, it may also play a role as an adjunct in the treatment of oesophageal and pancreatic cancer. Neo-adjuvant systemic therapy has resulted in a greater proportion of patients able to undergo operative resection. Chemotherapeutic regimes have not as yet been standardised in the treatment of gastric cancer. Most regimens use 5-fluorouracil (5FU) in combination with other agents. Systemic chemotherapy does confer a survival advantage in advanced disease as compared to best supportive treatment but the overall survival is only improved by a matter of months and it is difficult to assess the impact on the patient's quality of life as the treatment may be attended by considerable toxicity (Saltz & Kelsen 1992, Gastrointestinal Tumour Study Group 1988).

There is little role for the systemic treatment of colon cancer in isolation. Adjuvant chemotherapy for patients with Dukes' C stage colon cancer appears to confer an improvement in survival. When several recent studies are combined the improvement is a reduction in the odds of death by 26% (Slevin & Gray 1991). Folinic acid is a biochemical modulator of the efficiency of 5FU and increases the response rate, but has a less certain effect on the survival rate in patients with advanced colon cancer. It may have a role with 5FU in adjuvant treatment.

Overall it is clear that there is a need to develop new treatment strategies aimed at improving the survival of patients with gastrointestinal malignancies. Surgery can effectively treat patients with localised disease and occasionally those with metastases but the treatment of metastatic disease remains unsatisfactory. Strategies that specifically target tumour cell populations regardless of dissemination is the ultimate aim of such treatments.

HORMONE TREATMENT

Principles of hormonal treatment of tumours

All tissues within the body are under the influence of systemically (endocrine) or locally (paracrine) secreted peptides. In addition steroid hormones, particularly the sex hormones, are also important regulators of cell proliferation. Growth factors are peptides that act in nanomolar concentrations to alter the growth or maturity of cells. Traditionally, peptide hormones act in an endocrine fashion but the activities of growth factors and hormones overlap considerably.

The benefit of hormone based therapy in the control of advanced malignancy was first demonstrated by the use of ovarian ablation in the treatment of advanced breast cancer in a premenopausal woman in 1896. The locally invasive tumour regressed after oophorectomy but unfortunately the woman succumbed to metastatic disease after a number of months. The ovary secretes a number of hormones but it is oestrogen that has the greatest effect on cellular proliferation within the breast and female genital tract. Similarly, the male genital tract is under the control of testosterone, another steroid hormone. Control of growth of androgen dependent tissues can be achieved by removal of testosterone producing tissues, this therapy is effective when used to treat prostatic carcinoma, the use of steroid hormone manipulations to treat cancer in these organs is widespread.

There are three main principles of action through which hormone dependency of tumours can be manipulated. The first is to deprive the tumour of the hormone either by removal of hormone producing tissue (oophorectomy or radiation induced menopause) or inhibition of the metabolic pathways that produce the hormone (aromatase inhibitors for steroid hormones). The second method is to blockade the hormone's receptor with antagonists and prevent its activity locally (tamoxifen in breast cancer). The third rather indirect method is to overload the system with a stimulatory signal which leads to receptor downregulation and inhibition of hormone production by the manufacturing organ (leutinising hormone releasing hormone therapy in both breast and prostate cancer). Unfortunately, many tumours arising from hormone sensitive tissue do not respond to hormone ablation usually because these tumours do not express the normal hormone receptor or its signal transduction mechanism. Similarly, many previously sensitive tumours lose their dependence on a hormone rich environment and continue to proliferate. This phenomenon is associated with the loss of hormone receptors and often with a rapid clinical deterioration. Treatment strategies should aim to prevent the escape from hormonal control of particular clones of cells, thus not conferring a survival advantage on these cell populations. The combination of a number of hormone based strategies may reduce the possibility of escape from control mechanisms.

Peptide hormones can also be manipulated in order to treat malignant disease. The thyroid gland is under the influence of thyroid stimulating hormone (TSH) secreted by the pituitary gland which promotes the production of thyroxine by the follicular cells of the thyroid and stimulates growth. Serum thyroxine has a negative feedback on the production of TSH. Thus, in order to reduce production of the growth promoting TSH, thyroxine can be administered therapeutically. This method of growth control is used in the treatment of well-differentiated papillary, mixed and follicular thyroid cancers (Clark 1981).

Peptide and steroid hormones can, therefore, be used to manipulate tumour proliferation with varying degrees of success. There is certainly much scope for their use in combination with other therapeutic regimes. It is also possible that concurrent manipulation of two or more hormone types may have a profound effect on tumour growth. The hormonal approach to cancer therapy may be of particular importance in the prevention of metastases, hormonal manipulation being most likely to inhibit early tumour development and the delicate process of establishment of metastases. In order to develop new treatment strategies, it is essential to identify which hormones and growth factors are important in the control of proliferation in the gastrointestinal tract.

The gastrointestinal tract as an endocrine organ

In order to develop hormonal treatment strategies of an organ, it is first important to demonstrate the dependence of that organ on a hormone for growth stimulation. The gastrointestinal tract is subject to both systemically secreted hormones and locally produced growth factors (Bloom & Polak 1981). Peptide hormones are produced in the gastrointestinal tract by specialised endocrine cells. A list of the peptides secreted both locally and systemically which affect gut proliferation is presented in Table 11.2. This list is by no means exhaustive but provides an indication of the complexity of hormonal interactions within the gut. Three examples of gut peptide hormones and their actions are given later. The effects of all peptide growth factors must be transmitted through high affinity cell surface receptors and these receptors are reduced in number when sustained high levels of growth factor are present. In order to determine the level at which these crucial signalling pathways can be manipulated, the mechanism of receptor signal transduction must be understood.

Cell surface receptors which modulate proliferation

Several classes of cell surface receptor modulate cell growth. They can be conveniently divided into two main classes. The first group, Type I or tyrosine kinase type, consist of a series of proteins encompassing an extracellular domain involved in ligand binding, a transmembrane and an intracellular domain which initiates signal transduction (Pawson & Schlessinger 1993). Many of these receptors, such as the epidermal growth factor receptor and the platelet derived growth factor receptor, have catalytic domains on the intracellular portion which have intrinsic tyrosine kinase activity. Activation results in the phosphorylation of target proteins on tyrosine residues including on the receptor itself. These changes, via a number of adaptor proteins, initiate a series of intracellular events, such as the activation of the *ras* oncogene and consequently a cascade of serine/threonine kinases, which ultimately result in gene transcription in the nucleus.

The second principal class of receptors, and the one most relevant to this chapter, is the seven transmembrane domain family of receptors. As the name implies, the receptor passes through the membrane not once but seven times. Ligand binding outside the cell results in conformational changes within the cell which cause the intracellular portion to become associated with a G protein (Birnbaumer & Brown 1990). G proteins are heterotrimers

Table 11.2 Gastrointestinal peptides that have a proliferative action on the gastrointestinal tract

Hormone	Stomach	Pancreas	Colon	Experimental data for proliferative response
Gastrin	Stimulated		Stimulated	Stimulates growth of gastric and colonic xenografts. Receptors internalised with prolonged stimulation - no increased incidence of gastric or colon cancers in Zollinger-Ellison syndrome or long-term H2 blockers
CCK	? Stimulated	Stimulated		Shares receptor with gastrin – these receptors increased on pancreatic cancer cells and stimulate rise in intracellular calcium
GRP et al	Stimulated	Stimulated	Stimulated	Autocrine mitogen in SCLC. High affinity binding sites for receptors found on ~50% stomach and ~30% colon cancers and not normal mucosa
Serotonin				Coupled to INsP3 stimulatory intracellular signalling pathway. Expression of receptor can lead to malignant transformation
Histamine				Both H1 and H2 receptors linked to stimulation of cAMP and intracellular calcium
Secretin	Inhibited	Stimulated	Inhibited	Gastrin stimulated proliferation inhibited.
Somatostatin	Inhibited	Inhibited	Inhibited	Inhibits adenylyl cyclase and activates protein phosphatases. Inhibits hormone and growth factor production, angiogenesis and proliferation. Downregulates tyrosine kinase receptors. Inhibits expression of c-jun and c-fos
VIP	? Stimulated	Inhibited	Inhibited	Stimulates cAMP but not growth most cell lines. Enhances NK activity against colon cancer cell lines
Peptide YY				Plasma levels correlate with proliferation (? significance)
Bradykinin				Mitogenic, induces expression of c-myc. Stimulates InsP3 pathway. Not known as growth factor
Vasopressin				Induces oncogene expression, acts as autocrine growth factor in SCLC
Neurotensin				Peptide locally secreted in gut. Acts as autocrine growth factor in SCLC. Increases gastric antral hyperplasia

H1, H2 = histamine type 1 and 2 receptors; CCK = cholecystokinin; GRP = gastrin releasing peptide; SCLC = small cell lung cancer; InsP3 = inositol trisphosphate; cAMP = cyclic adenosine monophosphate; and NK = natural killer cells.

consisting of α, β and γ subunits and are named because of their ability to hydrolyse GTP to GDP. The G protein bound to GTP associates with the receptor and is dissociated to a GTP bound α subunit and the βγ subunits. It is principally, but not exclusively, the GTP α complex which is involved in signal transduction which occurs through a number of effector proteins. There are at least 15 classes of G proteins which, under different circumstances, can associate with different receptors leading to considerable complexity in the system. In terms of peptide hormones and cancer, the most relevant signal transduction pathways involving G protein coupled receptors are activation of phospholipase C and adenylyl cyclase. The first of these pathways involves the generation of inositol phosphates, the elevation of intracellular calcium, the formation of diacyl glycerol and the activation of the serine-threonine kinase, protein kinase C. This leads to a cascade of intracellular events which ultimately lead to gene transcription and mitogenesis. Adenylyl cyclase activation leads to the production of cAMP which may also, but less certainly, lead to proliferation. Formation of cAMP is mediated by a stimulatory G protein (Gas) and inhibition of its formation is mediated by an inhibitory protein (Gai). Some G protein coupled receptors activate protein phosphatases, effectively damping proliferative signals.

Therapeutic strategies using growth factor receptors

The principal mechanisms by which peptide hormone receptors may be used in the treatment of gastrointestinal cancers are as follows:

Direct utilization of the expression of hormone receptors on tumour cells

This may involve using antagonists to stimulatory peptides or agonists of inhibitory peptides.

Indirect hormone antagonism

These may alter the endocrine environment of a tumour, for example by the inhibition of the endocrine or paracrine production of other hormones or growth factors.

Other use of hormone receptors

These are rapidly internalised by the cell when bound to the ligand. Coupling a cytotoxin such as ricin, which has no natural cell receptor, to a peptide hormone analogue may allow specific targeting and tumour cell lysis.

Most of these strategies depend on the tumour universally expressing hormone receptors and normal tissue being relatively unaffected by the treatment. There is some evidence that, in certain situations, receptors may be selectively expressed by tumours (see below) but it is unclear if this is a universal phenomenon.

The preliminary studies to ascertain the viability of growth factor manipulation as a strategy for treatment of gastrointestinal malignancies must first of all determine the peptides of influence and the distribution of their receptors. The nature of receptor–ligand interaction and the effector response in specific tissues must also be ascertained and the intracellular response to analogues must be predictable.

Gastrin and cholecystokinin

Gastrin is a 17 amino acid peptide that stimulates gastric acid secretion, gastric motility and contraction of the lower oesophageal sphincter. It acts as a neurotransmitter in the hypothalamus and pituitary, and is secreted by the neuroendocrine cells of the gastric antrum and proximal duodenum. Gastrin has an identical carboxyl terminus to cholecystokinin (CCK) and shares a common receptor. The receptor is of the G-protein coupled type and is linked to the stimulation of cAMP production and an increase in intracellular calcium. CCK is secreted by I cells of the duodenum and ileum, promotes pancreatic exocrine secretion and growth, and causes gall bladder contraction. CCK-A receptors respond only to CCK, while CCK-B/gastrin receptors respond to both ligands. Receptor distribution is quite distinct.

In vivo experiments suggest that gastrin exerts a trophic effect on normal pancreas and gastrointestinal mucosa. When given exogenously, gastrin stimulates DNA synthesis in fundic gastric mucosa and increases pancreatic weight. If gastrin production is decreased by surgical antrectomy or antigastrin antibodies, DNA synthesis is decreased in pancreatic, duodenal and colonic mucosal and oxyntic glands. These effects can be reversed by pentagastrin treatment (Bloom & Polak 1981). Growth of gastric, pancreatic and colonic cancer cell lines in vitro is enhanced by the addition of gastrin or pentagastrin to the medium and is reduced by its withdrawal (Palmer Smith & Solomon 1988). Similarly, the growth of xenografts of human and animal cancer cells lines in nude mice can be stimulated by any treatment that increases serum gastrin levels. Carcinogen-induced colon and pancreatic cancers have their growth stimulated by surgical vagotomy or pentagastrin administration.

Receptors for gastrin have been shown to be present on both normal gastrointestinal tissues and malignant tissues and cell lines. Some of these cells have been shown to produce both receptor and ligand, providing evidence for an autocrine loop (Finley et al 1993). The prognosis for colonic tumours which express gastrin receptors is better than for those which do not (Upp et al 1989). However, the converse is true for the prognosis of gastric tumours expressing gastrin receptors (Kumamoto 1988) and there is some experimental evidence to suggest that the intracellular response to gastrin is different in colonic and gastric tissues.

Clinical hypergastrinaemia occurs in a number of disease states (Zollinger-Ellison syndrome, pernicious anaemia and continuous use of the H2-receptor antagonists) and after surgical vagotomy. There is no evidence to suggest that these states have an excess of colon or stomach cancers (Goodlad & Wright 1990). Chronic atrophic gastritis is associated with chronic *Helicobacter pylori* infection and a moderate hypergastrinaemia and this is associated with an increase in gastric cancer incidence. The time from infection with *Helicobacter* to the development of gastric cancer is thought to be at least 20 years and so considerable long-term follow up is required before a link can be refuted. Hypergastrinaemia does cause an increase in proliferation of both the fundic parietal cells and the enterochromaffin cells. There is no evidence that this hyperplasia leads to the development of malignancy and it regresses when gastrin levels normalise (Baldwin & Whitehead 1994). Further studies found increased serum concentrations of gastrin in cancer subjects compared to those with polyps who had higher levels than normal subjects. There are a number of variables in this study that may have confounded the results and it appears that the endocrine microenvironment is of more significance than serum concentrations in venous blood.

Cholecystokin has also been shown to have growth promoting effects on pancreatic cancer cells fines in vitro on xenografts and on the normal pancreas (Smith et al 1987). However, clinical trials by Abbruzzese et al (1992) using CCK antagonists in the treatment of advanced pancreatic cancer showed no benefit. CCK has been implicated as an autocrine growth factor in small cell lung cancer lines (Sethi et al 1993). It does not appear to have growth promoting effects on gastric or colonic mucosa indicating that, although gastrin and CCK share a common receptor, the effector response produced is different.

Bombesin-like peptides

Bombesin is a bioactive tetradecapeptide first isolated from the skin of a frog by Anastasi et al (1971). Subsequent work identified three subfamilies of bombesin; the bombesin group, ranatensin group and the pyllolitorin group. Mammalian counterparts were later discovered – gastrin–releasing peptide (GRP) which is related to the bombesin group and neuromedin B (NMB), related to the ranatensin group. No ligand corresponding to the pyllolitirin group has been identified.

The bombesin-like peptides function as growth factors, neurotransmitters and paracrine hormones. Most work has been performed on GRP. Its functions include stimulation of gastric acid secretion; pancreatico-biliary stimulation; disruption of peristaltic activity; modification of renal blood flow; hypothermia; hyperglycaemia and satiety. It stimulates the release of gastrin, glucagon, insulin and pancreatic polypeptide.

NMB is involved in smooth muscle contraction. There are no recognised hypersecretion syndromes in man and, therefore, no natural models to study. Extensive in vitro studies have confirmed the mitogenic effects of bombesin in cell cultures. Bombesin-like peptides are mitogenic to Swiss 3T3 fibroblasts (Rozengurt & Sinnett-Smith 1983), small cell lung cancer cell lines (Carney et al 1983), as well as several gastrointestinal cancer cell lines. It may also play a role in medullary thyroid cancer (Sunday et al 1988). Corresponding high affinity receptors have been demonstrated and in certain cases the cells have also been shown to produce the ligand. An autocrine loop was first demonstrated in small cell lung cancer lines and subsequently in gastrointestinal cancer lines (Cuttitta 1986). The mitogenic effect of bombesin/GRP can be blocked by specific bombesin receptor antagonists. Studies on human cancer cell lines transplanted into nude nice showed that bombesin stimulated tumour growth and that this could be inhibited by an antagonist. Similar results were found with azaserine induced cancer in rats (Lohste & Longnecker 1987) but, conversely, bombesin had no effect on the growth of nitrosamine–induced pancreatic cancer in hamsters (Szepezhasi et al 1993).

Bombesin receptors

Three distinct receptors have been characterised and sequenced. They all belong to the G-protein coupling seven times membrane spanning family. GRP receptors have been demonstrated on guinea pig pancreatic acinar cells (Jenson et al 1978), rat brain membranes (Moody et al 1978), pituitary tumour cells (Westendorf & Schonbrunn 1983), and certain human small cell lung cancer cell lines. NMB receptors are present in the muscularis mucosa of rat oesophagus (Von Schrenck et al 1989), certain lung cancer cell lines (Corjay et al 1991) and in rat brain (Landerheim et al 1990). Bombesin receptor subtype 3 has only recently been isolated and so far it has only been detected in humans in some small cell lung cancer cell lines (Fathi et al 1993).

Studies have shown receptors for bombesin on between 25–40% of human colon cancers and the majority of gastric cancers. The receptors cannot be detected in normal mucosa (Preston et al 1993, 1995).

Bombesin–related therapy

There is currently a trial in progress involving human subjects, using the murine monoclonal anti-GRP/bombesin antibody 2A11 (Kelly et al 1993). One of 12 patients achieved full remission but the small cell lung cancers recurred after 5 months and did not respond to further treatment. GRP receptors were not demonstrated on the tumours so the mechanism of tumour response remains unclear.

From the studies performed so far, the bombesin-like peptides have been shown to act as mitogens. Their receptors seem to be overexpressed in cancer as opposed to normal mucosa and, therefore, may be a potential target for the development of new treatments. There is a need to define clearly the distribution and the mechanism of action in order to design a potential therapeutic agent.

Somatostatin

In mammalian species, somatostatin exists in two forms with 14 or 28 amino acids. Somatostatin-14 (S14) and -28 (S28) have inhibitory effects on a wide variety of cell types. Somatostatin-14 mainly inhibits glucagon and gastric acid secretion, in contrast to somatostatin-28 which inhibits the secretion of growth hormone, insulin and the exocrine pancreatic enzymes (Schulkes 1994). Somatostatin has neurotransmitter and neuromodulator activity both in the central nervous system and in the myenteric plexus of the gastrointestinal tract (Bloom & Polak 1981). The effect of ligand binding on an individual cell is in part determined by the subtype of receptor that is being expressed on the cell surface. So far, five human somatostatin receptor (hSSTR) subtypes have been isolated and sequenced.

Somatostatin analogues have been used to treat a variety of hypersecretory disorders, particularly acromegaly. They have also been successfully used to relieve the symptoms of gastrointestinal endocrine tumours. During the treatment of these including carcinoids, VIPomas and insulinomas, it was noted that somatostatin analogues had an antiproliferative action and biopsies of metastases revealed an increase in the number of cells undergoing apoptosis. In transplantable tumours in animals, somatostatin and its analogues have been shown to decrease tumour growth as demonstrated by a reduction in tumour volume and inhibition of DNA and RNA synthesis (Bloom & Polak 1981). Further reports of the antiproliferative effects of somatostatin were reported in the treatment of breast, prostate, colon, pancreatic and small cell lung cancer both in vivo and in vitro (Lehy et al 1979).

The half life of somatostatin in serum is very short and it has to be administered by continuous infusion. A number of analogues have been developed. The octapeptide analogue octreotide (SMS 201-995) is a longer acting and more potent peptide than native somatostatin and has been in clinical use for a number of years. Octreotide considerably reduces the secretion of gastrointestinal peptides from gut endocrine tumours. Nearly all the studies on somatostatin analogues in cancer treatment in humans have used this preparation (Lamberts 1990). However, only a small percentage of colorectal cancers have been to express somatostatin receptors using radiolabelled ligand. This, in part, may be due to low copy numbers of receptor protein.

Three studies on the growth response of colon lines to somatostatin have confirmed its antiproliferative potential. Octreotide was shown to inhibit pentagastrin stimulated growth of a mouse colon cancer cell (for review see Lewin 1992). Similarly, two human colon cancer cell lines transplanted into nude mice and treated with another analogue (MK-678) demonstrated significant growth reduction (Milhoan 1988). A further study on three human cancer cell lines showed that octreotide inhibited tumour growth in two of the cell lines (Stewart et al 1994, van Eijck et al 1994). Inhibition of tumour growth by octreotide is greatest if the agent is administered as soon as possible after xenograft transplantation. A phase II study of octreotide in pancreatic and gastrointestinal malignancies was disappointing (Klijn et al 1990).

Thirty-four patients with metastatic disease were treated with subcutaneous octreotide until objective tumour progression. There were no complete or partial responses to treatment and most patients had no slowing of the progression of their disease. Another somatostatin analogue, RC-160, has been developed for its specific anticancer activity. It has been shown to inhibit the growth of colon cancer cell lines in nude mice (Qin et al 1992, Radulovic et al 1993). It has little effect on growth hormone release.

Figure 11.1 shows a number of possible mechanisms by which somatostatin may exert its effects. Each of somatostatin's activities are dependent on interaction with a specific high affinity receptor. Five receptor subtypes have been isolated and the ligand affinities characterised. Somatostatin receptors (hSSTR)1–4 prefer SS14 and hSSTR5 prefers SS28 (Yamada et al 1992a, 1992b, O'Carroll et al 1994). The somatostatin receptors also have different preferences for the many synthetic analogues. For example octreotide preferentially binds to hSSTR2 which appears to be the receptor that is principally involved in inhibition of endocrine activity (Raynor et al 1993).

The somatostatin receptors are part of the family of seven transmembrane receptors and are coupled to the trimeric G-proteins. Coupling is principally to G-proteins with an inhibitory alpha subunit and, in appropriate systems, all receptors inhibit adenylyl cyclase. Somatostatin has also been shown to inhibit the induction of the 'early' nuclear oncogenes *c-jun* and *c-fos* and the expression of the gastrin gene (Todisco 1994). Perhaps of most relevance to therapeutic oncology is the coupling of somatostatin receptors to protein phosphatases. Protein phosphatases catalyse the removal of phosphate residues from activated proteins thus reducing their activity. Proteins that can be deactivated in this manner include proteins of the intracellular signalling cascade and cell surface receptors. Somatostatin has been shown to dephosphorylate the EGF and FGF receptors as well as other intracellular phosphoproteins (Liebow 1989). This clearly provides a mechanism for antiproliferative activity and possibly also the induction of apoptosis in cancer cells. Octreotide appears to have no activity to induce protein phosphatases and this may explain its lack of effect on tumour growth. RC-160 has a very marked effect on phosphatase activity (Buscail et al 1995) and this may be a promising analogue for use in the treatment of cancer. It is clearly important to determine the subtype of receptor expressed by the target tissue in order to determine which analogues will be effective. In addition, the nature of the intracellular response to that analogue may be dependent on the G-protein subtype expressed by the target cell population. Our preliminary results have indicated that over 97% of tumour-mucosa pairs express at least one somatostatin receptor subtype. Gastric tissues allways express hSSTR1 and usually hSSTR2. Almost no tissues expressed hSSTR4. The SS28 preferring subtype, hSSTR5, was found on approximately 45% of all colonic specimens. A number of metastases have been studied and all express hSSTR2 (Laws 1996, in press). Elucidation of receptor subtype expression may allow appropriate clinical trials using the corresponding analogue.

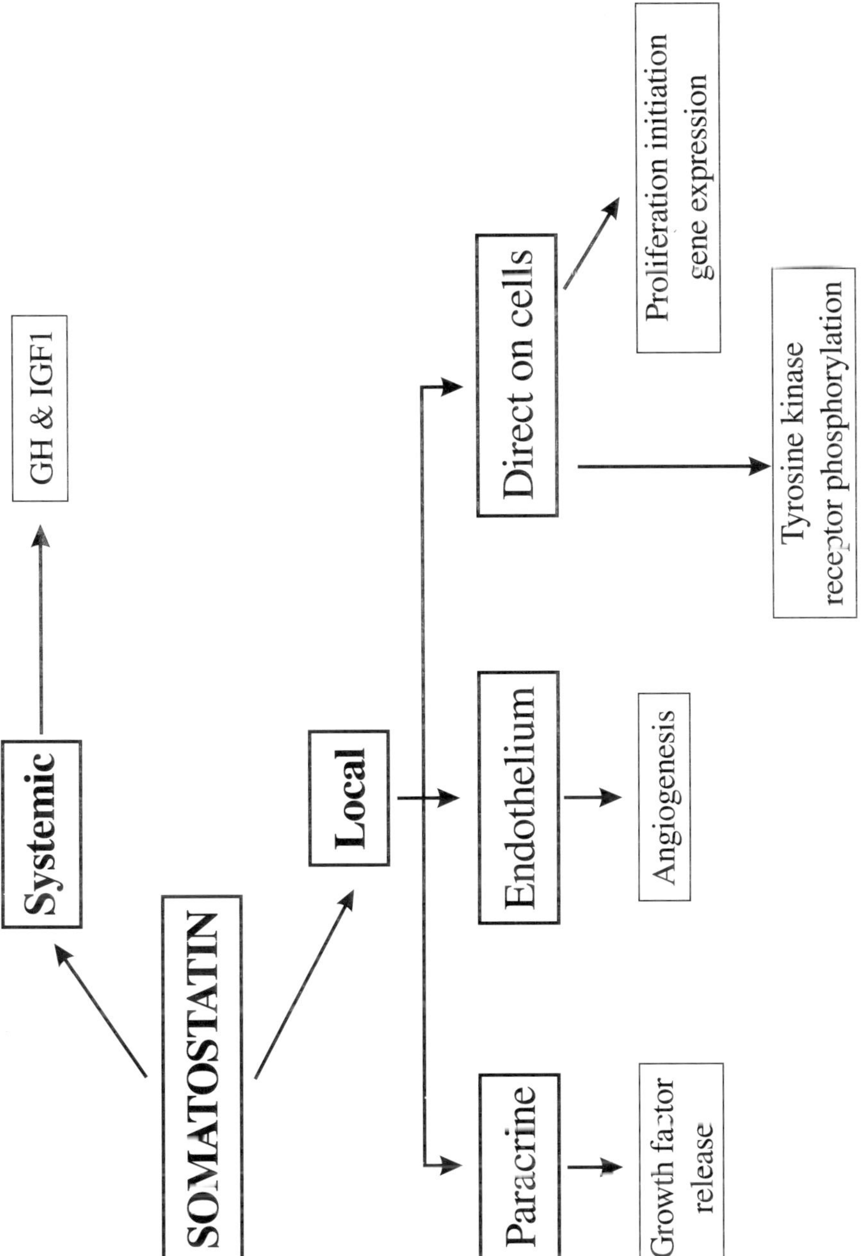

Fig. 11.1 Inhibitory pathways of somatostatin's anticancer activity.

KEY POINTS FOR CLINICAL PRACTICE

- The incidence and prevalence of gastrointestinal cancers is increasing and curative treatment is limited.
- The study of the molecular mechanisms of carcinogenesis and tumour progression leads to the development of novel treatment strategies. Manipulation of the gastrointestinal hormone/peptide axis may represent such a strategy.
- Detailed understanding of peptide receptor expression and coupling in normal and malignant tissues is required before clinical trials can be devised.

ACKNOWLEDGEMENTS

The authors would like to thank Professor J. N. Primrose for help in the preparation of this manuscript.

REFERENCES

Abbruzzese JL, Gholson CF, Daugherty K et al 1992 MK-329 A pilot clinical trial of the cholecystokinin receptor antagonist in patients with advanced pancreatic cancer. Pancreas 7: 165-171

Abulafi, Williams 1994 Local recurrence of colorectal cancer: the problems, mechanisms, management and adjuvant therapy. Br J Surg 81: 7-19

Anastasi A, Erspamer V, Bucci M 1971 Isolation and structure of bombesin and alyteoin, two analogous active peptides from the skin of the european amphibians *Bombina* and *Alytes*. Experientia 27: 166-167

Baldwin GS, Whitehead RH 1994 Gut hormones: growth and malignancy. Baillieres Clin Endocrinol Metab 8: 185-214

Birnbaumer L, Brown AM 1990 G proteins and the mechanism of action of hormones, neurotransmitters and autocrine and paracrine regulatory factors. Am Rev Respir Dis 141: S106-S114

Bloom SR, Polak JM 1981 Gut hormones. 2nd Edn. Churchill Livingstone, Edinburgh

Buscial L, Esteve J-P, Saint-Laurent N et al 1995 Inhibition of cell proliferation by the somatostatin analogue RC-160 is mediated by somatostatin receptor subtypes SSTR2 and SSTR5 through different mechanisms. Proc Natl Acad Sci USA 92: 1580-1584

Callam J 1994 *Helicobacter pylori*. Eur J Clin Invest 24: 501-510

Carney D, Oie H, Moody T, Gazdar A, Cuttitta F, Minna J 1983 Bombesin: an autocrine growth factor for human small cell lung cancer lung cancer cell lines. Clin Res 31: 404A

Cancer Research Campaign 1991 Factsheet 1.1

Clark OH 1981 TSH suppression in the management of thyroid nodules and thyroid cancer. World J Surg 5: 39-47

Corjay MH, Dobrzanski DJ, Way JM et al 1991 Two distinct bombesin receptor subtypes are expressed and functional in human lung carcinoma cells. J Biol Chem 266: 18771-18779

Cuttitta F, Carney DN, Mulshine J et al 1986. Bombesin-like peptides can function as autocrine growth factors in human small-cell lung cancer. Nature 316: 823-826

Fathi Z, Corjay M, Shapira H et al 1993 BRS-3: a novel bombesin subtype selectively expressed in testes and lung carcinoma cells. J Biol Chem 268: 5979-5984

Finley GG, Koski RA, Melhem W, Pipas JM, Meisler AI 1993 Expression of the gastrin gene in the normal human colon and colorectal adenocarcinoma. Cancer Res 53: 2919-2926

Gastrointestinal cancer study group 1987 Further evidence of elective adjuvant combined radiation and chemotherapy following curative resection of pancreatic cancer. Cancer 59: 2006-2010

Gastrointestinal cancer study group 1988 Treatment of locally unresectable cancer of the pancreas: comparison of combined modality therapy (chemotherapy plus radiotherapy) to chemotherapy alone. J Natl Cancer Inst 80: 751-755
Goodlad RA, Wright NA. 1990 Growth control factors in the gastrointestinal tract. Baillieres Clin Gastroenterol 4: 97-118
Jeekel JJ, Treurniet-Donker 1991 Treatment perspectives in locally advanced unresectable pancreatic cancer. Br J Surg 78: 1332-1334
Jenson RT, Moody T, Pert C, Rivier JE, Gardner JD 1978 Interactions of bombesin and litorin with specific membrane receptors on pancreatic acinar cells. Proc Natl Acad Sci USA 75: 6139-6143
Kalser MH, Ellenberg SS 1985 Pancreatic cancer: adjuvant combined radiation and chemotherapy following curative resection. Arch Surg 120: 899-903
Kelly MJ, Avis I, Linnoila RI et al 1993 Complete response in a patient with small cell lung cancer (SCLC) treated on a phase II trial using a murine monoclonal antibody (2A11) directed against gastrin releasing peptide (GRP). Proc Am Soc Clin Oncol 12: 339
Klijn JGM, Hoff AM, Planting AST et al 1990 Treatment of patients with metastatic pancreatic and gastrointestinal tumours with the somatostatin analogue sandostatin: a phase II study including endocrine effects. Br J Cancer 62: 627-630
Kumamoto T 1988 Gastrin receptors in human gastric scirrhous carcinoma. Gastroenterol Jpn 23: 284-389
Lamberts SWJ, Krenning EP, Klijn JGM, Reubi J-C 1990 The clinical use of somatostatin analogues in the treatment of cancer. Baillieres Clin Endocrinol Metab 4: 29-49
Landerheim EE, Jensen RT, Mantey SA, McHugh PR, Moran TH 1990 Receptor heterogeneity for bombesin-like peptides in the rat central nervous system. Brain Res 537: 233-240
Lehy T, Debrasquet M, Bonfils S 1979 Effect of somatostatin on normal and gastric-stimulated cell proliferation in the gastric and intestinal mucosae of the rat. Digestion 19: 99-109
Laws SAM, Gough AC, Primrose JN 1996 Expression of somatostatin receptor subtype mRNA in human colon cancer and normal mucosa. (in press)
Lewin MJM 1992 The somatostatin receptor in the GI tract. Annu Rev Physiol 54: 455-468
Liebow C, Reilly C, Serrono M, Schally AV 1989 Somatostatin analogues inhibit growth of pancreatic cancer by stimulating tyrosine phosphatase. Proc Natl Acad Sci USA 86: 2003-2007
Lohste EF, Longnecker DS 1987 Effect of bombesin and caerulein on early stages of carcinogenesis induced by azaserine in the rat pancreas. Cancer Res 47: 3273-3277
Milhoan RA, Milhoan LH, Trudel JL et al 1988 Somatostatin and α-difluoromethylornithine (DFMO) have additive inhibitory effects on the growth of human colon carcinoma (HCC) in vivo. Biomed Res 9: A-36
Moody TW, Pert CB, Rivier J, Brown MR 1978 Bombesin: specific binding to rat brain membranes. Proc Natl Acad Sci USA 75: 5372-5376
O'Carroll A, Raynor K, Lolait SJ, Reisine T 1994 Characterisation of cloned human somatostatin receptor SSTR5. Mol Pharmacol 46: 291-298
Palmer Smith J, Solomon TE 1988 Effects of gastrin proglumide and somatostatin on growth of human colon cancer. Gastroenterology 95: 1541-1548
Pawson T, Schlessinger J 1993 SH2 and SH3 domains. Curr Biol 3: 434-442
Preston SR, Woodhouse LF, Jones-Blackett S, Wyatt JI, Primrose JN 1993 High affinity binding sites for gastrin releasing peptide on human gastric cancer and Menetrier's mucosa. Cancer Res 53: 5090-5092
Preston SR, Woodhouse LF, Jones-Blackett S, Miller GV, Primrose JN 1995 High affinity binding sites for gastrin releasing peptide on human colorectal cancer tissue but not uninvolved mucosa. Br J Cancer 71: 1087-1089
Qin Y, Schally AV, Willems G 1992 Treatment of liver metastases of human colon cancer in nude mice with somatostatin analogue RC-160. Int J Cancer 52: 791-796
Radulovic S, Comaru-Schally AM, Milovanovic S, Schally AV 1993 Somatostatin analogue RC-160 and LHRH antagonist SB-75 inhibit growth of MIA PaCa-2 human pancreatic xenografts in nude mice. Pancreas 8: 88-97
Raynor K, Murphy WA, Coy DH et al 1993 Cloned somatostatin receptors: identification of subtype selective peptides and demonstration of high affinity binding of linear peptides. Mol Pharmacol 43: 838-844

Rozengurt E, Sinnett-Smith J 1983 Bombesin stimulation of DNA synthesis and cell division in cultures of Swiss 3T3 cells. Proc Natl Acad Sci USA 80: 2936-2940
Saltz L, Kelsen D 1992 Combined-modality therapy in the treatment of local-regional oesophageal cancer. Ann Oncol 3: 793-799
Sethi T, Herget T, Wu SV, Walsh JH, Rozengurt E 1993 CCK(A) and CCK(B) receptors are expressed in small cell lung cancer lines and mediate Ca^{2+} mobilization and clonal growth. Cancer Res 53: 5208-5213
Shulkes A 1994 Somatostatin: physiology and clinical applications. Baillieres Clin Endocrinol Metab 8: 215-237
Slevin ML, Gray R 1991 Adjuvant therapy for cancer of the colon. BMJ 302: 1100-1101
Smith JP, Barrett B, Solomon TE 1987 CCK stimulates growth of five human pancreatic cancer cell lines in serum-free medium. Gastroenterology 92: 1646-1650
Stewart GJ, Lawson JA, Morris DL 1994 Octreotide inhibits development of hepatic metastases from a human colonic cancer cell line. Br J Surg 81: 1332
Sunday ME, Kaplan LM, Motoyama E, Chin WW, Spindel ER 1988 Gastrin releasing peptide (mammalian bombesin) gene expression in health and disease. Lab Invest 59: 5-24
Szepeshazi K, Schally AV, Groot K, Halmos G 1993. Effect of bombesin, gastrin-releasing peptide (GRP) (14–27) and bombesin/GRP receptor antagonist RC3095 on the growth of nitrosamine-induced pancreas cancer in hamsters. Int J Cancer 54: 282-289
Todisco A, Seva C, Dickinson CJ, Yamada T 1994 Somatostatin inhibits AP-1 function via multiple protein phosphatases. Gastroenterology 106: A846
Upp JR, Singh P, Townsend CM, Thompson JC 1989 Clinical significance of gastrin receptors in human colon cancer. Cancer Res 49: 488
van Eijck CHJ, Slooter GD, Hofland LJ, Jeekel WKJ, Lamberts SWJ, Marquet RL 1994 Somatostatin receptor-dependant inhibition of liver metastases by octreotide. Br J Surg 81: 1333-1337
Von Schrenck T, Heinz-Erian P, Moran T, Mantey SA, Gardener JD, Jensen RT 1989 Neuromedin B receptor in the oesophagus: evidence for receptor subtypes of bombesin receptors. Am J Physiol 256: G747-G758
Westendorf JM, Schonbrunn A 1983 Characterization of bombesin receptors in a rat pituitary cell line. J Biol Chem 258: 7527-7535
Yamada Y, Post SR, Wang K, Tager HS, Bell GI, Seino S 1992a Cloning and functional characterisation of a family of human and mouse somatostatin receptors expressed in brain, gastrointestinal tract and kidney. Proc Natl Acad Sci USA 89: 251-255
Yamada Y, Reisine T, Law SF et al 1992b Somatostatin receptors, an expanding gene family: cloning and functional characterisation of human SSTR3, a protein coupled to adenyl cyclase. Mol Endocrinol 6: 2136-2142

12

Surgical treatment of obesity

J-C. Gazet

The management of obesity is difficult and surgical intervention controversial. Garrow (1994) in noting the adverse disabilities associated with obesity, such as decreased longevity, increased risk of cardiovascular disease, hypertension, diabetes, osteoarthritis, and some forms of cancer sensitive to sex hormones (Table 12.1) has asked two crucial questions. First, is it physiologically possible for a severely obese patient to achieve normal weight and health? and if so, is the cure less distressing to the patient than the disease? Unless the answer is **yes** to both, he believes one should not treat obesity.

It is possible for obese people to achieve normal weight and the ideal is a loss of 1 kg/week. Woolley and Garner (1994) feel that dietary treatments for obesity are ineffective and demand for treatment is not a justification. Rubins (1994), in a commentary on both articles, suggests that one should leave obesity alone in healthy and happy people. However, the problem of obesity is rapidly increasing in many countries, including the UK, and the demand for treatment is consumer-led. This begs the question of how obesity is defined.

MEASUREMENT OF OBESITY

Obesity is simply defined as the accumulation of excess adipose tissue and implies an optimum weight for any individual but weight is a variable in which there is a continuum between excessive low and excessive high weight within a normal range. Accurate measurement of body fat is time consuming and cumbersome. Thus, the accepted clinical method which is convenient depends on height and weight. Relative weight is the weight expressed as a percentage of the optimal standard weight for a person, related to sex and height. The standard weight depends on actuarial tables devised by life insurance companies for weights for men and women, according to height and age, but not necessarily to race. The desirable weight is the weight range with the least morbidity, and the standard weight usually means the average weight. This may depend upon whether the person is considered to have a large or small frame. Although these tables are derived from very large samples, life insurance applicants are a selected group even within one country and these tables must be treated with caution.

In reviewing the whole problem, MacFarland (1986) felt that the Body Mass Index (BMI) is the preferred formula. This is calculated as weight (W) in kg divided by the square of the height (H) in metres (W/H^2).

Table 12.1 Disorders associated with obesity (after McFarland 1986)

- Cardiovascular
  - Ischaemic heart disease
  - Myocardial infarction
  - Angina pectoris*
  - Arrhythmias
- Fluid retention*
  - Heart failure
  - Increased filling pressures
- Hypertension*
  - Stroke
  - Venous thrombosis, embolism and stasis ulcer
- Respiratory
  - Sleep apnoea*
  - Pickwickian syndrome*
  - Secondary polycythemia*
  - Cor pulmonale
- Diabetes mellitus*
- Cholelithiasis
- Osteoarthritis*
- Gout*
- Nephrotic syndrome*
- Hyperlipidaemia
- Skin diseases and immune complex disorders*
- Menstrual disorders subfertility and obstetric problems
- Cancer
- Psychosocial incapacity*
- Surgical and anaesthetic complications
- Accidental death

*Likely to improve with weight loss.

In clinical practice, a range of acceptable weights has to be defined and for this the American data are commonly used. Relative weight is expressed as a percentage of average or desirable weight. Obesity is defined arbitrarily as, for example, 120% of standard weight. BMI assumes no standard but has a desirable range of 20–25 kg/m^2 and obese (120% above standard weight) is equivalent to a BMI above 30 kg/m^2. Garrow (1981) divided all subjects into four broad categories using BMI:

- Grade 0 – desirable weight, minimal mortality (20–25 kg/m^2)
- Grade I – mild obesity, health risk detectable (25–30 kg/m^2)
- Grade II – moderate obesity, transition range (30–40 kg/m^2)
- Grade III – severe obesity, unequivocal health risk (> 40 kg/m^2)

It is generally accepted that morbid obesity is defined as 45 kg (100 lb) over desirable weight. This is approximately equivalent to a BMI of 40 kg/m^2, though a figure of 35 kg/m^2 and above is acceptable as an appropriate level for treatment.

TREATMENT

Genetic engineering aside, which is for the future, there are three main methods of treatment, namely diet, drugs which suppress appetite or increase metabolic rate, and surgery. The scope of this review is to discuss surgery only.

In 1985, the American Society for Bariatric Surgery adopted guidelines for selection of patients for surgical treatment for obesity based on the serious sequelae of massive obesity. Criteria for operation included:

- Presence of serious sequelae of morbid obesity.
- Greater than 45 kg overweight or twice ideal weight for more than 5 years.
- Failure of sustained weight loss on exhaustive supervised dietary and conservative regimens for more than 5 years.
- Absence of endocrine causes.
- Willingness to co-operate with long-term follow up.
- Acceptable operative risks.
- No history of alcoholism or major psychiatric disorder.

To this may be added further requirements. It is essential that patients be cared for within a multidisciplinary team of psychiatrist, physician, surgeon, dietician and dedicated staff, all interested in the management of obesity. One of the highest priorities is to protect the patients from blame for their condition and the enormous cost to them of fat prejudice.

A successful obesity operation must induce a negative energy balance. It is well known that patients who have lost functional small bowel length, due to inflammatory bowel disease, surgery or vascular accidents, had difficulty maintaining weight as well as electrolyte and nutritional balance. They, in fact, suffer from a malabsorbtion syndrome. In 1956, Payne, De Wind and Commons (1963) performed the first 10 intestinal bypass operations by dividing the jejunum 50 cm beyond the duodenojejunal flexure and anastomosing it end to side to the transverse colon. This procedure was unacceptable due to progressive loss of weight, diarrhoea and electrolyte imbalance.

Eventually, after many trials and errors, a jejunoileal bypass was devised which excluded all but 35 cm of small bowel, the usual limits being 10 cm of proximal jejunum anastomosed to the terminal 25 cm of ileum. However, in our experience, the easiest method was a 7/7, that is 17.5 cm (7 inches) of jejunum as measured on the anti-mesenteric border from the duodeno-jejunal flexure to 17.5 cm (7 inches) of ileum as measured from the ileocaecal sphincter (McFarland 1986). The jejunum was anastomosed end to side to the ileum (Fig. 12.1). The problems of the blind loop were later dealt with by anastomosing the cut proximal end of the jejunum to the fundus of the gall-bladder (Hallberg & Holmgren 1979).

At or about this time, the standard operation for complicated peptic ulcer was sub-total gastrectomy with a Billroth II type anastomosis. It was noted that due to the restricted gastric remnant, many patients failed to gain weight due to reduced intake. In 1966, Mason (1967) experimented with restrictive gastric surgery and the first procedure suggested was a gastric bypass using a loop gastrojejunostomy (Fig. 12.2). The difficulties associated with the subsequent variations on this theme were such that jejunoileal bypass became the standard procedure. It was quick and simple to perform with a low immediate postoperative mortality and morbidity.

The introduction of stapling devices aided gastric surgery which then developed along two specific lines. Gastric operations had two important objectives, the formation of a very small upper gastric pouch and the formation of a very small outlet. Pouch emptying should thus be slow and the feeling of satiety after a meal should persist for a long time. A small gastric pouch restricted the intake and thus reduced the nutritional value of the food taken in. Gastric operations could then be classified into two broad groups, namely gastric bypass and gastroplasty. In gastric bypass operations, the stomach was divided into two segments by staples, sutures or surgical sec-

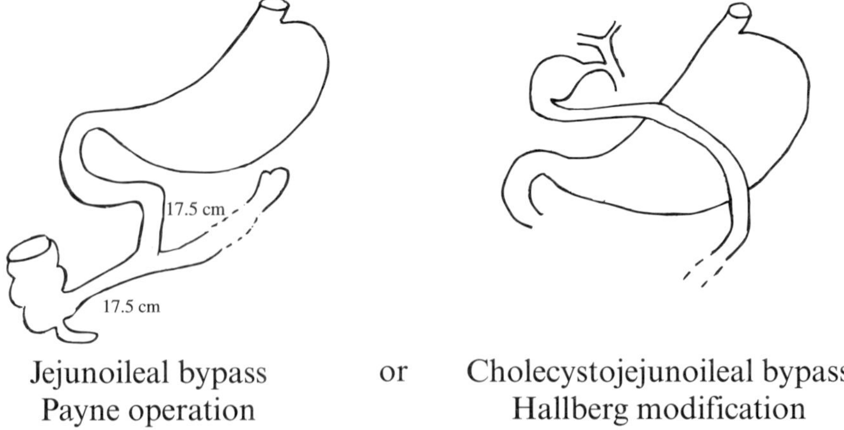

Fig. 12.1 The standard jejunoileal bypass was based on Payne's operation with variations on length of jejunum and ileum included in the anastomosis. Hallberg's variation was to anastomose the proximal end of the cut ileum to the fundus of the gallbladder to avoid a blind-loop syndrome.

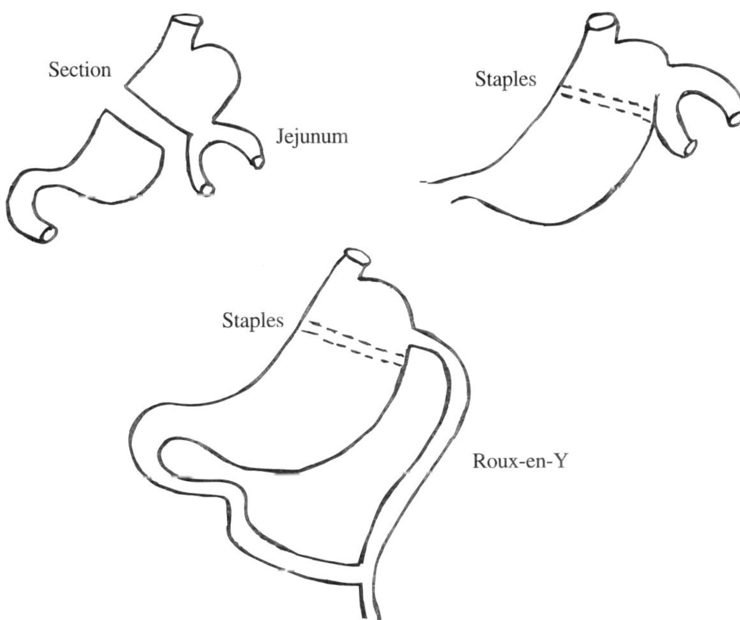

Fig. 12.2 These three variations show gastric bypass operations which exlcuded all but the fundus of the stomach with an associated jejunal bypass. All were difficult to perform.

tion. Thereafter, some type of anastomosis was constructed between the upper gastric pouch and the jejunum.

In gastroplasty, however, there was no need for intestinal bypass as the gastric segments remained in continuity though they were divided by staples or sutures. A small outlet was constructed between the small upper gastric pouch and the rest of the stomach. This could either be by a frank gastrogastrostomy (Buckwalter operation 1982) or removing staples to allow a small dehiscence in the staple line (Pace or Gomez operation 1979) (Fig. 12.3).

In the following two decades, intensive investigations and research were performed on intestinal bypass and gastric surgery, each with its own advocates. One of the serious flaws in the study of the effects of bariatric surgery was the failure to appreciate the importance of long-term follow-up. In most series, detailed analysis was made of the short-term mortality and morbidity without assessing the long-term follow-up mortality and morbidity associated with these procedures. These are not only metabolic or mechanical but also psychosexual and are associated with the changes in body image after major weight loss

Jejunoileal bypass

Many jejunoileal bypass operations were performed worldwide up to 1980.

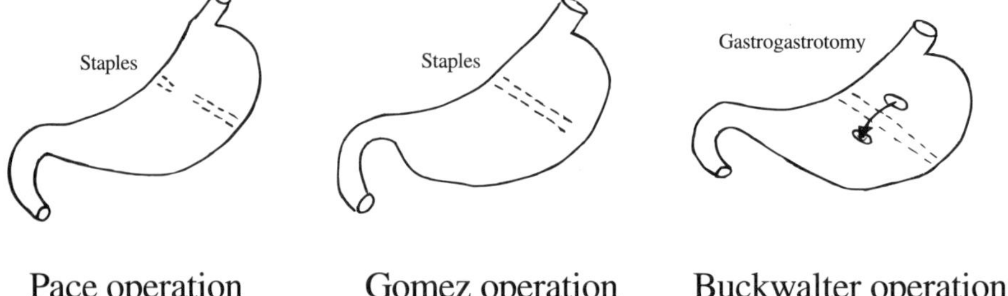

Fig. 12.3 Horizontal gastric partition was a simplification of a gastric bypass but it was difficult to control stoma size by staple removal only.

MacFarland (1986) reporting on 182 cases noted only 11 after this date. Experience showed that with 35 cm of small bowel in continuity, i.e. 17.5 cm of jejunum anastamosed to 17.5 cm of terminal ileum, weight loss was excellent whether cholecystojejunostomy was added to the procedure or not. The majority of patients stabilised their weight 2 years postoperatively and remained static at 5 years. The mean fall in BMI was 30–45 kg/m^2, but this was related to the original BMI. The fatter or more obese patient lost more but remained proportionally heavier. If gastric restrictive procedures had not developed so successfully, it is possible but unlikely that jejunoileal operations would still be performed. However, this procedure had the potential for serious sequelae and continuing follow-up showed that it is mandatory to institute close surveillance on these patients. Patients who have had a jejunoileal bypass become a full time ongoing responsibility for the bariatric surgeon (Table 12.2).

Anderson et al in 1994 reviewed the 19 year follow-up of our series of 182 patients and noted that by this time 60 (33%) had had to be reversed. The compelling reasons for reversal were life-threatening metabolic failure, severe electrolyte disturbance, immune complex disease, renal oxalate stones and osteomalacia. At the time of reversal in 12 patients, a vertical banding gastroplasty was performed. There were significant complications from the reversal procedure including sepsis, incisional hernia, ileus and pulmonary emboli but no deaths. All regained weight, some exceeding their pre-operative weight before bypass. They were generally freed from their bypass associated symptoms and complications with the exception of arthralgia and arthritis.

Our policy now is that they should all be converted to a Mason's vertical banded gastroplasty and in the 12 patients in which this was done, 10 remained within the obesity grades I and II. Riding's and Sugerman's (1994) commentary on this report was that failure of jejunoileal bypass was the result of a poor operation now obsolete and they converted their patients to a Roux en Y gastric bypass rather than a gastroplasty.

Table 12.2 Early and late complications of jejunoileal bypass in a personal series of 182 patients (after McFarland 1986)

Complications			
Early		Late	
Wound infection	13%	Intestinal obstruction	4%
Burst abdomen	2%*	Cholecystitis	4%
Chest infection	14%	Incisional hernia	21%
Urinary infection	7%		
Anastomotic leak	3%		

*One death

Late deaths (6)	
3 months	Pulmonary embolism after cholecystectomy
8 and 9 months	Metabolic derangement, liver failure
8 months	Viral pneumonia
2 years	Miliary tuberculosis
8 years	Sudden death? metabolic derangement

Reasons for reversal in 60 of these patients (after Anderson 1994. In most patients there were multiple indications)	
Fluid and electrolyte imbalance	21
Metabolic failure	23
Immune complex problems	27
Oxaluria and urinary calculi	9
Recurrent bowel obstruction	4
Osteomalacia	3
Patient's request	10
Failure to lose weight	6
Psychological disturbance	6

Thus, although this procedure is no longer performed, bariatric surgeons must follow up their patients and be constantly aware of their problems.

Gastric bypass

Following Mason's suggestion, it seemed that morbid obesity could be treated by gastric bypass using a loop gastrojejunostomy. The problem with this procedure was that it was technically difficult to perform in the morbidly obese patient with a significant and worrying anastomotic leak rate. Two factors became apparent in producing a satisfactory outcome, namely the size of the residual pouch which should not exceed 50–100 ml and the size of the outlet stoma which should not exceed 7–10 mm in diameter. The introduction of the stapling devices confirmed that it was unnecessary to divide the stomach but to ease the anastomotic problems, many surgeons preferred to perform a Roux en Y procedure (Fig. 12.2) . Significant complications occurred with these procedures including subdiaphragmatic abscess, atelectasis of the lung, infection and peptic ulceration. Late complications included narrowing of the gastrojejunostomy, obstruction, stomal ulceration and bleeding. The mortality in experienced hands did not exceed 0.5%. The weight loss was satisfactory and as a procedure it was acceptable, but, due to its technical requirements, it has been superseded by simpler procedures.

Biliopancreatic bypass

The satisfactory weight loss obtained by jejunoileal bypass but marred by serious complications and blind loop syndrome, suggested the possibility of combining it with a gastric bypass operation. Duodenoileal bypass was no better than a jejunoileal bypass, but Gourlay and Cleator (1989) described a variation on the Salman type bypass. In this procedure, a jejunoileal bypass of 25 cm of jejunum, measured from the duodenojejunal flexure, was anastomosed end to end to 50 cm of terminal ileum measured from the ileocaecal sphincter. The divided end of the distal ileum was then anastomosed to the fundus or body of the stomach, and the distal divided end of the jejunum was closed (Fig. 12.4). The aim was to eradicate the blind loop syndrome. Though this novel procedure was never popular, it stimulated the development of alternative procedures to produce a malabsorption syndrome without the undesirable effects of jejunoileal bypass.

Scopinaro et al (1979) reported a biliopancreatic bypass procedure which has been developed and used by others and is based on a Billroth II gastrec-

Jejunoileal bypass
with ileogastrostomy

Biliopancreatic bypass

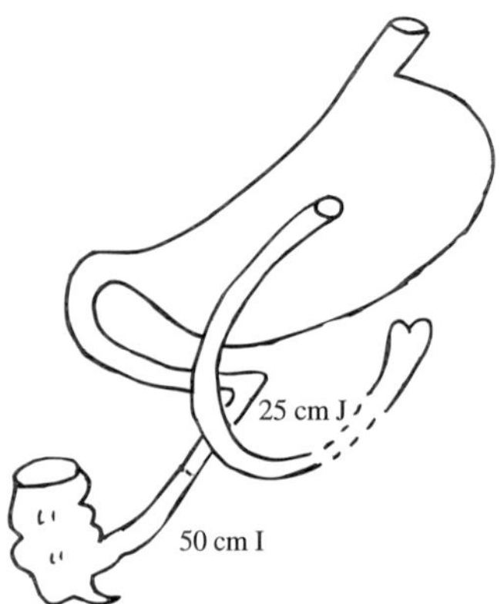

250 cm
50 cm

Gourlay & Cleator operation

Scopinaro operation

Fig. 12.4 Both operations attempt to prevent blind-loop syndrome with either the jejunoileal bypass or partial gastrectomy.

tomy with a Roux en Y loop. A high gastrectomy is performed leaving a gastric pouch no greater than 200 ml. After cholecystectomy, the ileum is divided 250 cm proximal to the ileocaecal sphincter and the distal end of the ileum anastomosed to the stomach forming a gastroileostomy. The proximal end of the ileum is anastomosed end to side to the terminal ileum 50 cm from the ileocaecal sphincter (Fig. 12.4). This operation is similar to the Mann-Williamson experimental gastric operation devised in 1923 to produce peptic ulceration in dogs. The peptic ulceration could then be reversed by either a partial gastrectomy or vagotomy.

Biliopancreatic bypass produces good permanent weight loss, but the sheer magnitude of the operation has prevented its greater acceptance as an alternative to jejunoileal bypass or indeed, gastric bypass. It has been suggested that stapling across the stomach as opposed to partial gastrectomy with the addition of a truncal vagotomy is a valid alternative, and Cuffaro et al (1994) reported a small pilot series of 40 patients treated since 1988 (Fig. 12.5). These were randomised to have vagotomy or not. The complications mimicked to a degree those found in jejunoileal bypass and a high but usually transient oxaluria was noted which led to renal calculus in one patient. This procedure though attractive is complex and has a higher mortality and early morbidity than the operation of choice which must be now Mason's vertical banded gastroplasty.

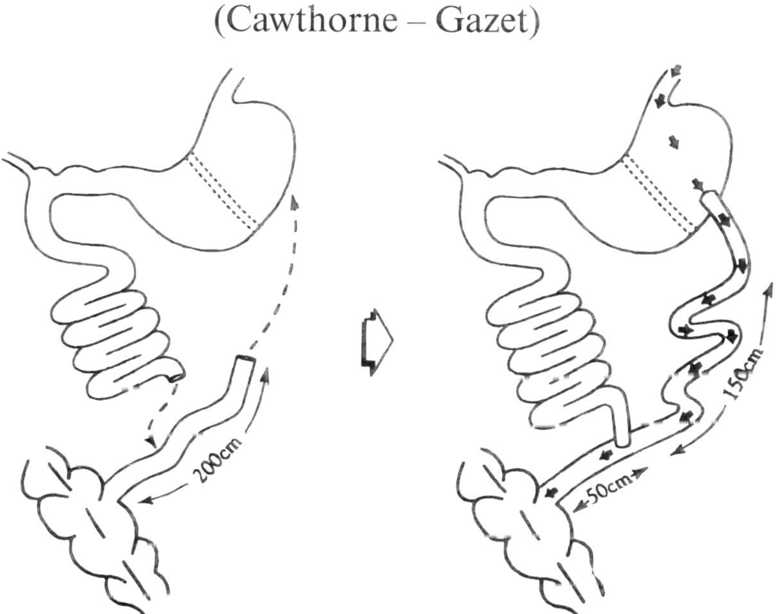

Fig. 12.5 The Cawthorne-Gazet operation was based on reducing the magnitude of the Scopinaro operation and allowing for reversal of the operation if necessary. To avoid antral and duodenal ulceration a truncal vagotomy could be performed or H2 antagonist given.

Vertical banded gastroplasty

Mason (1982), in 1980, described the procedure which with few modifications has become the standard primary procedure for morbid obesity. This technically simple operation carries a low risk, produces minimal disturbance and good weight loss. However, like all procedures, it has some complications.

After a mid-line laparotomy, a 30° French diameter nasogastric tube is passed. The oesophagogastric junction is mobilised using a finger for blunt dissection without vascular division through the lesser omentum behind the stomach up to the greater curve at the oesophagogastric junction. A circular stapler (EEA) producing an end to end anastomosis is used to cut a window in the stomach close to the lesser curve halfway down the lesser curve. This stapled window can be reinforced with sutures to minimise the possibility of a leak.

A linear stapler is then inserted through the gastric window up to the oesophagogastric angle on the greater curve which has been previously mobilised. A TA 90B stapler delivering 4 equidistant rows of staples is then fired to close off the stomach between the window and the oesophagogastric angle (Fig. 12.6).

A teflon tape 1.5 cm wide is wrapped around the channel between the lesser curve and the gastric window and is sutured to prevent stomal dilatation.

A further development, described by Willbanks (1987), is the use of a notched TA90 in which the stapler is placed across the stomach from lesser curve to gastro-oesophageal angle on the greater curve. In the notch of the instrument within the lumen of the stomach lies a nasogastric tube. Once the stapler has been fired a length of silastic tube can be sutured around the lesser curve channel in a similar manner to the tape which was placed through the gastric window. This obviates the production of a gastric window which is a potential site for an anastomotic leak (Fig. 12.6).

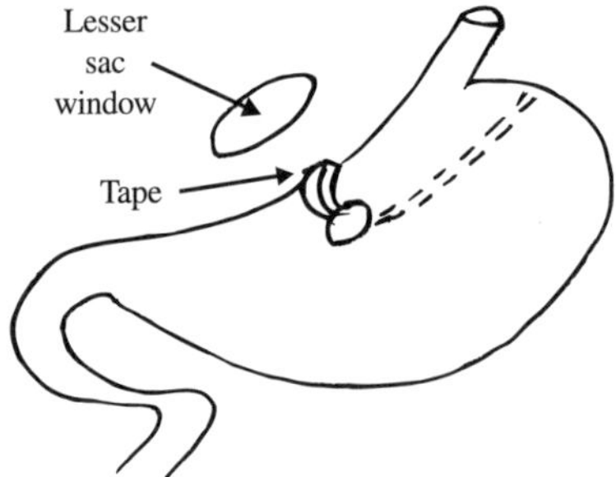

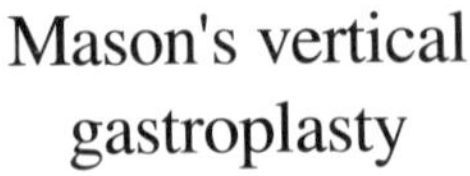

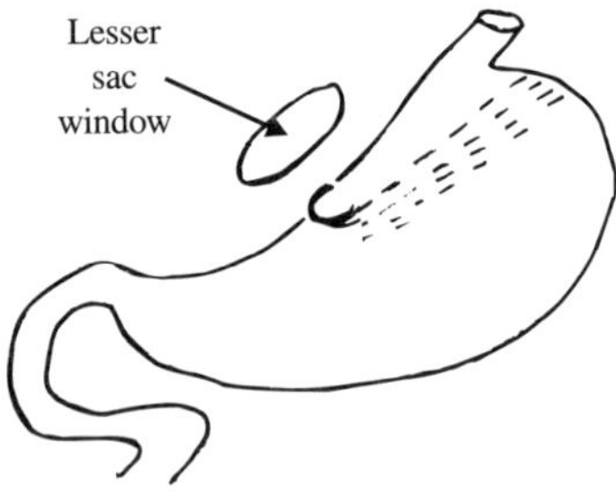

Willbanks' vertical ring gastroplasty

Fig. 12.6 Mason's vertical gastroplasty is the definitive procedure at the present time. Willbrank's notched stapler avoids the gastric window (a site of gastric leaks) and improves the safety and speed of the vertical gastroplasty.

The postoperative management of these patients on a general surgical unit requires a well-motivated and physically strong nursing team. Occasionally pulmonary support is required.

After operation, patients require a liquid diet for the first 6 weeks slowly supplemented by purèed or liquidised food for the succeeding 6 weeks. In effect, it requires a period of 3 months before a light diet can be introduced. This is best supervised by a dedicated dietician as it is essential to add minerals and vitamin supplements to prevent the patients having a too low calorific or mineral intake and developing vitamin deficiency.

The commonest complication in the immediate postoperative period is excess intake of fluid or food which causes repeated vomiting with the possibility of aspiration pneumonia. Excess intake stresses the suture line and must be avoided.

Vertical banded gastroplasty satisfies all the criteria which are required for good bariatric surgery. It produces a small gastric pouch with a small gastric outlet. This leads to a reduced calorie intake. This in all respects is better than a malabsorption syndrome. Needless to say, numerous different techniques have been suggested, but this basic procedure has stood the test of time. Complications include stenosis with ulceration of the gastric outlet, stomal ulceration and bleeding. Gastric leakage, the most serious complication, is uncommon (Table 12.3). Occasionally, erosion of the tape into the lumen has been noted. Stapled dehiscence is an ever present risk but with four rows of staples is rare. The operation can be easily reversed and is basically sound in design provided the execution is meticulous in every aspect.

Table 12.3 Vertical banded gastroplasty. Complications reported in 11 papers and 827 patients selected from the literature in the last 15 years

		Average
Early		
	Death (30 days)	0.5%
	Splenectomy	1.5%
	Gastric haemorrhage	1.0%
	Anastomotic leak	0.5%
	Infection	5.5%
	Pulmonary embolism	0.5%
	Vomiting (in-patient treatment)	8.0%
	Subphrenic abscess	7.0%
Late		
	Staple line failure	3.4%
	Stomal erosion/ulcer	14.1%
	Stomal dilatation	15.0%
	Stomal stenosis	6.0%
	Anaemia	8.0%
	Revision	15.0%
	Incisional hernia	7.0%
	Band erosion	2.0%
	Band removal	9.0%
	Occasional vomiting	76.0%

Table 12.4 Possible operative procedures

- Small bowel
  - Jejunocolic bypass
  - Jejunoileal bypass with ileogastric drainage
  - Jejunoileal bypass with cholecystojejunostomy
  - Duodenoileal bypass
- Stomach gastric bypass
  - Horizontal gastric partition
  - Vertical banded gastroplasty
- Stomach and small bowel
  - Biliopancreatic bypass
- Miscellaneous
  - Teeth wiring
  - Intragastric balloon
  - Vagotomy
  - Gastric banding
  - Gastric wrap
  - Gastroclip gastroplasty

Miscellaneous procedures

Certain procedures need to be discussed if only to be disregarded from future discussion (Table 12.4).

Teeth wiring

This is an effective procedure and will produce a satisfactory weight loss in the short term. Towers (1980) reported that 101 of 104 patients completed periods of jaw fixation resulting in an average loss of 52.6 kg when followed up for a mean fixation of 9 months. It depends upon wiring the teeth as for a fracture of the mandible. The wiring inserted around the teeth in both jaws is kept together by wires or elastic bands. Few patients will continue with the wiring for more than 6 months due to the social stigmata of difficulty of speech and eating. Clearly, it is possible to cheat by sucking in liquidised food but as a preamble to laparotomy in the compromised patient unfit for primary bariatric surgery, it is a useful adjunct. In itself, as a permanent method of producing weight loss, it is useless, as, if it is the only operation suggested, all patients will regain weight as soon as the wires are removed.

Intragastric balloon

The intragastric balloon was a plausible idea as gastric distension had been recognised as a satiety mechanism for many years. Trichobezoars and phytobezoars can present as weight loss in otherwise healthy subjects. However, MacFarland (1986) reviewed 12 grossly obese patients who weighed 121 kg (SD 22 kg) and had a free-floating balloon made of silicone inserted via an oesophagoscopy. These were followed up for up to 2 years. Nine patients lost up to 21 kg (11 ± 6.4 kg) over 3 months after which they reached a plateau. By 1 year, only one patient had maintained her weight loss. Three patients could not tolerate the balloon. There were no complications. The procedure, in his opinion, was useless. Lieber et al (1989), in 1987, reported 45 personal cases in which complications were seen in all but one case. These included persistent pain, nausea and vomiting, gastritis, spontaneous deflation, etc. The overall weight loss was 12% of excess weight (9 kg).

Vagotomy

This was suggested as a bariatric procedure because gastric stasis was noted in patients treated by truncal vagotomy without a drainage procedure in the management of peptic ulceration. In the morbidly obese patient, it is only of value as an adjunct to associated procedures and has never by itself found a useful place.

Gastric wrap, band or clip

A gastric wrap is based on the fundoplication operation for hiatus hernia and is an extension of that procedure. It involves an anterior and posterior mobilisation of the stomach wall and suture of the stomach around the lesser curve, over a gastrointestinal tube. It is, in effect, a reduction of the gastric reservoir.

A whole series of ingenious procedures has been suggested. The stomach may be wrapped in a restrictive cover of teflon or marlex mesh. A further suggestion has been that it is possible to put an external band around the body of the stomach or a plastic clip similar to the Angelchick prosthesis used for treatment of gastro-oesophageal reflux. All these procedures have the well-known problems associated with the introduction of foreign material, such as infection, obstruction, ulceration and haemorrhage.

The extended fundoplication which would appear to be the most satisfactory procedure has not proven its value as the loss of weight is usually less than 10%.

Horizontal gastric partition

A horizontal gastric partition (Gomez or Pace Operation 1979) is an excellent concept, but tends to be ineffective. It has a high failure rate and should not be performed. The concept is to leave an upper pouch of up to 50 ml using a transverse double row of staples across the stomach. The staples are prepared by having three staples removed, two from the upper and one from the lower row, allowing a 9 mm central dehiscence. We performed this procedure 31 times between 1979 and 1982. Overall weight loss was poor (17% at 1 year) and this, in part, was related to the size of the pouch which, when measured radiologically at 1 year following the procedure, averaged 220 ml

(SD 165). Complications were serious with three subphrenic abscesses, one haemorrhage, three outlet stenosis and three incisional hernias in addition to one deep vein thrombosis and one late death. Martin, in 1979, claimed a 75% success in 239 patients over a 2-year period. However, this has not been substantiated by other authors. Furthermore, having removed some staples and not reinforced the opening, staple breakdown is a common complication with subsequent enlargement of the stoma, which defeats the object of the operation. An alternative procedure known as a gastric gastroplasty only complicated what should be a simple procedure. However, Buckwalter and Herbst (1982) have compared the two procedures using greater curvature gastroplasty (GP) in 47 patients and gastroplasty (GG) in 144 patients. Postoperative complications occurred in 25.5% of the GP and 10.4% of the GG patients. No deaths occurred. Re-operation for stomal obstruction was necessary in 14.9% of the GP patients compared with 1.4% of the GG patients. The difference in weight loss following GP and GG were not significantly different and both were equally satisfactory.

ASSESSMENT OF RESULTS

At present, there are no agreed objective standards on how to assess the results of surgery for morbid obesity.

Weight loss is the key, and if reduced to within a 50% range of an ideal body weight will be effective in reducing the sequelae of massive overweight (Table 12.1). Weight loss may be reported as percentage change in relation to original body weight, excess body weight or ideal body weight. It is unsatisfactory to have a report only of kg lost and desirable to record changes in BMI. Most papers report weight loss at 1 or 2 years follow-up.

With regard to the operation, it is difficult to standardise the residual gastric pouch in gastric operations. Neither in the literature or in our experience has a close association been noted between the volume of the gastric pouch and weight loss. There is a closer relationship between the stoma size and rate of pouch emptying with weight loss. Although it is felt that weight loss after gastric procedures is maintained in the long-term, most reports deal with complications and short-term follow up of 1 or 2 years.

Finally, in the literature there are very few long-term follow-up series of any specific procedures and certainly none comparing various surgical procedures in a randomised clinical trial.

PROBLEMS OF BARIATRIC SURGERY

Patients undergoing bariatric surgery, require constant lifelong supervision. Our experience in over 600 patients treated over 20 years was that their attendance was erratic to say the least. Life-threatening complications must be looked for and the surgeon must be ready to reverse the procedure at all times. Failure to lose weight needs to be investigated; in our experience in over 100 vertical gastric bandings, the commonest cause was staple failure.

The follow-up of jejuno-ileal bypass patients continues and suggests that though a third do require urgent reversal, very few of the rest are keen to be converted to a vertical gastric banding whilst they feel well. Except in clinical trials, we have abandoned all procedures apart from the vertical gastric banding.

It has to be accepted that a stable weight is always relative to the original weight and is not related to an ideal weight. When this has been achieved, then redundant skin may require to be excised. An apronectomy is a relatively simple cosmetic procedure and, where necessary, may be combined with repair of an incisional hernia. In women, refashioning of the breast is not so much a breast reduction as a reconstruction of a smaller 'skin brassiere' for the remaining breast. Removal of excessive skin in the thighs will produce unsightly thigh scars; this is much more apparent in arm flaps which, in our view, should not be performed. After bariatric surgery the patient may have developed a satisfactory body image for external appearances but the resultant skin redundancy may severely limit body self esteem.

Follow-up requires routine liver and renal function tests in addition to a full blood profile. It is also necessary to assess from time to time, vitamin B12 absorption, folate absorption and the rare magnesium and zinc levels (Table 12.5). Oxaluria must always be watched for and anaemia is not an uncommon complication. These patients are rewarding to treat but constant surveillance is the key word in their management.

Table 12.5 Clinical investigations

- Before operation
  - Full blood count
  - Liver function test
  - Chest radiograph
  - Electrocardiogram
  - Serum calcium, magnesium, zinc and copper
  - Serum vitamin B12 and folate
  - Vitamin D
  - Serum iron
  - Urinary oxalates
- Follow-up
  - Full blood count
  - Liver function test

These should be performed every 6 months; with anaemia then B12 and folate. All other investigations at 12-monthly interval for 3 years or until stable. Barium studies and gastroscopy as required.

KEY NOTES FOR CLINICAL PRACTICE

- Bariatric surgery is a major undertaking which requires a specialised multidisciplinary team.
- Careful pre-operative assessment and counselling are essential.
- Vertical banded gastroplasty is now the operation of choice.
- Lifelong follow-up is advised to detect and deal with late metabolic and psychological complications.

REFERENCES

Anderson PE, Pilkington TRE, Gazet J-C 1994 Reversal of jejunoileal bypass in patients with morbid obesity. Br J Surg 81: 1015-1017

Buckwalter JA, Herbst CA 1982 Gastric partition for morbid obesity. Greater curvature gastroplasty or gastrogastrostomy World J Surg 6: 403-411

Cuffaro J, Cawthorne S, Gazet J-C 1994 The modified Scopinaro (biliopancreatic bypass) operation: a report of 40 patients. RCSEd/RSM Clinical & Scientific Meeting Workshop on the Surgery of Morbid Obesity, Edinburgh

Garrow JS 1981 Treat obesity seriously. Churchill Livingstone, London

Garrow JS 1994 Should obesity be treated? BMJ 309: 654-655

Gomez CA 1979 Gastroplasty in morbid obesity. Surg Clin North Am 59: 113-120

Gourlay RH, Cleator IGM 1989 Jejunoileal bypass with drainage of the bypassed small bowel into stomach (ileogastrotomy). In: Deitel M (ed) Surgery for the morbidly obese patient. Lea & Febiger, Philadelphia, 91-98

Hallberg D, Holmgren U 1979 Bilio-intestinal shunt: a method and a pilot study for treatment of obesity. Acta Chir Scand 145: 405-408

Lieber CP, Seinige UL, Sataloff DM et al 1989 Intragastric balloon. In: Deitel M (ed) Surgery for the morbidly obese patient. Lea & Febiger, Philadelphia, 289-298

Martin EW, Ellison CE, Tetirick CE, Mojzisik CM, Carey LC, Pace WG 1980 Stapled gastric partitioning. In: Maxwell JD, Gazet J-C, Pilkington TR (eds) Surgical management of obesity. Academic Press, London, 41-52

Mason EE, Ito C 1967 Gastric bypass in obesity. Surg Clin North Am 47: 1345-1352

Mason EE 1982 Vertical banded gastroplasty. Arch Surg 117: 701-706

McFarland RJ 1986 Surgery for obesity with particular referral to jejunoileal bypass, gastric partition and the intragastric balloon. M Chir Thesis, University of Cambridge

Pace WG, Martin EW, Tetirick CE 1979 Gastric partitioning for morbid obesity. Ann Surg 190: 392-401

Payne JH, DeWind LT, Commons PR 1963 Metabolic observations in patients with jejunocolic shunts. Am J Surg 106: 273-289

Riding R, Sugarman HJ 1994 Reversal of jejunoileal bypass in patients with morbid obesity. Br J Surg 81: 18-28

Rubins PC 1994 Commentary: leave obesity alone in healthy and happy patients. BMJ 309: 656.

Scopinaro N, Gianetta E, Civalleri D et al 1979 Biliopancreatic bypass for obesity. II. Initial experience in man. Br J Surg 66: 618-620

Towers JF 1980 Jaw fixation in massive obesity. In: Maxwell JD, Gazet J-C, Pilkington TR (eds) Surgical management of obesity. Academic Press, London, 57-66

Willbanks OL 1987 Longterm results of silicone elastomer ring vertical gastroplasty for the treatment of morbid obesity. Surgery 101: 606-610

Wooley SC, Garner DM 1994 Dietary treatments for obesity are ineffective. BMJ 309: 655-656

13

The surgical management of cutaneous malignant melanoma

D. S. Soutar

Surgeons entering the twenty-first century should not forget the advantages they have over their predecessors. This is not confined to our improved understanding of the biological behaviour and the natural history of malignant melanoma, but includes advances in medicine, anaesthesia, surgery, histopathology and investigative radiology which have increased our ability to stage disease accurately.

The role of surgery in the management of cutaneous malignant melanoma is not confined to excision of the primary lesion with or without the regional lymph nodes in continuity or discontinuity. It now includes complicated procedures involving extra-corporeal circulation, as in isolated limb perfusion, and surgical techniques capable of dealing with distant metastases to other organs. With this increasing role, surgery continues to be the major therapeutic option for cutaneous malignant melanoma.

NATURAL HISTORY OF CUTANEOUS MALIGNANT MELANOMA

In common with other malignant conditions, complete surgical excision can result in cure. All too often, however, the tumour recurs locally or spreads to involve the regional lymph nodes or appears as subcutaneous nodules between the primary and the draining lymph node basin (intransit metastases) or is disseminated through the body to appear as distant metastases in lung, liver and brain (Fig. 13.1). There is no evidence of a linear progression through all the stages of malignant melanoma and even small seemingly innocuous lesions can give rise to widespread distant metastases and death.

A significant advance in staging came with the realisation that superficial or thin melanomas had a better prognosis than thick melanomas (Allan & Spitz 1953). This subsequently led to a classification based on the depth of invasion of melanoma which was developed by Clark et al (1969). The following year, Breslow (1970) described what is probably a more reproducible measurement where the actual thickness is measured from the top of the granular layer of the epidermis to the deepest level of invasion of melanoma cells.

Many series have pointed to the importance of tumour thickness in predicting survival. Recently, a multivariate study of over 4500 patients com-

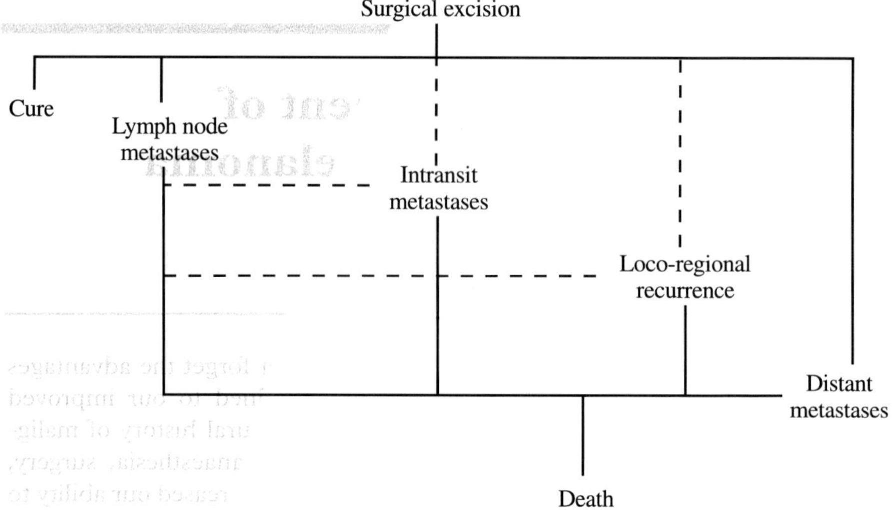

Fig. 13.1 Schematic representation of the natural history of cutaneous melanoma.

bining two large series from the University of Alabama at Birmingham (UAB) and the Sydney Melanoma Unit (SMU) demonstrated that tumour thickness at diagnosis is the single most important prognostic indicator for all outcomes (Soong et al 1992). This includes not only survival but local recurrence, regional recurrence and distant metastases. This study also identified other factors which correlated well with the overall survival for some of the tumour thickness sub-groups (Table 13.1).

The vital importance of tumour thickness has now been adopted in the staging system for melanoma by both the International Union Against Cancer (UICC) and the American Joint Committee on Cancer (AJCC). Both Clark level and Breslow thickness are now included in the T-staging (Table 13.2: UICC 1992).

Unfortunately, there have been many staging systems devised and revised over the past 20 years so that no single system has been universally accepted. Most research groups have, therefore, had to make arbitrary decisions when defining good, intermediate and poor prognosis categories. The Scottish

Table 13.1 Factors predicting melanoma recurrence and death

Prognostic Factor	Disease free interval			
	Diagnosis–2 years	2–5 years	5–10 years	10 years +
Tumour thickness	++++	++++	++++	++++
Ulceration	++++		++	
Lesion localisation	++++	++++		++

Modified from Soong et al 1992.

Table 13.2 TNM classification of cutaneous malignant melanoma (Hemanek & Sobin 1992)

Primary Tumour			
PT_1	≤ 0.75 mm	Level II	
PT_2	0.75–1.5 mm	Level III	
$PT3_a$	1.5–3.00 mm	Level IV	
$PT3_b$	3.00–4.00 mm	Level IV	
$PT4_a$	> 4.00 mm	Level V	
$PT4_b$	Satellite(s) within 2 cm of primary tumour		
Stage grouping			
Stage I	PT_1	N_0	M_0
	PT_2	N_0	M_0
Stage II	PT_3	N_0	M_0
Stage III	PT_4	N_0	M_0
	Any PT	N_1N_2	M_0
Stage IV	Any PT	Any N	M_1

Melanoma Group, for example, has adopted three arbitrarily selected thickness groups, namely 0–1.49 mm, 1.5–3.49 mm and over 3.5 mm (Mackie et al 1992). There is no worldwide agreement over the classification of thin, intermediate and thick melanomas and it is important in reviewing the literature to be aware of differences. These problems with staging remain a hindrance to progress. There is perhaps a natural reluctance amongst surgeons to plan their treatment on one single prognostic factor. Park et al (1993) in a study of thin melanomas less than 1.5 mm thickness showed 30 recurrences in a series of 555 cases: 4 recurrences were local, i.e. within 2 cm of the primary complete excision, and 26 were metastatic, including 2 intransit metastases and 24 regional lymph node metastases. This study also showed no evidence of recurrence in any tumour less than 1 mm in thickness which was completely excised and this was irrespective of the width of excision.

Local recurrence

The major concern about local recurrence is that it is associated with a poor prognosis. Cruse et al (1992), in a retrospective series of 382 patients with stage I and stage II disease, looked at actuarial survival curves taken from the day of diagnosis of the primary tumour. There was a significant decrease in survival in those patients who developed local recurrence as the initial recurrence compared with patients that remained disease free. Furthermore, 10-year actuarial survival curves of patients with local recurrence were the same as those who developed regional or systemic recurrence as the first recurrence when survival was calculated from the date of diagnosis of the primary malignant melanoma.

Intransit metastases

Intransit metastases are located in the subcutaneous tissue between the primary site and the regional nodes. They are thought to originate from melanoma cells trapped in lymphatic vessels. Sometimes intransit metastases appear in the skin as intracutaneous metastases which are termed satellites. The presence of satellites, or intransit metastases, has now been incorporated into the staging system (see Table 13.2). Satellites within 2 cm of the primary tumour are staged as if part of the primary tumour (PT_4). Intransit metastases are staged as for nodal metastases (N_2). Isolated intransit metastases are exceedingly rare and usually occur in conjunction with metastases to the regional lymph nodes. The incidence of intransit metastases is probably in the region of 2%. It has been suggested that intransit metastases are related to lymphoedema following lymphadenectomy or to entrapment in the lymph channels between the primary site and the regional nodal basin. There is little scientific evidence for this, however, since the patients at risk for intransit metastases are the same as those at risk of developing lymph node metastases, namely those with thick primary tumours showing ulceration (Milton et al 1980, Roses et al 1983).

Lymph node metastases

The importance of regional lymph node metastases cannot be overemphasised. It is the most common presentation of metastatic melanoma and is associated with a poor prognosis. Woods (1989) believes that the presence of nodal metastases is the single most important determinant in outlook for melanoma. When nodal metastases are present, the patients' survival may be less than half that of patients without nodal involvement. It is estimated that somewhere between 70–85% of patients will have distant metastases by the time regional nodes are detected clinically and that, in such cases, 10-year survival falls to approximately 10% (Balch et al 1981). More recently, the major determinant of survival has been shown to be the pathological stage (PS) of disease with stage III disease leading to survival of 39% at 5 years falling to 32% at 10 years and stage IV having 9% survival at 5 years (Coit et al 1991).

There are obviously common factors which relate to local recurrence, regional lymph node metastases, intransit metastases and their recurrences. In looking at the natural history of malignant melanoma, somewhere in the region of 30–40% of patients with stage I or stage II disease will suffer a relapse of melanoma (Cruse et al 1992, Griffiths & Briggs 1984) and this increases with the increasing thickness of the tumour, the presence of ulceration, increasing age and specific anatomical sites. Loco-regional disease is by far the commonest site of first relapse and it is reported that 87.5% of recurrences in extremity melanomas occur in the local/regional area, either as local recurrence, intransit metastases or regional node metastases (Reintgen et al 1987).

Distant metastases

A recent analysis of 144 patients with distant metastases has demonstrated that survival is dependent on the anatomical site of the metastases and also the number of metastases resected with single metastases doing best (Wong et al 1993). The overall 5-year survival is quoted as 20%, with the overall 10-year survival as 14%. In the management of distant metastases from cutaneous malignant melanoma, surgery does have a role to play. Solitary subcutaneous, nonregional lymph nodes and lung metastases are the most likely to benefit from excisional surgery. Treatment should be regarded, however, as palliative and is often carried out in conjunction with other modalities of treatment, such as systemic chemotherapy or local radiotherapy.

More recently, a retrospective multivariate analysis of 114 cases of distant metastases has shown a median survival of 19 months (Karakousis et al 1994). Factors of prognostic significance with regard to survival include location of metastases with subcutaneous lesions being better than metastases in vital organs, such as liver or brain, thickness of the primary tumour and the presence or absence of prior regional disease.

DILEMMAS IN SURGICAL MANAGEMENT

It is the unpredictable nature of primary cutaneous malignant melanoma that continues to pose problems in surgical management. Clinicians are desperately seeking prognostic indicators and predictors of outcome that will enable them to counsel their patients and institute appropriate investigation and treatment. The natural history of cutaneous melanoma previously discussed highlights some of the problems that the surgeon will face.

Diagnosis and prognostic indicators

Biopsy

Excision biopsy is the mainstay of diagnosis and should be encouraged in preference to incision biopsy. There is conflicting evidence regarding the risk of incision biopsy with regard to overall prognosis but complete excision avoids any sampling errors and allows the histopathologist the whole specimen for detailed investigation. Histopathology plays a key role in determining prognostic indicators and the natural history of a particular melanoma. As mentioned previously, the thickness of the melanoma (Breslow or Clark level) is essential in staging the disease.

The type of melanoma, whether it is nodular, superficial spreading, lentigo maligna, or acral, is not thought to have any significance in survival. It is noted that lesions of the hands and feet have a generally unfavourable prognosis (Schmueckel et al 1983) and these are the sites commonly of acral lentiginous melanoma. Lentigo maligna melanoma previously thought to have a good prognosis has shown no difference in 5-year mortality compared to other histogenetic types of melanoma of equal thickness (Cox et al 1987).

Apart from tumour thickness, no other pathological feature of melanoma has been consistently shown to be a reliable prognostic indicator. Features studied include mitotic rate, phase of tumour growth, evidence of vascular or lymphatic invasion, lymphocytic response and the presence or absence of abnormal melanoyctes adjacent to the tumour.

The size of the primary tumour and the presence of regression, particularly in thin melanomas (Breslow < 1.5 mm) have been shown to be associated with a poor prognosis (Park et al 1993). The presence of ulceration does appear to be an independent variable of poor prognosis (Soong et al 1992, Yeung 1993).

Site

Anatomical site does play a major part in influencing surgical decisions. Where there is plenty of tissue available and no reconstruction is required, then it is a simple procedure to perform a fairly wide local excision. There is also some debate as to whether some sites in the body have a better prognosis. Recently, in an analysis of 8500 patients, a correlation between anatomical site and survival has been shown. The arm has the best prognosis; this gets worse on the leg and the trunk and is worst of all in the head and neck (Balch et al 1992).

Other features

Women appear to have a survival advantage in melanoma when one compares thickness for thickness but increasing age is associated with a poorer prognosis (Mackie et al 1992, McHenry et al 1992). At the present time, the commonest features liable to influence surgical decisions are:

- Tumour thickness
- Ulceration
- Anatomical location
- Sex of patient
- Age of patient

Resection margins for primary cutaneous melanoma

In the past, local recurrence has been seen as surgical failure to excise the primary disease adequately. Combined with the poor prognosis associated with patients developing local recurrence, it is not surprising that surgeons advocated wide excision margins for cutaneous melanoma.

A variety of studies have now shown that local recurrence in melanomas less than 1 mm in thickness is rare and that the risk of local recurrence increases with the thickness of melanoma (Breslow 1970, Balch et al 1979, Milton et al 1980, Griffiths & Briggs 1986).

The World Health Organization (WHO) Melanoma Group undertook a retrospective study of 593 patients with stage I cutaneous malignant melanoma (Cascinelli et al 1980). This study caused great controversy when it reported a 9.3% local recurrence rate in lesions greater than 1 mm thickness when excision was less than 3 cm, compared to a 3.2% local recurrence rate when excision was equal to or greater than 3 cm; but when the patients were divided arbitrarily into groups of thickness greater than 2 mm and less than 2 mm and resection margins were divided into greater than 2 cm and less than 2 cm, there was no significant difference between narrower and wider excisions. Rampen (1981), in reviewing the figures, noted that local recurrence following excision of melanomas more than 2 mm thick was significantly higher with excision margins of 2 cm or less when compared to margins in excess of 2 cm. Milton et al (1985) also expressed doubts about the safety of narrow excisions and reported an unacceptable local recurrence rate in malignant melanomas of greater than 3 mm thickness when narrow excision margins (1 cm) were used. The local recurrence rate was reported at 27% and compared unfavourably with the recurrence rate of 7% when similar tumours were treated with a 2–3 cm margin. Evans and McCann (1990) have suggested basing excision on Breslow thickness and the Clark level (Table 13.3) and reported the interim results in 806 cases. Hughes and his co-workers (Neades et al 1993) have advocated a rather ingenious surgical method of determining the excision margin based on whether the lesion is impalpable, palpable or frankly nodular and have suggested a 1 cm, 2 cm and 3 cm margin, respectively. They have shown an overall local recurrence rate of 2.5% in a series of 434 patients and demonstrated the accuracy of clinical examination relating to Breslow thickness. They now advocate a policy of 2 cm margins for palpable and nodular lesions and a 1 cm excision margin for impalpable lesions.

In an attempt to clarify the situation, the World Health Organization Melanoma Group organised a prospective, randomised study which began in 1980 (Veronesi & Cascinelli 1991). The study comprised 612 patients who had a stage I cutaneous malignant melanoma not greater than 2 mm in thickness; 305 patients underwent excision with a 1 cm margin and 307 patients had excision with a 3 cm margin. 84 patients (13.7%) subsequently had relapse of their disease (see Table 13.4). Although survival was better in the

Table 13.3 Protocol for the treatment of stage I cutaneous melanoma

Risk group	Staging		Excision margin
Low	< 0.76 mm	Clark II or III	2 mm (i.e. biopsy)
Medium	< 0.76 0.76–1.5 mm	Clark IV All	20 mm
High	> 1.5 mm All	Clark IV Clark V	50 mm

Modified from Evans and McCann 1990.

Table 13.4 WHO melanoma programme trial 10, site of first relapse

	Narrow excision 1 cm (n = 305)	Wide excision 3 cm (n = 307)
Local recurrence	4	0
Intransit metastases	2	2
Regional node metastases	21	24
Distant metastases	17	14
TOTAL	44	40

Modified from Veronesi and Cascinelli 1991.

thin melanomas less than 1 mm when compared to the remainder, the wider excision did not improve disease free or overall survival times. Critics of this study have pointed to the fact that local recurrences occur in the narrow excision group and that in fact the number of local recurrences has now increased with longer follow-up (Marsden 1993). Of equal importance is the fact that of the four local recurrences reported, two died of melanoma, one developed lymph node metastases and in transit metastases and one patient underwent wide local excision and showed no evidence of disease at the time of writing. A progress report of this trial was given in June 1993 (Marsden 1993), by which time local recurrence in the narrow excision group had risen to six and there had been one local recurrence in the wide excision group. The total number of relapses had also increased to 53 in the narrow excision and 51 in the wide excision groups.

Another prospective randomised multi-centre trial has looked at the effectiveness of 2 cm excision margins in dealing with intermediate thickness melanomas (1–4 mm thickness). This prospective trial comprised 486 patients with melanomas confined to the trunk and proximal extremities. The patients were randomised into two groups to have 2 cm excision or 4 cm excision. The need for skin grafting was reduced from 46% to 11% in the smaller excision group and hospital stay was reduced. There was no difference between the two groups in local recurrence rate, intransit metastases or overall survival but the study was complicated by further randomisation to receive elective lymph node dissection (ELND) or a 'wait and see' policy (Balch et al 1993).

Currently, there appears to be a significant balance of evidence to support narrowing the excision margins in malignant melanoma. Despite this, there is no uniformity of surgical opinion with widely varying protocols for surgical management (Timmons 1993). There is, however, good evidence that in thin melanomas a simple local excision with narrow margins is sufficient treatment and there is no clear evidence that increasing excision margins improves survival. The incidence of local recurrence, however, increases with tumour thickness and therefore tempts the surgeon to use a wider excision margin for thicker lesions. It is the arbitrary division into thin, intermediate

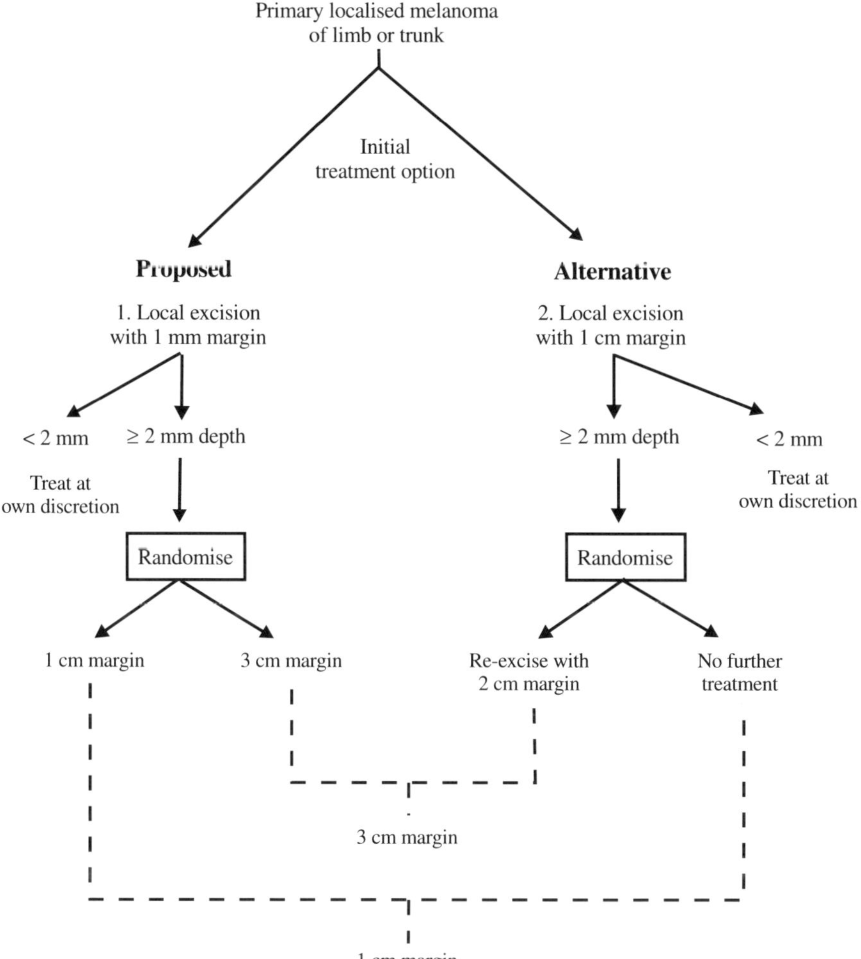

Fig. 13.2 Randomised trial of width excision of thick cutaneous malignant melanoma (1 cm vs 3 cm margin). Melanoma Sudy Group and British Association of Plastic Surgeons.

and thick melanomas that remains a problem in surgical management. The British Melanoma Study Group in conjunction with the British Association of Plastic Surgeons are currently undertaking a randomised controlled trial of 1 and 3 cm excision margins for primary cutaneous melanomas 2 mm or more in thickness. Recruitment in the trial is progressing satisfactorily and the outline is shown in Figure 13.2.

On a cautionary note, we must remember that even thin melanomas can be fatal (Park et al 1993). In an attempt to identify patients at risk, Slingluff et al (1988) have designed a prognostic model based on risk factors which they have identified as a male patient, axial sited lesions, lesions showing severe regression and Clark level IV. Other authors have identified high risk categories for developing local recurrence, particularly tumour thickness, ulceration and increasing age with particularly high recurrence rates in the foot and hand (Urist et al 1985).

One further complication of looking at the safety margins for excision of melanoma concerns the incidence of late recurrence which varies from 1–7%. In the largest series (Shaw et al 1985), none of the factors of prognostic significance in the treatment of the primary lesion, such as thickness, ulceration, anatomical site, sex and age proved to be of any value in determining those at risk of developing late recurrence. The importance of local recurrence lies in its effect on overall prognosis. Local recurrence is usually associated with a poorer prognosis. Parallel to this is the fact that local recurrence rates rise with increasing thickness of melanoma ranging from about 0–2% for tumours less than 1 mm thick to approximately 10% for tumours 4 mm thick or more (Milton et al 1980, Milton et al 1985, Griffiths & Briggs 1986, Ames et al 1992). In the current state of our knowledge, there is no evidence that wide excision margins confer any survival advantage on patients with malignant melanoma. There is similarly no clear evidence that wide margins diminish the incidence of intransit metastases, regional lymph node metastases or distant metastases. Current opinion favours narrow excision for thin melanomas, certainly of those less than 1 mm and probably for melanomas less than 1.5 mm in thickness. Whether narrow excision is a safe option for thicker melanomas is a subject of continued controversy and will require analysis of ongoing prospective randomised trials. Currently, however, there is no evidence that excision wider than 3 cm confers any advantage in controlling local recurrence.

Regional lymph nodes

Despite the poor prognosis of patients who develop clinically positive regional lymph nodes, there is a surgical consensus that the best treatment for such involved nodes is surgical removal. It is perhaps debatable as to whether such treatment is therapeutic or palliative but it does appear to be a reasonable surgical principle to reduce the tumour burden, to attempt to gain regional control of the disease, and to assist in accurate staging of the disease.

Furthermore, the extent of involvement of regional lymph nodes also seems to be an important prognostic indicator. A favourable outcome may be achieved if there is microscopic nodal involvement or where the number of positive nodes is less than 3. Extranodal disease and extracapsular spread are poor prognostic signs (Woods 1989, Coit 1991).

Although there is no controversy about the role of therapeutic lymph node dissection in clinically positive nodes, there is considerable debate about the value of elective lymph node dissection (ELND) in the treatment of clinically node negative patients. The importance of the thickness of the primary tumour and the presence or absence of ulceration, in predicting lymph node metastases has been confirmed by many series.

Melanomas less than 1 mm thick are not usually prone to developing lymph node metastases and cure rates in excess of 95% are reported after local excision alone. The risk of developing nodal metastases increases with the thickness of the primary cutaneous melanoma such that in primary melanomas of greater than 4 mm, there is a 60% incidence of regional nodal metastases and possibly greater than 70% incidence of occult distant metastases at presentation (Stankard 1992).

There is general surgical agreement that such elective lymph node dissection is not warranted in thin malignant melanomas (< 0.76 mm) where the risk of lymph node metastases is small and the prognosis is so good that any benefit of ELND would not be demonstrable. Similarly, for thick melanomas (≥ 4 mm) where the risk of lymph node metastases is over 60% and where there is a high association with occult distant disease, there again would be no therapeutic benefit in ELND.

Controversy has, therefore, centred around the intermediate thickness melanomas (0.76–4 mm) staged as clinically node negative at the time of presentation. Several extensive retrospective studies have purported to show a distinct survival advantage in this group of patients with intermediate thickness melanomas who underwent elective lymph node dissection (Balch et al 1985, McCarthy et al 1985). Taking an opposing view are the results of two randomised prospective clinical trials, one performed by the World Health Organization (Veronesi et al 1982a) and the other from the Mayo Clinic (Sim et al 1986). Despite all the arguments that surround the problems of retrospective versus prospective trials, methods of statistical analysis, randomisation, and control populations for comparison, there is as yet no clear evidence of the value of elective lymph node dissection (Harris et al 1995). Perhaps one of the problems is that the grouping of 0.76–4 mm as a classification for intermediate thickness melanoma appears to some authors, including this writer, to be too broad a category. It is likely that further subdivisions on the basis of known prognostic indicators such as tumour thickness, ulceration, sex, site and age, will need to be taken into account. We await with interest the results of prospective randomised controlled trials that are in progress in the hope that the role of elective lymph node dissection can be elucidated.

Unfortunately, there are other problems that surround the surgical management of regional lymph nodes. Lymphatic drainage patterns for particular sites can be difficult to determine but may be defined using lymphoscintigraphy (Loong & Balch 1985, Berman et al 1992). In addition to accurately defining lymphatic drainage and regional lymph nodes, there is also the question of morbidity associated with regional node dissection. It is perhaps not surprising that there has been a natural reluctance amongst surgeons, particularly in Europe, to carry out elective lymph node dissection.

Node sampling

An appealing compromise is node sampling, which would allow identification of occult metastases, and when these are present, a full regional node dissection could be performed. Wong et al (1991) demonstrated that after injection of isosulfan blue intradermally, the dye was taken up to a first stage lymph node which he termed the sentinel node. This technique was applied clinically by Morton et al (1992) and they reported the successful identification of sentinel nodes in 194 of 237 cases. They also showed positive metastases in 21% with a false positive rate of less than 1%. This paper also quoted survival rates as 27% higher for patients undergoing elective lymph node dissection for occult metastases when compared to patients undergoing therapeutic lymph node dissection for palpable lymph nodes.

Dye directed selective lymphadenectomy has further been refined. A recent protocol highlights high risk primary cutaneous malignant melanoma of Clark level III, Breslow thickness greater than 0.65 mm, tumours showing regression and cases where there is incomplete excision (Cochran et al 1992). The sentinel node is identified using an injection dye technique and the node is examined at frozen section by haematoxylin and eosin stains and immunohistochemical techniques. Where the node is positive for metastatic disease (approximately 20%), a complete en bloc lymph node dissection is performed. These authors report that 29% of melanoma patients regarded as stage I by standard clinical evaluation actually prove to have lymph node metastases.

This technique offers surgeons who are reluctant to carry out radical lymphadenectomy the opportunity to biopsy the sentinel node and to undertake appropriate treatment on the results of histological examination.

Recurrent malignant melanoma

The term recurrence implies the reappearance of malignant disease at the site of previous treatment. Recurrence may occur locally, either at the site of primary excision, or in the regional nodes, or in the tissue between these two sites.

Local recurrence

Recurrence within a scar or graft at the site of primary excision of a malignant melanoma is undoubtedly local recurrence. Also included is tumour adjacent to such scars within a radius that varies between 1–5 cm. The risk of local recurrence increases with increasing thickness of melanoma, being exceptionally rare in thin melanomas less than 0.76 mm (0–0.2%) and much more common in thick tumours of 4 mm or greater (10–13.2%). In addition to tumour thickness, ulceration, increasing age, and certain sites such as hand and feet, are highly significant predictors of recurrence. Local recurrence does not appear to be influenced by the width of excision of the primary tumour, particularly in thin melanomas and possibly in intermediate thickness melanomas, although this is currently undergoing further study in prospective randomised trials. There is also no evidence that excision margins greater than 3 cm reduce the incidence of local recurrence (Milton et al 1980, Ames et al 1992).

Such reports indicate that in completely excised malignant melanoma, subsequent local recurrence is not a factor related to excision but indicates the aggressive nature of the primary tumour. In considering the surgical management of local recurrence, one has to think in terms of the disease already being disseminated. A wider excision can be carried out to excise completely the local recurrence and attention should be focused on the regional lymph nodes if they have not previously been surgically excised. Lymphoscintigraphy might help in identifying the drainage lymphatic systems and dye directed sentinel node biopsy might also be of value. In the management of recurrent melanoma in limbs, isolated limb perfusion becomes an important surgical option.

Recurrent lymph node disease

Even in patients undergoing lymphadenectomy, whether therapeutic or elective, there is an incidence of further relapse of disease. In a retrospective analysis of 4323 patients (Calabro et al 1989), 26% of patients developed lymph node metastases. Of these, 1001 consecutive patients were available for study to assess the patterns of relapse. Recurrence within the nodal basin occurred in 15% of cervical node dissections, 15% of axillary dissections and 17% of the inguinal dissections. Such recurrence was related to extranodal spread and to the number of lymph nodes involved at the primary operation. In this series, it was also noted that 10% of patients developed intransit metastases after lymph node dissection and the incidence of intransit metastases was dependent on the number of positive nodes and also the presence of extranodal spread. Distant metastases arose in 68% and again this appeared to be related to the extent of the tumour burden, namely the number of positive nodes and the presence or absence of extranodal disease. In another series of 1019 patients who underwent lymphadenectomy, 40% were found to show evidence of further disease (Gadd & Coit 1992). This review was confined to melanomas of the extremity and trunk and 72% showed evidence of recurrent disease at a single site with a median survival of 11 months, whereas the remaining 28% showed disease at multiple sites and had a median survival of only 3 months.

The surgical treatment for recurrent nodal metastases is further excision. Where there has been an incomplete previous lymph node dissection then a complete radical lymphadenectomy can be performed. In cases where there has previously been a complete clearance, recurrence is usually very close to the site of previous surgery and in such situations wide local excision of the melanoma deposits can be undertaken. Frequently, in such situations, surgery is combined with other modalities of treatment, either in the form of chemotherapy and/or radiotherapy.

Intransit metastases

As previously stated, intransit metastases are most frequently seen in combination with disease in lymph nodes, and together with local recurrence and lymph node recurrence, common prognostic factors pertain. In addition, intransit metastases found in 10% of patients who underwent lymph node dissection were found to be related to both the number of positive nodes and the presence of extranodal spread (Calabro et al 1989).

Isolated limb perfusion

The high incidence of loco-regional problems in extremity melanomas prompted surgeons to investigate methods of giving high dose chemotherapy to the affected limb. Thus the techniques of isolated limb perfusion were developed. This technique has been described in a previous edition of *Recent Advances in Surgery* (Rosin 1991).

Isolated limb perfusion is currently the treatment of choice for recurrent melanoma which is confined to an extremity and has proved useful in dealing with local and intransit metastases. Krementz et al (1994) have published their experience in isolated limb perfusion over the past 35 years. This includes 1139 patients with malignant melanoma. In common with many centres reporting the results of isolated limb perfusion, they have used the MD Anderson Cancer Center staging which is very useful in defining loco-regional recurrence. The cumulative 10-year and 20-year survival rates for limb melanomas are shown in Table 13.5. In the light of their experience, they list as their indications for isolated limb perfusion:

- Definitive treatment of intransit metastases, non-resectable recurrences or non-resectable tumours.
- Adjunct to surgical excision for regionally confined poor prognosis melanoma.
- To convert advanced non-resectable lesions to operability.

Table 13.5 Cutaneous melanoma of limbs (n = 1088) treated by regional limb perfusion

Stage (MD Anderson)		Number of cases	Cumulative survival 10 years	20 years
Stage I	Localised primary tumour	458	70%	56%
Stage II	Local recurrence/satellites	36	61%	42%
Stage IIIA	Intransit metastases	143	30%	18%
Stage IIIB	Removal node metastases	180	39%	30%
Stage IIIAB	Intransit & regional metastases	145	17%	10%
Stage IV	Distant metastases	126	8%	8%
	TOTAL	1088		

Modified from Krementz et al 1994.

- Palliation to maintain a functional limb even in the presence of systemic metastases.

Regrettably, there has to date been only one prospective randomised study in which 107 patients with extremity melanomas were randomised to have either wide local excision and regional lymph node dissection or wide local excision, regional lymph node dissection and hyperthermic isolated perfusion with melphalanan. With stage I, stage II and stage III disease, there was a considerable advantage in the perfused group which showed a much lower rate of recurrence (Ghussen et al 1984, 1989).

Recently, a preliminary report of a randomised trial of prophylactic isolated limb perfusion for stage I high risk (greater than 1.5 mm thickness melanoma) has been reported (Krementz et al 1994). The initial results of this study showed that while perfusion may reduce the incidence of locoregional disease in the form of lymph node metastases, local recurrence or intransit metastases, the overall survival appears to remain the same.

In the current state of our understanding, isolated limb perfusion does appear to be of use in controlling recurrent disease in extremities and may improve survival in this group of patients. There is, as yet, no definitive evidence that adjuvant isolated limb perfusion confers any advantage over traditional surgical treatments for extremity melanomas as far as survival is concerned.

It is worth considering repeat isolated perfusion in cases that continue to show residual and recurrent disease. This can often be used in palliation to preserve a functioning limb since there is a high probability that such cases have distant metastases.

Distant metastases

The management of distant metastases requires the involvement of other disciplines. In the surgical field, this may involve neurosurgeons, cardiothoracic surgeons and abdominal surgeons with a special interest in liver diseases. Subcutaneous non-regional lymph nodes and single lung metastases are the most likely to benefit from excisional surgery. Karakousis et al (1994) concluded that excision of distant metastases has an application in approximately 25% of patients with disseminated malignant melanoma.

Adjuvant treatments

There is a natural tendency when dealing with high risk primary tumours to seek ancillary treatments in an attempt to lessen the risk of recurrence following definitive surgery. Such adjuvant treatments include radiotherapy, isolated limb perfusion, chemotherapy and more recently immunotherapy and targeted gene therapy.

Adjuvant isolated limb perfusion does not appear to confer any survival advantage. Similarly, most randomised trials looking at adjuvant chemotherapy have failed to demonstrate improved survival (Fisher et al 1981, Veronesi et al, 1982, Meisenberg et al 1993).

Melanoma is not a particularly radiosensitive tumour and therefore adjuvant radiotherapy is not commonly advocated. It is, however, used in cases with nodal metastases where complete surgical excision has been in doubt, particularly in the head and neck region, but its effect on improving survival is as yet unproven. Newer therapies incorporating the use of vaccines and gene targeted therapy are in their infancy and may hold promise for the future. This is an area requiring a high level of expertise and control and patients should only be submitted to this type of treatment in a carefully controlled study.

Barth and Morton (1995) have reviewed a variety of adjuvant treatment protocols including chemotherapy, radiotherapy, isolated limb perfusion and immunotherapy. They concluded that none of the published prospective randomised trials so far has clearly demonstrated a significant benefit of adjuvant treatment in patients with a high risk of recurrence.

Palliative treatment

Many of the above treatments may be used in palliation and these include radiotherapy, chemotherapy, isolated limb perfusion and excisional surgery. Laser ablation is an increasingly popular treatment for palliation, particularly of subcutaneous and cutaneous deposits which often worry patients. There have been recent encouraging reports of laser ablation of subcutaneous deposits using a carbon dioxide laser (Lingham & McKay 1994).

Resource management

When looking at the natural history of malignant melanoma, there are significant resource implications for the National Health Service.

In addition to the surgical aspects of malignant melanoma, there is also the question of follow-up. It is clear that high risk groups have to be identified for regular and continuous follow-up. This is difficult in melanoma because of the unpredictable nature of the disease and the incidence of late recurrences (Shaw et al 1985). On the other hand, by far the majority of relapses occur within the first few years of diagnosis and treatment of the primary cutaneous lesion; 90% of all first tumour recurrences occur within 5 years (Griffiths & Briggs, 1984). It is also reported that 65% of all recurrences occur within the first 3 years of follow-up but it should be noted that relapses after 5 years can occur in up to 20% of patients ((Cruse et al 1992). Unfortunately, we cannot use the normal prognostic parameters to identify patients who should be followed up for longer periods of time. The high risk group patients will probably recur or metastasise within the 3–5 year follow-up and, therefore, do not help us define the problem satisfactorily. The single most important prognostic indicator throughout remains tumour thickness

(Table 13.1). Patient education is vitally important and regular follow-up in the early postoperative period should alert patients to look for and identify specific signs or symptoms. Regan et al (1985) demonstrated that 69% of patients with recurrence detected this themselves prior to attending a review clinic.

Prevention and early diagnosis

The importance of patient education with regard to the dangers of sun exposure cannot be over-emphasised. Elder (1995) has recently reported a dramatic increase in skin cancers over a 15-year period. He did, however, notice increasing survival rates for individual cases suggesting patients were presenting earlier for diagnosis and treatment. His series also reported a 600% increase in *in situ* melanomas, again suggesting earlier presentation.

All efforts in the direction of preventative medicine and patient education are to be actively encouraged and perhaps in the future, although the incidence is increasing, we will see a gradual improvement in survival as patients present with early, thin lesions which are readily amenable to surgical excision.

KEY POINTS FOR CLINICAL PRACTICE

- The incidence of malignant melanoma of the skin is increasing in virtually every country where records are kept for epidemiological study.
- There is an increasing number of early melanomas suggesting that patient education is leading to earlier diagnosis. Resection margins are becoming narrower, particularly for thin melanomas.
- Increasing resection margins beyond 3 cm confers no survival advantage.
- Direct wound closure and avoidance of skin grafts have significant impact on hospital resources.
- The case for elective lymph node dissection has still to be proven. Dye injected sentinel node biopsy is a useful alternative to a 'wait and see' policy.
- Adjuvant treatments have yet to show significant improvement in survival. Important questions remain to be answered and require controlled trials with uniform protocols.
- Isolated limb perfusion is an established technique with a good record in the control of loco-regional disease.
- Laser ablation using a CO_2 laser is an effective tool for surgical palliation.
- Distant metastases may benefit from surgical excision.

REFERENCES

Allan AC, Spitz S 1953 Malignant melanoma: a clinicopathological analysis of the criteria for diagnosis and prognosis. Cancer 6: 1-45

Ames FC, Balch CM, Reintgen D 1992 Local recurrences and their management. In: Balch CM, Houghton AN, Milton GW, Sober AJ, Soong S-J (eds) Cutaneous melanoma 2nd edn. Lippincott, Philadelphia, 287-294
Balch CM, Murad TM, Soong S-J et al 1979 Tumour thickness as a guide to surgical management of clinical stage I melanoma patients. Cancer 43: 883-888
Balch CM, Soong S-J, Murad TM et al 1981 A multifactorial analysis of melanoma. III Prognostic factors in melanoma patient with lymph node metastases (stage II). Ann Surg 193: 377-388
Balch CM, Cascinelli N, Milton GW, Sim FH 1985 Elective lymph node dissection: pros and cons In: Balch CM, Milton GW (eds) Cutaneous melanoma. Clinical management and treatment results worldwide. Lippincott, Philadelphia, 131-157
Balch CM, Soong S-J, Shaw HM, Urist MM, McCarthy WH 1992 An analysis of prognostic factors in 8500 patients with cutaneous melanoma. In: Balch CM, Houghton AN, Milton GW, Sober AJ, Soong S-J (eds). Cutaneous melanoma 2nd edn. Lippincott, Philadelphia, 165-187
Balch CM, Urist MM, Karakousis CP et al 1993 Efficacy of 2 cm surgical margins for intermediate thickness melanoma (1 to 4 mm). Results of a multi-institutional randomised surgical trial. Narrow excision (1 cm). Ann Surg 218: 262-267
Barth A, Morton DL 1995 The role of adjuvant therapy in melanoma management. Cancer 75: 726-734
Berman CG, Norman J, Cruse CW et al 1992 Lymphoscintigraphy in malignant melanomas. Ann Plast Surg 28: 29-32
Breslow A 1970 Thickness, cross-sectional areas and depth of invasion in the prognosis of cutaneous melanoma. Ann Surg 172: 902-908
Calabro A, Singletary SE, Balch CM 1989 Patterns of relapse in 1001 consecutive patients with melanoma nodal metastases. Arch Surg 124: 1051-1055
Cascinelli N, Van der Esch EP, Breslow A et al 1980 Stage I melanoma of the skin: the problem of resection margins. Eur J Cancer 16: 1079-1085
Clark WH, From L, Bernardino EA, Mihm MC 1969 The histogenesis and biologic behaviour of primary human malignant melanomas of the skin. Cancer Res 29: 705-726
Cochran AJ, Wen DR, Morton DL 1992 Management of the regional lymph nodes in patients with cutaneous malignant melanoma. World J Surg 16: 214-221
Coit DH, Rogatko A, Brennan MF 1991 Prognostic factors in patients with melanomas metastatic to axillary or inguinal lymph nodes. Ann Surg 214: 627-636
Cox NH, Jones SK, Mackie RM 1987 Malignant melanoma of the head and neck in Scotland: an eight year analysis of trends in prevalence, distribution and prognosis. Q J Med New Series 64 244: 661-670
Cruse CW, Wells KE, Schroer KR, Reintgen DS 1992 Etiology and prognosis of local recurrence in malignant melanoma of the skin. Ann Plast Surg 28: 26-28
Elder DE 1995 Skin cancer – melanoma and other specific non-melanoma skin cancers. Cancer 75: 245-256
Evans J, McCann BG 1990 A new protocol for the treatment of stage I cutaneous malignant melanoma: interim results of the first 806 patients treated. Br J Plast Surg 43: 426-430
Fisher RI, Terry WD, Hodes RJ et al 1981 Adjuvant immunotherapy or chemotherapy for malignant melanoma. Surg Clin North Am 61: 1270-1277
Gadd MA, Coit DG 1992 Recurrence patterns and outcome in 1019 patients undergoing axillary or inguinal lymphadenectomy for melanomas. Arch Surg 127: 1412-1416
Ghussen F, Nagel K, Groth W et al 1984 A prospective randomised study of regional extremity perfusion in patients with malignant melanoma. Ann Surg 200: 764-768
Ghussen F, Kruger I, Smalley RU, Groth W 1989 Hyperthermic perfusion with chemotherapy and melanoma of the extremities. World J Surg 13: 598-602
Griffiths RW, Briggs JC 1984 Long term follow up in cutaneous malignant melanoma. The relationship of maximal tumour thickness to disease free survival, disease recurrence and death. Br J Plast Surg 37: 507-513
Griffiths RW, Briggs JC 1986 Incidence of locally metastatic ('recurrent') cutaneous malignant melanoma following conventional wide excisional surgery for invasive clinical stage I tumours: importance of maximal tumour thickness. Br J Surg 73: 349-353
Harris MN, Shapiro RL, Roses DF 1995 Malignant melanoma: primary surgical management (excision and node dissection) based on pathology and staging. Cancer 75: 751-725
Hemanek P, Sobin LH eds 1992 TNM classification of malignant tumours. 4th edn, 2nd rev. Springer Verlag, Berlin

Karakousis CP, Velez A, Driscoll DL, Takita H 1994 Metastasectomy in malignant melanoma. Surgery 115: 295-302
Krementz ET, Carter DL, Sutherland CM et al 1994 Regional chemotherapy for melanomas. A 35-year experience. Ann Surg 220: 520-538
Lingham MK, McKay AJ 1994 Carbon dioxide laser – a new treatment modality for limb recurrence in malignant melanoma. Melanoma Res 4 Suppl 2: 52-53
Loong JR, Balch CM 1985 Defining lymphatic patterns with cutaneous lymphoscintigraphy. In: Balch CM, Milton GW eds Cutaneous melanoma. Clinical management and treatment results worldwide. Lippincott, Philadelphia, 159-170
Mackie R, Hunter JAA, Aitchison TC et al 1992 Cutaneous malignant melanoma, Scotland, 1979–89. Lancet 339: 971-975
Marsden JR. 1993 Malignant melanoma excision margins (letter) Lancet 341: 184
McCarthy WH, Shaw HM, Milton GW 1985 Efficacy of elective lymph node dissection in 2347 patients with clinical stage I malignant melanoma. Surg Gynec Obstet 161: 575-580.
McHenry PM, Hole DJ, MacKie RM 1992 Melanoma in people aged 65 and over in Scotland, 1979–1989. BMJ 34: 746-749
Meisenberg BR, Ross M, Vredenburgh JJ et al 1993 Randomised trial of high dose chemotherapy with autologous bone marrow support as adjuvant therapy for high risk multi node positive malignant melanoma. J Natl Cancer Inst 85: 1080-1085
Milton GW, Shaw HM, Farago GA, McCarthy WH 1980 Tumour thickness and the site and time of first recurrence in cutaneous malignant melanoma (stage I). Br J Surg 67: 543-546
Milton GW, Shaw HM, McCarthy WH 1985 Resection margins for melanoma. Aust NZ J Surg 55: 225-226
Morton DL, Wen DR, Wong JH et al 1992 Technical details of intraoperative lymphatic mapping for early stage melanoma. Arch Surg 127: 392-399
Neades GT, Orr DJA, Hughes LE, Horgan K 1993 Safe margins in the excision of primary cutaneous melanoma. Br J Surg 80: 731-733
Park KGM, Blessing K, McLaren KM, Watson ACH 1993 A study of thin (< 1.5 mm) malignant melanomas with poor prognosis. Br J Plast Surg 46: 607-610
Rampen F 1981 Melanoma of the skin: the problem of resection margins (letter). Eur J Cancer 17: 589-590
Regan MW, Reid CD, Griffiths RW, Briggs JC 1985 Malignant melanoma. Evaluation of clinical follow up by questionnaire survey. Br J Plast Surg 38: 11-14
Reintgen DS, Vollmer R, Tso CY, Seigler FH 1987 Prognosis for recurrent stage I malignant melanoma. Arch Surg 122: 1338-1342
Roses DF, Harris MM, Rigel D et al 1983 Local and intransit metastases following definitive excision for primary cutaneous malignant melanomas. Ann Surg 198: 65-69
Rosin RD 1991 Treatment of cutaneous malignant melanoma. Recent Adv Surg 14: 117-137
Schmueckel C, Bockelbrink A, Bockelbrink H, Braun-Falco O 1983 Low and high risk malignant melanoma II. Multivariate analysis for a prognostic classification. Eur J Oncol 19: 237-243
Shaw HM, Beattie CW, McCarthy WH, Milton GW 1985 Late relapse from cutaneous stage I malignant melanoma. Arch Surg 120: 1155-1159
Sim FH, Taylor WF, Pritchard DJ et al 1986 Lymphadenectomy in the management of stage I malignant melanoma: a prospective randomised study. Mayo Clin Proc 61: 697-705
Slingluff CL, Vollmer RT, Reintgen DS, Seigler HF 1988 Lethal 'thin' malignant melanoma. Identifying patients at risk. Ann Surg 208: 150-153
Soong S J, Shaw HM, Balch CM et al 1992 Predicting survival and recurrence in localised melanoma: a multivariate approach. World J Surg. 16: 191-195
Stankard C, Cruse CW, Cox C et al 1992 The concept of lymph node dissections in patients with malignant melanoma. Ann Plast Surg 28: 33-38
Timmons MJ 1993 Malignant melanoma excision margins: plastic surgery audit in Britain and Ireland, 1991, and review. Br J Plast Surg 46: 525-531
Urist MM, Balch CM, Soong S-J et al 1985 The influence of surgical margins and prognostic factors: predicting the risk of local recurrence in 3445 patients with primary cutaneous melanomas. Cancer 55: 1398-1402
Veronesi U, Adamus J, Aubert C 1982 A randomised trial of adjuvant chemotherapy and immunotherapy in cutaneous melanoma. N Engl J Med 307: 913-916
Veronesi U, Adamus J, Bandiera DC et al 1982a Delayed regional lymph node dissection in stage I melanoma of the skin of the lower extremities. Cancer 49: 2420-2430

Veronesi U, Cascinelli N 1991 Narrow excision (1 cm margin): a safe procedure for thin cutaneous melanoma. Arch Surg 126: 438-441

Wong JH, Cagle LA, Morton DL 1991 Lymphatic drainage of skin to a sentinel lymph node in a feline model. Ann Surg 214: 637-641

Wong JH, Skinner KA, Kim KA et al 1993 The role of surgery in the treatment of non regionally recurrent melanoma. Surgery 113: 389-394

Woods JE 1989 Malignant melanoma: an update. Adv Plast Reconstr Surg 5: 1-4

Yeung RSW 1993 Recurrent cutaneous melanoma: a surgical perspective. Semin Oncol 20: 400-418

14

What's new in general surgery – a review of the journals

I. Taylor

In this chapter, I review interesting and significant developments in the field of gastrointestinal surgery (both upper and lower), pancreaticobiliary surgery, hepatic surgery, breast and emergency surgery. Constraints on space inevitably limit inclusions, but I hope the selection covers most of the innovations during the last year.

OESOPHAGUS

Reflux

Nissen's fundoplication for the surgical treatment of gastro-oesophageal reflux disease was initially devised in 1956. It has been a constant source of controversy since then. However, recently, it has generated increasing interest because of laparoscopic techniques.

Jamieson et al (1994) have described the technique of laparoscopic Nissen fundoplication in 155 patients followed up for three or more months. Ten patients required subsequent surgery and there was one postoperative death; 133 of the patients were well and free from reflux. Their view was that this is a useful technique which might gain increasing enthusiasm. Similar results have been obtained by Hinder et al (1994) and Watson et al (1994). Complications of oesophageal perforation, pneumothorax and sepsis are described. The operating time is greater than with the open repair but the median hospital stay of 3 days is clearly an advantage. Collard et al (1994) were unable to demonstrate a reduced postoperative complication rate and discomfort and even questioned whether there was an earlier return to work following laparoscopic surgery. A randomised trial is clearly required in this disease and several centres have initiated such a study. Interestingly, in a randomised trial, the Angelchik prosthesis was found to be equally effective to a Nissen fundoplication although three patients required removal of the prosthesis (Hill et al 1994). If re-operation is required after failed anti-reflux surgery, Rieger et al (1994) have reported that repeat anti-reflux procedures can actually provide results almost as good as those of the primary procedure.

Carcinoma

Carcinoma of the oesophagus continues to be a dreadful disease. Earlier diagnosis and prevention would clearly be extremely important. With regard to adenocarcinoma arising in Barrett's oesophagus, Hardwick et al (1994) have demonstrated that p53 dysfunction may participate in the progression from dysplasia to carcinoma. This observation requires further investigation.

As an illustration of the poor results of treatment for carcinoma of the oesophagus, Sagar et al (1994) have performed an audit on 316 patients from the Yorkshire Cancer Registry. Operative mortality was 27% in the 134 patients who underwent surgical exploration. Median survival in 106 patients who underwent surgical resection was 292 days and 7% survived 5 years. Few studies have shown any benefit for either adjuvant chemotherapy or radiotherapy. Chung et al (1994) in a review of surgical therapy for squamous cell carcinoma recommend treatment in a specialist unit and, as a result of experience in Hong Kong, advise the Ivor-Lewis procedure. Bolton et al (1994) have reported trans-hiatal oesophagectomy with a decreased morbidity and a significant reduction in operative mortality. They achieved an encouraging 30% disease-free survival at 3 years.

Selection of patients suitable for either curative or palliative resection is most important and new techniques have attempted to achieve this. Peters et al (1994) have reported that pre-operative endoscopic ultrasonography is a reliable method for staging and particularly for determining wall penetration. However, whether more extensive resection provides better disease-free survival compared to the increased complication rate has been questioned (van Lanschot et al 1994).

GASTRODUODENAL DISEASE

Studies relating the effect of *Helicobacter pylori* infection to upper GI disease are ever more frequent. The previously reported association of *H. pylori* infection with peptic ulcer disease and possibly gastric carcinoma has led to a search for non-invasive methods for diagnosis of infection. Patel et al (1994) have described a study to detect salivary immunoglobulins to *H. pylori* in screening patients, under 45 years of age, for endoscopy. This study detected all peptic ulcers in their series while saving 39% of endoscopies. There is undoubtedly inappropriate use of upper gastrointestinal endoscopy and this has been discussed in a prospective audit (Quine et al 1994).

Duodenal ulcer

Two recent studies have reported the long-term effects of parietal cell vagotomy (PCV) in patients with duodenal ulceration. Undoubtedly the recurrence rate after PCV is proportional to the duration of follow-up. Meisner et al (1994) have reported 350 patients followed up for a median duration of 140 months; 21.9% developed recurrent ulceration, frequently occurring as late as 17 years after surgery and 80% of the recurrences occurred after 10 years of follow-up. Jordan et al (1994) have reported results 20 years after either PCV or selective vagotomy and antrectomy. There were no operative deaths and no difference in the frequency of diarrhoea. Recurrence rates following PCV of 16.5% at 10 years were reported. Recent attempts at laparoscopic highly selective vagotomy (HSV) have been described. Dallemagne et al (1994) reported 35 patients undergoing laparoscopic HSV. There was no mortality or morbidity and the operating time was a mean of 110 min. The main advantage appears to be a 70% reduction in hospital stay and 50% in the overall recovery period compared to open surgery. However, randomised trials are required to establish whether this procedure is indicated.

The most effective management for bleeding peptic ulcer is still actively debated. Conservative treatment is reasonably effective if managed correctly. Indeed, in a prospective audit of 126 patients, Mueller et al (1994) described conservative treatment in 80%, the remainder having early surgery because they bled further or because they were considered to be at high risk for further bleeding. Hypovolaemic shock, a non-bleeding visible vessel and adherent clot on an ulcer base are of independent significance in predicting re-bleeding (Hsu et al 19914). Two randomised trials have investigated the role of injection treatment. Choudari and Palmer (1994) compared endoscopic injection of adrenaline alone and adrenaline plus ethanolamine oleate. The addition of a sclerosant conferred no advantage over injection with adrenaline alone. Similarly, Carter and Anderson (1994) compared adrenaline injection with laser photocoagulation; injection of adrenaline achieved similar results to laser photocoagulation and is simpler.

The optimum management for perforated peptic ulcer has been debated over several years. A vogue for conservative treatment was in place some years ago, but many regard this as dangerous. Svanes et al (1994) have reported significantly more adverse effects in delaying treatment for perforated peptic ulcer. There was an increased complication rate and prolonged hospital stay. They suggest every effort should be made to operate within 12 hours, particularly in elderly patients.

Three recent studies have investigated whether there is an increased instance of malignancy following surgery for benign ulcer disease. Macintyre and O'Brien (1994) reviewed 2241 patients who had surgery between 1947 and 1968. There was no evidence to support an increased incidence of malignancy and no evidence for routine endoscopic screening after surgery for duodenal ulceration. Similarly, Lundegardh et al (1994a) were unable to demonstrate any increased risk of gastric cancer in the first 10 years after surgery in some 7198 patients, although in a subsequent paper by the same group an increased risk of lung and oesophageal cancer was recognised (Lundegardh et al 1994b). The significance, however, of this is not apparent at present.

Carcinoma

The results of treatment for gastric carcinoma are poor. Attempts to recognise and resect early gastric cancers in the hope of improving prognosis have continued over a number of years. The Japanese experience would suggest that radical D2 gastrectomy for cancer is desirable in this condition. McCulloch (1994) has described the technique in detail, but undoubtedly it is associated with increased postoperative morbidity. This has been demonstrated in a prospective randomised trial in which a D1 sub-total gastrectomy was compared to a D3 total gastrectomy for antral carcinoma in 55 patients. There were no complications in the D1 group, but 14 patients in the D3 group developed a left subphrenic abscess. Overall survival was significantly better in the D1 group (Robertson et al 1994). Similarly, Heesakkers et al (1994) has assessed the benefit of D2 gastrectomy for patients with early gastric cancer. Resection margins in all 46 patients were free from tumour. They obtained a 91%, 5-year survival in patients undergoing conventional R1 gastrectomy and did not consider the need for D2 gastrectomy with its higher morbidity and mortality. These two studies suggest that further assessment of D3 gastrectomy is indicated before it is routinely used in patients with early gastric cancer.

Whether adjuvant therapy is of benefit in patients following resection is doubtful. The second British Stomach Cancer Group Trial utilising radiotherapy or cytotoxic therapy with mitomycin, doxorubicin and fluorouracil has been reported (Hallissey et al 1994). No survival advantage was found for patients receiving adjuvant therapy compared to surgery alone. In Japan, however, standard adjuvant treatment following resection is intravenous mitomycin and oral fluorouracil. A recent study has demonstrated that the addition of protein-bound polysaccharide was beneficial and improved the 5-year survival rate (Nakazato et al 1994). Jones et al (1994) have discussed a phase 2 trial evaluating intra-peritoneal cisplatin in patients at high risk of relapse. However, the incidence and pattern of relapse was similar to that expected. It is doubtful whether this form of adjuvant therapy will prove to be beneficial in the long-term.

The management of primary gastric non-Hodgkin's lymphoma has undergone changes in recent years. Pytel et al (1994) described the outcome and treatment of 36 such patients. Their policy is surgical resection where feasible, and adjuvant therapy in addition. According to the stage, the overall 5-year survival is between 75–100%. However, they make the point that surgical resection is probably important in all stages in order to ensure a high cure rate and avoid life threatening complications.

Another relatively rare tumour is adenocarcinoma of the duodenum. Scott-Coombes and Williamson (1994) have published their personal series of 22 patients operated on between 1979 and 1993. 17 underwent 'curative' resection with one hospital death and a 5-year survival of 40%. It has a better prognosis than pancreatic cancer after radical resection. Similar data have been described by Rotman et al (1994) who described actual 3- and 5-year survival rates of 59% and 45% respectively. None of the standard prognostic factors appeared to influence survival and they recommend radical resection whenever possible.

COLORECTAL SURGERY

Inflammatory bowel disease

The relationship between inflammatory bowel disease (both ulcerative colitis and Crohn's disease), and subsequent development of malignancy remains a highly controversial topic. Bernstein et al (1994) have reviewed 10 prospective studies and suggest clinicians should treat dysplasia more aggressively. Up to 29% of patients with untreated low grade dysplasia progressed to a dysplasia-associated mass or lesion. Jonsson et al (1994) have carried out a prospective study of some 130 patients with ulcerative colitis undergoing regular colonoscopy and biopsy. Both colorectal carcinoma and dysplasia were diagnosed mainly in the left colon and almost always in patients with total colitis. Clearly this should be considered in any surveillance programme. Although there is an increased risk of developing colorectal cancer in extensive ulcerative colitis, the number of patients with Crohn's disease who develop colorectal cancer is small because these patients tend to undergo colectomy at an earlier stage. However, Gillen et al (1994) have demonstrated that such patients have a risk of developing cancer which is very similar to that in ulcerative colitis. A similar observation has been made by Connell et al (1994) who observed that the development of malignancy applies particularly to those patients who have complicated anorectal disease. Carcinomas complicating Crohn's disease and ulcerative colitis have strikingly similar clinicopathological features which tend to suggest a common underlying process (Choi & Zelig 1994). It would appear that whatever form of surveillance is carried out in patients with ulcerative colitis, a similar programme should be performed in patients with Crohn's disease.

Two controversial surgical procedures in Crohn's disease are colectomy with ileorectal anastomosis and strictureplasty of the small bowel. Chevalier et al (1994) have described the results in 83 patients undergoing ileorectal anastomosis for Crohn's disease. There were two postoperative deaths and seven leaks. The cumulative proportion of patients with a functioning ileorectal anastomosis was 77% and 63% at 5 and 10 years, respectively. Patients presenting with perforated Crohn's disease had an increased risk of anastomotic failure. Tjandra and Fazio (1994) have looked at the efficacy of 250 strictureplasty procedures in 54 patients with obstructive Crohn's disease. There were no postoperative deaths and only two patients developed serious postoperative complications. Weight gain was satisfactory after the procedure and the recurrent stricture rate was 3%. These are satisfactory results and should be taken into account in determining selection of patients undergoing surgery for small bowel Crohn's disease.

Diverticular disease

Complications arising from diverticular disease of the colon are common and frequently require surgical intervention. Tudor et al (1994) reported a national audit of complicated diverticular disease. The overall mortality rate was 11.3% but up to 27% when purulent peritonitis occurred and 46% in the presence of faecal peritonitis. Management of purulent peritonitis generally involves a Hartmann's procedure (62%) or resection and primary anastomoses (15%). After 5 years, a significant proportion of patients developed further complications and of the 10 patients who died from recurrent diverticular disease, 9 had not undergone sigmoid colectomy at or after the original admission (Farmakis et al 1994).

Sarin and Boulos (1994) looked at the long-term outcome in 164 patients with diverticular disease who presented with acute complications. Conservative treatment was successful in 85% with a recurrence rate of 2% per patient year follow-up. Patients requiring colonic resection had a mortality of 12% but no further admissions with complications. They conclude that after successful conservative treatment of the acute complications subsequent elective surgery is not justified. Ambrosetti et al (1994) have compared the outcome of left colonic diverticulitis with age. Patients less than 50 were significantly more prone to recurrences and complications after conservative treatment of diverticulitis. Older patients required surgery significantly more often during their first hospitalisation. McGuire (1994) has looked at the natural history of bleeding colonic dieverticula in 78 patients and, in his series, 75% of episodes stopped spontaneously with all but one patient requiring less than 4 units of blood. He observed that re-bleeding is rare and that blind resection was unsafe.

Colorectal cancer

The role of screening for colorectal cancer still occupies a good deal of interest. The topic has recently been reviewed by Austoker (1994a). However, until the present studies are completed, it is difficult to recommend routine screening although the role of flexible sigmoidoscopy is generating some enthusiasm. Certainly dietary restriction has an effect on compliance with haemoccult screening (Robinson et al 1994a). A recent study has also demonstrated that the immunological occult blood test (hemeselect) is more sensitive for symptomatic colorectal cancer although it does have a high positive rate (Robinson et al 1994b).

A number of studies have investigated specific markers as prognostic factors in colorectal cancer. For example, CD44v6 may reflect propensity for metastases after curative surgery (Mulder et al 1994); lymphatic dissemination appears to be related to the presence of mutated p53 whereas haematogenous dissemination was apparently the result of absent functional wild-type p53 (Goh et al 1994); urokinase-type plasminogen activator in epithelium is associated with a poor prognosis for Dukes B disease (Mulcahy et al 1994a).

Another factor which was thought to be related to prognosis is age. However, a study by Mulcahy et al (1994b) disputes this and demonstrates that allowing for population mortality, age had no effect on long-term survival of elderly patients with large bowel cancer. Similarly Heys et al (1994) found that survival rates in a group of patients under the age of 45 were comparable to those of older patients when considering the equivalent Dukes stages. Patients with previous extra-colonic cancer have a prognosis somewhat better than that of the general colorectal cancer population (Varty et al 1994a). It would appear that the Dukes stage is still the most single important prognostic indicator particularly in association with tumour differentiation. Nevertheless, the overall results of surgery for colorectal cancer remain static. Allum et al (1994) have reviewed the outcome of patients in the West Midlands between 1957 and 1981. The overall 5-year survival is approximately 30% although curative and palliative resection rates have increased especially for anterior resection. The results overall have improved over the years but, in general, there is much room for improvement.

It is still not known how intensive follow-up should be following surgery for colorectal cancer. Bruinvels et al (1994) have performed a meta-analysis of CEA assays. There is some evidence that regular assays may identify treatable recurrence at a relatively early stage although this is by no means certain compared to other randomised studies. Similarly, asymptomatic recurrences detected during hospital follow-up were initially suspected after clinical examination alone or following additional blood tests in a study by Wyatt and Aitken (1994). There is certainly a wide variation in clinical practice with regard to follow-up. Lautenbach et al (1994) reported results in 290 patients who had colonoscopy performed regularly in the postoperative period. Overall, 31 patients developed recurrent disease and 13 asymptomatic patients had curative resections for localised recurrent disease. They suggest that colonoscopy may be a useful modality in the early detection of recurrence.

Surgical technique is the major single factor determining outcome in patients with colorectal cancer. Postoperative morbidity, particularly the presence of sepsis, has been regarded by several as a poor prognostic factor in long-term survival of colorectal cancer. However a study by Varty et al (1994b) showed no significant difference in 5-year survival between patients who had postoperative intra-abdominal sepsis and those without.

Another long held concept has been questioned. Burke et al (1994) have demonstrated in a prospective randomised trial that mechanical bowel preparation does not influence the incidence of postoperative complications, particularly dehiscence, in patients undergoing surgery for colorectal cancer.

Although mesorectal excision is now regarded as the treatment of choice in rectal cancer, it should, however, be noted that this results in a higher incidence of postoperative leakage. Karanjia et al (1994) recommend defunctioning colostomy in patients undergoing a low anterior resection with mesorectal excision. In their series there was a major anastomatic leak in 11% of patients.

Local recurrence in rectal cancer is a significant problem. Abulafi and Williams (1994) have reviewed the mechanisms and management of this condition in a comprehensive review. Whether radiotherapy, either pre- or postoperatively, has an effect in reducing the incidence of rectal recurrence is still highly controversial. Holm et al (1994) described a randomised trial of 849 patients with a minimum follow-up of 4 years. 156 patients developed local recurrence and curative treatment was rarely possible. Survival was only 1 year irrespective of adjuvant therapy. Ogiwara et al (1994) believes that adjunctive radiotherapy and chemotherapy should be considered in patients with rectal cancer who have lesions greater than 2 cm in diameter with serosal involvement irrespective of lymph node metastases. It is apparent that the actual dose of radiotherapy is important, Sause et al (1994) were unable to detect any improvement in recurrence rate with low dose pre-operative radiotherapy although many studies have demonstrated a reduction in local recurrence rate (although not necessarily overall survival) with both pre- and postoperative radiotherapy. Nevertheless, Kollmorgen et al (1994) have looked at the long-term effects of postoperative chemoradiotherapy and, in a study involving several regimes, have concluded that adjuvant postoperative chemoradiotherapy does have a detrimental effect on bowel function, both in the short- and long-term. Many of these studies, however, have reviewed relatively small numbers of patients and in order to demonstrate a moderate improvement both in survival and recurrence rates, large studies are indicated (Wils et al 1994). In the UK, the AXIS study is investigating radiotherapy and portal vein infusion and has now accrued over 2500 patients. In a preliminary report of the first 2000 patients (AXIS Steering Group 1994), no increased toxicity or morbidity was found in treated patients compared to control groups. Interestingly, Nossal et al (1994) have reviewed a trial of chemo-immunotherapy in Dukes C disease. This utilises a monoclonal antibody 17-1A directed against an epithelial cell surface glycoprotein. The initial results from this study are encouraging and deserve further investigation.

Laparoscopic assisted colectomy continues to generate interest, although it should be said that some less enthusiastic reports have appeared. Hoffman et al (1994) described their experience in 80 consecutive laparoscopic assisted colectomies with a 23% conversion rate. The length of operating time, operating room charge and total hospital charge were greater for patients undergoing laparoscopic assisted colectomy. One major complication, which is now becoming increasingly appreciated, is the incidence of abdominal wall metastases following laparoscopy. This has been reported by Nduka et al (1994). In their review article, they indicate that the most likely mechanism is direct implantation of viable exfoliated tumour cells, but manipulation and close contact are also important.

ANORECTAL SURGERY

Rectal evacuatory disorders resulting in severe intractable constipation are a major problem. Williams et al (1994a) have described a continent colonic conduit for rectal evacuation in 10 patients. This relatively simple procedure results in significant improvement and should be considered in selected cases.

The most effective method for dealing with rectal prolapse is also controversial. Deen et al (1994) have reported a randomised trial comparing abdominal resection rectopexy with pelvic floor repair and perineal rectosigmoidectomy. In a small study, the former technique gave better function and physiological results. Novel et al (1994) have compared Ivalon sponge with suture rectopexy for rectal prolapse. The medium term results of rectopexy by suture alone were equivalent to those obtained using Ivalon. In view of the potential problems with Ivalon, they suggest Ivalon rectopexy should now be abandoned. Cuschieri et al (1994) have described laparoscopic mobilisation and posterior fixation to the presacral fascia using Marlex mesh in 5 patients. No recurrence of the prolapse occurred during the period of follow-up of 4–27 months. However, the operating times were between 2–4.5 hours.

Haemorrhoids result in significant problems and the aetiology is still disputed. An excellent review of the pathology, pathophysiology and aetiology has been carried out by Loder et al (1994) and the importance of displacement of the distal anal cushions is emphasised. A very extensive comparison of emergency and elective haemorrhoidectomy by Eu et al (1994) has been reported. In over 704 patients operated on in a 2-year period, 204 were carried out as an emergency for prolapse, thrombosis or gangrenous change within the haemorrhoids. The main complications were secondary haemorrhage, and anal stenosis after emergency procedure in 5.9% of patients.

The management of anal intraepithelial neoplasia is uncertain. This is mainly because of the natural history and controversy about its malignant potential. Scholefield et al (1994) have described the treatment of 27 patients by surgical excision; frequently excision of the whole of the epithelium and application of split skin grafts. Low grade lesions often require no treatment. There is no doubt that there is an increased risk of anal cancer among patients with AIDS at and after AIDS diagnosis (Melbye et al 1994).

The management of anal squamous cell carcinoma is controversial. This tumour is probably best treated by radiotherapy and studies involving the role of chemotherapy are in progress (Deans et al 1994, Mendenhall et al 1994). With regard to recurrent anal carcinoma, a multivariate analysis of 405 patients has revealed that the stage of diagnosis and method of treatment were the sole predictors of recurrence. Salvage abdominoperineal resection is probably the most important treatment (Longo et al 1994).

BILIARY DISEASE

Gallstones

Laparoscopic cholecystectomy is now established as the treatment of choice for patients with gallstones, however some controversies still remain. There is no doubt that the most important issue is the prevention of bile duct injury.

A recent audit by the Royal College of Surgeons suggests that morbidity and mortality are low but in a series of 3319 attempted laparoscopic cholecystectomies, bile duct injury was more common than after open cholecystectomy (11 cases, 0.33%) (Dunn et al 1994). A smaller series from Leicester, (Birdi et al 1994) showed similar findings, although major complications occurred in 4.7% including 2 deaths, two of whom had major pre-existing morbidity. Bile duct injury was low (0.18%). How does laparoscopy compare with open cholecystectomy? There have been two interesting randomised trials. Berggren et al (1994), in a selected group of patients, demonstrated that postoperative analgesia was less common, the duration of postoperative hospital stay was reduced and sick leave was also significantly less following laparoscopic cholecystectomy. Compared to minilaparotomy cholecystectomy, laparoscopic cholecystectomy was also associated with a lower pain score, and improvement in postoperative pulmonary function (McMahon et al 1994a, 1994b). What about the relative costs of open and laparoscopic cholecystectomy? Fullarton et al (1994) have estimated the cost per patient of open cholecystectomy to be £2102 compared to £2026 following laparoscopic cholecystectomy. However, the costs do drop with experience. Mean hospital stay in this series for laparoscopic cholecystectomy was 4.8 days compared to 3.4 days in the open group. It should be noted that laparoscopic cholecystectomy also has a role in biliary pancreatitis (Tate et al 1994). Although early surgery in this situation is safe, the technical difficulty is increased and cystic duct dilatation in particular must be anticipated.

Another controversial topic of importance is the management and imaging of the common bile duct in patients undergoing laparoscopic cholecystectomy (Hainsworth et al 1994). Should ERCP be used pre-operatively for patients with a high risk of duct stones? Certainly not all surgeons perform pre-operative cholangiography. Watkin et al (1994) have relied on a selective policy and suggest that pre-operative assessment of the bile duct with ultrasonography and liver function tests obviates the need for routine cholangiography. This is probably the most popular regime at the moment in the UK. A similar study from Barkun et al (1994) has shown that the presence of common bile duct stones in patients older that 55 years of age could be predicted in 94% of cases by the presence of an elevated bilirubin and positive ultrasonography. This model, initially developed retrospectively, was validated prospectively in a subsequent series of 49 patients. Recently, the advent of laparoscopic ultrasonography has suggested another method of detection of common bile stones. In a prospective comparative study, Greig et al (1994) evaluated operative cholangiography and laparoscopic ultrasonography. Their initial data suggest that this method might be useful in a patient with a suggestion of small common bile duct stones. There is still great controversy with regard to the management of bile duct stones and this has been reviewed extensively by a working party (Perissat et al 1994). This review deals with all the possible permutations of management in patients with common bile duct stones. Whether these should be removed endoscopically either pre- or postoperatively or by laparoscopic common bile duct exploration depends very much upon experience of the available individuals.

Whereas endoscopic sphincterotomy is the treatment of choice for common bile duct stones in elderly patients, in some this fails and surgery is indicated. Davidson et al (1994) have demonstrated, in a carefully audited study, that open surgery can be performed both safely and effectively in elderly patients with retained bile duct stones.

The introduction of laparoscopic cholecystectomy has significantly affected and raised doubts about the future role of extracorporeal shock wave lithotripsy (ESWL). Darzi et al (1994) in a series of 67 patients undergoing ESWL have demonstrated that this is a costly procedure with a high failure and high recurrence rate compared to laparoscopic cholecystectomy. It is unlikely, therefore, to be a significant therapeutic option for the future. Nicholl et al (1994) have also looked at the cost effectiveness of adjuvant bile salt treatment following ESWL in the treatment of gall bladder stones. The additional cost is high and this does not appear to be a particularly effective treatment option.

Malignancy

Carcinoma of the biliary tree and gall bladder are associated with a poor prognosis. Boerma (1994) has reviewed the treatment results for gall bladder cancer and is led to the conclusion that only en-bloc resection of the complete area of gall bladder and adjacent liver can result in better results for patients with gall bladder stages T1, N0, M0 to T3, N1. Perhaps such patients should be referred to centres with experience in this technique.

Symptom relief and palliation for patients with malignant bile duct obstruction and unresectable hilar cholangiocarcinoma is a most important topic. Ballinger et al (1994) have demonstrated significant improvement in quality of life after stenting for malignant bile duct obstruction suggesting that this is a worthwhile intervention even though survival is measured in terms of weeks. Nordback et al (1994) have similarly demonstrated that operative placement of large-bore transhepatic stents reduces cholangitis, hepatic failure and prolongs survival. These techniques are certainly worthwhile in patients who require palliative procedures and are perhaps more beneficial than operative intervention in selected cases.

PANCREATIC DISEASE

Cancer

The results of surgery for pancreatic cancer remain poor. A large multicentre retrospective study described the short and long-term results of 787 pancreatic resections (Baumel et al 1994). Postoperative mortality was 10% and morbidity was 35%. In those patients who survived more than 30 days, the actuarial 5-year survival was 12% and the median survival was 12 months.

Operative mortality was higher after total pancreatectomy than pancreatico-duodenectomy. The results in patients over 70 were particularly poor and suggest that resection in this age group should be avoided. The results of radical resection for ampullary carcinoma, however, are somewhat better with overall 5- and 10-year survival rates of 56% and 36%, respectively. Certainly, radical resection in selected patients can be curative (Sperti et al 1994). Novel treatments for periampullary malignancy continue to be reported. Somatostatin analogues inhibit the growth of some pancreatic cancers probably by direct receptor mediated mechanisms. It has been suggested that somatostatin analogues may have a role in adjuvant therapy following curative resection (Poston 1994). Unfortunately, postoperative parenteral nutrition following major pancreatic resection does not benefit patients and indeed in one randomised trial (Brennan et al 1994) suggested that patients receiving TPN did worse as a result of infectious complications.

What is the best form of treatment in patients unsuitable for resection? Palmer et al (1994) in a small study have suggested that chemotherapy may improve overall survival from a median of 15 weeks to 33 weeks. They suggest that chemotherapy should be considered in this group of patients although many other authorities would dispute this. Smith et al (1994) have published an important randomised trial comparing endoscopic stenting with surgical bypass in patients with malignant lower bile duct obstruction. The majority of patients had a probable primary carcinoma of the pancreas. There was a lower procedure related mortality in stented patients and the median hospital stay was also lower (20 versus 26 days). However, late gastric outlet obstruction occurred in 17% of stented patients compared to 7% in the surgical group. There was no difference in overall survival in the two groups.

Pancreatitis

The diagnosis and treatment of complications of pancreatitis still generate much interest within the literature. For alcoholic acute pancreatitis Jaakkola et al (1994) have demonstrated the importance of the lipase/amylase ratio index and serum carbohydrate deficient transferrin.

Deaths still occur from acute pancreatitis and a prospective audit in the North West Thames region which recruited 631 patients over 54 months showed a 9% death rate. Of 26 patients who died from infection related complications, 15 had computed tomography, but only 9 underwent a necrosectomy or surgical drainage. There is a suggestion that improved diagnosis and management might improve the overall survival in this group of patients: in general, the outcome remains extremely poor (Mann et al 1994). With regard to chronic pancreatitis, Izbicki et al (1994) have reviewed duodenum preserving resection of the head of the pancreas in chronic pancreatitis. This technique was demonstrated to be effective in the treatment of severe disease with predominant involvement of the pancreatic head.

LIVER SURGERY

Metastases

There has been increased understanding of the factors affecting liver tumour growth in metastatic colorectal disease. Blood flow is particularly important in relation to cytotoxic drug uptake following locoregional infusions. Sitzmann et al (1994) have demonstrated a loss of angiotensin II receptors on the neovasculature of hepatic tumours and Hennigan and Allen-Mersh (1994) have demonstrated the role of vasoconstriction in increasing cytotoxic drug uptake within tumours. Two studies have demonstrated the possible therapeutic role of inhibition of somatostatin receptors in liver metastases. This has been demonstrated both in animal and human colorectal cancer lines (van Eijck et al 1994a, Stewart et al 1994). It is also likely that molecular genetic changes determine whether primary colorectal cancer metastasises to the liver. Ding et al (1994) have demonstrated that the frequency of allele loss is associated with prognostic factors such as the number and size of liver metastases.

There is great interest in liver resection for metastatic disease. Several groups have reported their results. However, in the absence of clinical trials, it is important to identify those specific factors which influence the natural history of colorectal liver metastases. Stangl et al (1994) have provided a very comprehensive review of this topic by examining 1099 consecutive patients. They have recognised independent significant factors and specifically looked at the percentage of liver volume replaced by tumour, grade of malignancy of the primary tumour and the presence of hepatic disease. It is clearly important to be able to predict accurately the feasibility of surgical resection. Vogel et al (1994) have compared two diagnostic techniques, arterial portography and hepatic arterial perfusion, with standard computed tomography. Unfortunately, false positive results of both techniques influence their ability to predict unresectability accurately. Similarly, it may be difficult to determine whether curative resection has been performed. Hohenberger et al (1994) measured carcinoembryonic antigen (CEA) levels to determine completeness of resection in 166 patients. They found that postoperative CEA was the most predictive factor with regard to survival and disease-free interval and recommend that this should be used as a criterion for adjuvant treatment.

There have been a number of studies providing further support for resection of liver metastases. Tsao et al (1994) have demonstrated a significant decrease in operative mortality, median peri-operative transfusion and length of hospital stay in the period 1986 to 1990, when operative mortality rates fell from 4.9% to 1.2%. Different groups have advocated specific technical aspects which they feel influence results. For example, Habib et al (1994a) advocate total vascular exclusion with a 30-day operative mortality rate of zero but a hospital mortality rate of 4%. This same group have described resection of the inferior vena cava as part of a resection for hepatocellular carcinoma in 4 patients. It is unlikely that this procedure will be commonly performed since it has as an indication occlusion of the IVC by tumour. Either autologous vein or primary repair can be used (Habib et al 1994b). In patients with multiple metastatic liver tumours who are thought suitable for extensive resection, Kawasaki et al (1994) advocate portal embolisation as a pre-operative manoeuvre to increase the safety of hepatectomy. There must be very few indications for this procedure and indeed only 5 patients are reported.

It was only a question of time before papers appeared on the results of repeated resection of colorectal metastases. Hemming and Langer (1994) feel that repeat resection is justified as the only hope of long term cure and in a review they report 5-year survivals of approximately 25% with an operative mortality of less than 9%. Several other groups have reported favourable data with a median survival of 19–23 months and postoperative mortality of 5–8% in a total of 59 patients (Briand et al 1994, Fong et al 1994, Que & Nagorney 1994). This must be a rare procedure but, nevertheless, in selected patients repeat resection deserves consideration. Gough et al (1994) also reported the results in 9 patients who underwent surgery for both liver and lung metastases from colorectal cancer. No operative deaths occurred and the postoperative hospital stay was 10 days. Median survival after completion of liver and lung surgery was 27 months.

Following resection, approximately 50% of patients develop recurrence outside the liver. Accordingly, there has been interest in adjuvant chemotherapy after surgical resection of liver metastases. Donato et al (1994) have reported 102 patients who received chemotherapy based on 5-fluorouracil (5FU). Although their results suggest a possible benefit with a reduction in metastatic disease, a multicentre prospective trial is required to confirm benefit.

Primary malignancy

The results of major hepatectomy in primary liver cancer and cirrhosis have improved significantly in recent years. Capussoti et al (1994) reported 33 cirrhotic patients who underwent major liver resection with a hospital mortality of 3%. Survival rate at 3 years was 37%. Cirrhotic patients with hepatic carcinoma and good liver function are regarded as suitable for major hepatectomy.

Numerous studies in recent years have advocated intrahepatic arterial chemotherapy in patients with multiple liver metastases unsuitable for resection. Modifications of this technique have appeared at frequent intervals. Civalleri et al (1994) have reported on the combination of mitomycin C and 5FU given both intraportally and intra-arterially and mixed with degradable starch microspheres to enhance uptake of the drugs into tumours. A high rate of complete and overall response in hypovascular tumours was demonstrated. It is important, however, to ensure that the quality of life following intrahepatic chemotherapy is acceptable. Allen-Mersh et al (1994) have reported a randomised trial of 100 patients receiving hepatic arterial infusion in which quality of life was measured. Survival benefit was noted, associated with a normal quality of life. This is a most important observation.

Varices

The emergency treatment of major variceal haemorrhage continues to provoke vigorous discussion. The creation of a transjugular intrahepatic portasystemic stent shunt (TIPSS) has become popular over the last few years. McCormick et al (1994) have reported 242 episodes of variceal bleeding over a 2-year period. The procedure was technically successful and controlled bleeding in all patients. Twelve patients died within 40 days from liver failure and sepsis. However, TIPSS must be regarded as an effective therapeutic option in acute variceal bleeding refractory to medical and endoscopic treatment. This technique should be compared to surgical transaction when other methods for controlling the bleeding have failed. Willson et al (1994) have reported their results with oesophageal transactions which, in a series of 30 patients, was effective at stopping variceal bleeding but did not modify the underlying disease. The overall 30-day mortality rate was 63%. It is likely that this technique will be used less frequently with the greater availability of TIPSS. Finally, Williams et al (1994a) reported the results of thrombin for the treatment of gastric varices in 11 patients. Variceal bleeding from this site is extremely difficult to deal with but injection with bovine thrombin produced haemostasis in all 11 patients. This appears to be a valuable method for the treatment of bleeding gastric varices.

BREAST DISEASE

Screening

Screening for breast cancer is now fairly well established in the UK. However, it still provokes controversy. Austoker (1994b) has reviewed the role of mammographic screening and confirmed benefits even though anxiety is raised in these women. Her review article does not demonstrate benefit from breast self-examination, although Mittra (1994) concludes that physical examination can be as effective as screening mammography in reducing mortality. He argues that mammography demonstrates predominantly lesions which are nonpalpable and non-infiltrating and do not threaten a woman's life. However, screening by physical examination may pick up smaller palpable tumours with a likely greater benefit. Nevertheless, with breast screening, smaller lesions are being demonstrated and the management of these remains controversial. Kerin et al (1994) have described the use of stereotactic localisation and fine needle aspiration in non-palpable abnormalities. In a series of 166 patients, cytology correctly diagnosed malignancy in 71. Clearly, this provides a valuable diagnostic test and can avoid repeat excisions in these patients. The techniques of fine wire localisation biopsy are now well established and with experience provide favourable results. For example, Allen et al (1994) accurately biopsied all of 212 patients during initial surgery and they were able to achieve breast conservation in 80%. These excellent results can also be achieved in smaller units as demonstrated by Beck et al (1994) with a benign to malignant ratio of 0.72:1.

This year has seen great interest in the recognition of BRCA1 gene mutations and its implications in selection of families for predictive testing for familial breast cancer (Evans et al 1994). Ford et al (1994) looked at 33 families with evidence of linkage to BRCA1 and estimated that risks of breast and ovarian cancer were increased. This is likely to be of clinical significance in certain families. Porter et al (1994) have demonstrated a lifetime disease penetrance of the BRCA1 gene at 88% and the plateau is reached earlier than estimated in segregation analysis. Five-year survival rate was significantly higher in BRCA1 carriers than in an age matched population. Inactivation of the p53 gene is known to occur in the majority of human malignancies. Green et al (1994) have found that auto-antibodies to p53 have a role in the molecular characterisation of familial breast cancer.

Prognosis

There is never a shortage of papers looking at prognostic factors in breast cancer. A particularly interesting one recently from Carnon et al (1994) has demonstrated differences in survival by category of socio-economic deprivation which cannot be accounted for by differences in tumour stage or biology. Generally speaking, however, the prognosis for breast cancer has improved over the years. Nab et al (1994) from the Dutch Cancer Registry have shown an improvement in all age groups and patients who survive for 19 years can be regarded as cured. Age probably does not affect breast cancer outcome although younger patients have more aggressive and advanced disease at presentation (Crowe et al 1994a). In an extensive study on pregnancy and prognosis, Guinee et al (1994) have shown that in patients, whose breast cancers were diagnosed during pregnancy, the risk of dying was significantly greater than that of women who had never been pregnant. Cytological grading of fine needle aspiration may also be used as a prognostic factor in patients being considered for neo-adjuvant therapy (Robinson et al 1994a).

There is continuing controversy on whether the timing of surgery in relation to the menstrual cycle has an effect in determining prognosis in patients with early breast cancer. Three studies illustrate the dilemma. Saad et al (1994), in a retrospective survey, observed large changes at 10 years in both disease-free and overall survival in patients whose initial surgery was 1–12 days after the start of the last menstrual period. These differences in survival remain significant at the time of both initial and definitive surgery. However, Kroman et al (1994) could not demonstrate any influence on survival related to the last menstrual period in their patients. Veronesi et al (1994) reviewing patients in a randomised trial showed that premenstrual patients with positive lymph nodes operated on during the luteal phase had a significantly better prognosis than patients operated on during the follicular phase. Clearly, this topic requires a major prospective study if it is to elucidate the role of the menstrual phase in determining outcome of breast cancer surgery.

Diagnosis

Two interesting nuclear medicine investigations have been reported in patients with breast cancer. van Eijck et al (1994b) reported positive results with somatostatin-receptor scintigraphy in 39 of 52 primary breast cancers. This technique has also been shown to be sensitive in the recognition of recurrences in somatostatin receptor positive breast cancer. Positron emission tomography was used in a series of 28 patients using fluoro-D-glucose to assess clinico-pathological characteristics in the primary tumour. This technique can distinguish malignant from benign lesions and the report suggests that further studies are indicated (Crowe et al 1994).

A tumour marker which has been used extensively is CA15.3. Barros et al (1994) have shown that this is a useful parameter in the management of patients with different stages of breast cancer. However, it does not appear to be particularly helpful in the pre-operative differential diagnosis of a breast lump. Other interesting predictive investigations include the role of plasma prolactin in predicting tamoxifen resistance in patients with advanced breast cancer (Bhatavdekar et al 1994) and immunocytochemical staining of pS2 protein in fine needle aspirates in elderly patients (Wilson et al 1994).

Treatment

There has been some dispute on the most effective method of management of elderly patients with breast cancer. Gazet et al (1994) reported a randomised trial comparing primary surgery and tamoxifen alone in elderly patients. 53 patients in the tamoxifen group had local relapse and were available for crossover to surgery. 36 patients in the surgical group developed local relapse only and were available for crossover to tamoxifen. The results tend to suggest that if a patient is fit and willing to undergo surgery this is the most effective treatment and tamoxifen can be used in other circumstances. Similar data have been reported by Dunser et al (1994) in a series of 37 patients who concluded that limited surgery with the addition of hormone therapy is effective. Surgical complications were minimal in this series. Other surgical procedures are also satisfactory in older women and indeed in a series of 242 patients over the age of 65 even breast reconstruction was found to be a safe option and should be considered (August et al 1994).

There are theoretical advantages to neo-adjuvant therapy compared to adjuvant chemotherapy in patients with large breast cancers. Scholl et al (1994) have reported the results of a prospective trial randomising patients to either neo-adjuvant chemotherapy or adjuvant chemotherapy after primary irradiation with or without surgery. There was improved survival in the neo-adjuvant treatment arm but the implications of this were difficult to interpret. There was a trend to a decreased incidence of metastases but local control was similar in both groups. No statistically significant improvement in survival was found. If neo-adjuvant therapy is to become popular, there needs to be a method of measuring breast tumour size. Forouhi et al (1994) have reported on the use of ultrasonography in this regard and demonstrated good correlation between pathological and clinical size in 31 of 35 patients. This appears to be a reasonably accurate method of assessing tumour responses to neo-adjuvant chemotherapy.

Preventative or prophylactic mastectomy is an extremely controversial topic and might be considered suitable for individual women (Bostwick 1994, Kinne 1994). However, there is no doubt that such techniques need to be considered very carefully as patients will have unnecessary breast removal on at least 75% of occasions. Similarly, many patients will be psychologically unable to accept this procedure; alternatively, they may be unable to accept the small risk of breast cancer in the contralateral breast. If bilateral mastectomy is considered to prevent disease in the contralateral breast then immediate breast reconstruction is feasible (Kroll et al 1994). This group have reported successful outcomes in 95 patients using TRAM flaps.

In conservation treatment for early breast cancer, it is important that complete wide excision with absence of residual disease is achieved. Recent studies have investigated both specimen scrape cytology and tumour bed biopsy to exclude residual disease (England et al 1994, Macmillan et al 1994) and intraoperative assessment of nodal status using contact cytology (Hadjiminas & Burke 1994). Both techniques allegedly provide useful information in determining optimum management. In order to determine axillary involvement, Guiliano et al (1994) have utilised intraoperative lymphatic mapping by injecting vital dye into the primary breast cancer site and identifying sentinel lymph nodes. They feel that this technique might enhance accurate breast cancer staging intraoperatively, although it is not clear how this would influence subsequent management.

An interesting new technique has been described in a preliminary review. This involves interstitial laser photocoagulation for the early treatment of breast cancer (Harries et al 1994). Clearly further studies are required to determine whether laser fibres inserted into tumours can adequately destroy the whole area.

With increasing emphasis on adjuvant treatment and particularly the role of tamoxifen in early breast cancer as well as in chemoprevention, there has been a great deal of interest in the long-term effects of tamoxifen, particularly on the uterus. Postmenopausal women taking tamoxifen who have not had a hysterectomy should be informed about potential endometrial hazards (Nevin et al 1994). There is certainly a risk of endometrial cancer both in patients treated for established disease (van Leeuwen et al 1994) as well as in chemoprevention (Kadar et al 1994).

Benign disease

Finally, there has been continuing interest in aetiological aspects of benign breast disease as they pertain to pre-malignant conditions. This has recently been reviewed by Bundred (1994). Interestingly, in a prospective study of nipple discharge, it has been demonstrated that this symptom in women who do not have positive findings on investigation is not associated with increased risk of the development of carcinoma and in nearly three-quarters of women with nipple discharge, symptoms spontaneously resolve over a 5-year period (Carty et al 1994).

EMERGENCY SURGERY

Although acute appendicitis continues to represent a high proportion of emergency surgery, nevertheless a recent report suggests that its incidence may be decreasing, particularly over the last 15 years (McCahy 1994). The natural history of appendicitis and its progression are clearly matters of importance. There are a number of interesting epidemiological features. For example, Andersson et al (1994) from a study in Sweden has demonstrated that the incidence of perforating appendicitis was independent of age, stable over time and uninfluenced by the rate of laparotomy, whereas the incidence of non-perforating appendicitis was age dependent, decreasing over time and is related to the diagnostic accuracy and rate of removal of a normal appendix. This suggests that perforating and non-perforating appendicitis appear to be separate entities. There is also an indication that appendicitis commonly resolves spontaneously.

There has been much interest recently in the laparoscopic approach to appendicectomy and a few randomised trials have appeared. Frazee et al (1994) randomised 75 patients into open or laparoscopic appendicectomy. There were no significant differences in the length of hospitalisation, interval until resumption of a regular diet or morbidity. Return to full activity was 25 days for open appendicectomy and 14 days for laparoscopic appendicectomy. Contrary to previous studies, this group suggests that laparoscopic appendicectomy is the procedure of choice for acute appendicitis.

Other roles for laparoscopy in the acute emergency have been reported. MacSweeney et al (1994) advocate second look laparoscopy in the management of acute mesenteric ischaemia in order to avoid morbidity in patients in whom no further procedure is indicated. Fernando et al (1994) have performed laparoscopy for triage in 33 patients with penetrating abdominal injuries. It effectively and safely detected patients with peritoneal penetration. Ultrasonography has also been advocated in the diagnosis of acute abdomen. This is particularly useful in confirming or excluding hepatobiliary disease, aortic aneurysms and in blunt abdominal trauma (Williams et al 1994b). It appears to be a technique which can easily be learnt by surgeons in training.

There are many surgical scoring schemes designed to predict morbidity and mortality. Kennedy et al (1994) have advocated a simple pre-operative assessment identifying high risks in elderly patients undergoing emergency surgery. The predictive parameters were hypotension on admission, presence of severe chronic disease and whether the patient was independent and self caring. Other authors have used prognostic scores to determine the length of administration of antibiotic therapy. Schein et al (1994) in 163 patients stratified into various groups demonstrated that antibiotics can be related to the score and a minimal postoperative antibiotic policy can be employed.

Finally, head injuries are both common and expensive. The resource implications on one acute surgical unit has been investigated by Williams et al (1994c). There is no doubt that this is an expensive injury and even patients admitted for a 24-hour overnight observation result in significant resource expenditure. This should be taken into account in determining hospital finances.

REFERENCES

Abulafi AM, Williams NS 1994 Local recurrence of colorectal cancer: the problem, mechanisms, management and adjuvant therapy. Br J Surg 81: 7-19

Allen MJ, Thompson WD, Stuart RC et al 1994 Management of non-palpable breast lesions detected mammographically. Br J Surg 81: 543-545

Allen-Mersh TG, Earlam S, Fordy K et al 1994 Quality of life and survival with continuous hepatic-artery floxuridine infusion for colorectal liver metastases. Lancet 343: 1255-1260

Allum WH, Slaney G, McConkey CC et al 1994 Cancer of the colon and rectum in the West Midlands, 1957–1981. Br J Surg 81: 1060-1063

Ambrosetti P, Robert JH, Witzig J-A et al 1994 Acute left colonic diverticulitis: a prospective analysis of 226 consecutive cases. Surgery 115: 546-550

Andersson R, Hugander A, Thulin A et al 1994 Indications for operation in suspected appendicitis and incidence of perforation. BMJ 308: 107-110

August DA, Wilkins E, Rea T 1994 Breast reconstruction in older women. Surgery 115: 663-667

Austoker J 1994a Screening for colorectal cancer. BMJ 309: 382-386

Austoker J 1994b Screening and self examination for breast cancer. BMJ 309: 168-174

AXIS Steering Group 1994 The AXIS colorectal cancer trial. Randomisation of over 2000 patients. Br J Surg 81: 1672

Ballinger AB, McHugh M, Catnach SM et al 1994 Symptom relief and quality of life after stenting for malignant bile duct obstruction. Gut 35: 467-470

Barkun AN, Barkun JS, Fried GM et al 1994 Useful predictors of bile duct stones in patients undergoing laparoscopic cholecystectomy. Ann Surg 220: 32-39

Barros ACSD, Fry W, Nazario ACP et al 1994 Experience with CA 15.3 as a tumour marker in breast cancer. Eur J Surg Oncol 29: 130-133

Baumel H, Huguier M, Manderscheid JC et al 1994 Results of resection for cancer of the exocrine pancreas: a study from the French association of surgery. Br J Surg 81: 102-107

Beck NE, Sampson M, Michell R et al 1994 Size isn't important; the Forrest Unit. Eur J Surg Oncol 20: 635-636.

Berggren U, Gordh T, Grama D et al 1994 Laparoscopic versus open cholecystectomy: hospitalisation, sick leave, analgesia and trauma responses. Br J Surg 81: 1362-1365

Bernstein CN, Shanahan F, Weinstein WM 1994 Are we telling patients the truth about surveillance colonoscopy in ulcerative colitis? Lancet 343: 71-74

Bhatavdekar JM, Patel DD, Karelia NH et al 1994 Can plasma prolactin predict tamoxifen resistance in patients with advanced breast cancer? Eur J Surg Oncol 20: 118-121

Birdi I, Hunt TM, Veitch PS et al 1994 Laparoscopic cholecystectomy in Leicester: an audit of 555 patients. Ann R Coll Surg 76: 390-395

Boerma E J 1994 Towards an oncological resection of gall bladder cancer. Eur J Surg Oncol 20: 537-544

Bolton JS, Ochsner JL, Abodoh AA 1994 Surgical management of oesophageal cancer. Ann Surg 219: 475-480
Bostwick J 1994 Preventative mastectomy. Ann Surg Oncol 1: 455-456
Brennan MF, Pisters PWT, Posner M et al 1994 A prospective randomised trial of total parenteral nutrition after major pancreatic resection for malignancy. Ann Surg 220: 436-444
Briand D, Rouanet P, Kyriakopoulou T et al 1994 Repeated hepatic resections for liver metastases for colon carcinoma. Montepelier Cancer Institute experience. Eur J Surg Oncol 20: 219-224
Bruinvels DJ, Stiggelbout AM, Keivit J et al 1994 Follow up of patients with colorectal cancer. Ann Surg 219: 174-182
Bundred NJ 1994 Aetiological factors in benign breast disease. Br J Surg 81: 788-789
Burke P, Mealy K, Gillen P et al 1994 Requirement for bowel preparation in colorectal surgery. Br J Surg 81: 907-910
Capussotti G, Borgonono G, Bouzari H et al 1994 Results of major hepatectomy for large primary liver cancer in patients with cirrhosis. Br J Surg 81: 427-431
Carnon AG, Ssemwogerere A, Lamont DW et al 1994 Relation between socioeconomic deprivation and pathological prognostic factors in women with breast cancer. BMJ 309: 1054-1057
Carter R, Anderson JR 1994 Randomised trial of adrenaline injection and laser photocoagulation in the control of haemorrhage from peptic ulcer. Br J Surg 81: 869-871
Carty NJ, Mudan SS, Ravichandran D et al 1994 Prospective study of outcome in women presenting with nipple discharge. Ann R Coll Surg 76: 387-389
Chevalier JM, Jones DJ, Ratelle R et al 1994 Colectomy and iliorectal anastomosis in patients with Crohn's disease. Br J Surg 81: 1379-1381
Choi PM, Zelig MP 1994 Similarity of colorectal cancer in Crohn's disease and ulcerative colitis: implications for carcinogenesis and prevention. Gut 35: 950-954
Choudari CP, Palmer KR 1994 Endoscopic injection therapy for bleeding peptic ulcer; a comparison of adrenaline alone with adrenaline plus ethanolamine oleate. Gut 35: 608-610
Chung SS, Stuart RC, Li AKC 1994 Surgical therapy for squamous cell carcinoma of the oesophagus. Lancet 343: 521-524
Civalleri D, Pector J-C, Hakansson L et al 1994 Treatment of patients with irresectable liver metastases from colorectal cancer by chemo-occlusion with degradable starch microspheres. Br J Surg 81: 1338-1341
Collard JM, de Gheldere CA, De Kock M et al 1994 Laparoscopic antireflux surgery. Ann Surg 220: 146-154
Connell WR, Sheffield JP, Kamm MA et al 1994 Lower gastrointestinal malignancy in Crohn's disease. Gut 35: 347-352
Crowe JP, Adler LP, Shenk RR et al 1994 Positron emission tomography and breast masses: comparison with clinical, mammographic and pathological findings. Ann Surg Oncol 1: 132-140
Crowe JP, Gordon NH, Shenk RR et al 1994a Age does not predict breast cancer outcome. Arch Surg 129: 483-488
Cuschieri A, Shimi SM, Van der Velpen G et al 1994 Laparoscopic prosthesis fixation rectopexy for complete rectal prolapse. Br J Surg 81: 138-139
Dallemagne B, Weerts JM, Jehaes C et al 1994 Laparoscopic highly selective vagotomy. Br J Surg 81: 554-556
Darzi A, Geraghty JG, Williams NN et al 1994 The pros and cons of laparoscopic cholecystectomy and extracorporeal shock wave lithotripsy in the management of gall stone disease. Ann R Coll Surg Engl 76: 42-46
Davidson BR, Lauri A, Horton R et al 1994 Outcome of surgery for failed endoscopic extraction of common bile duct stones in elderly patients. Ann R Coll Surg Engl 76: 320-323
Deans GT, McAleer JJA, Spence RAJ 1994 Malignant anal tumours. Br J Surg 81: 500-508
Deen KI, Grant E, Billingham C et al 1994 Abdominal resection rectopexy with pelvic floor repair versus perineal rectosigmoidectomy and pelvic floor repair for full-thickness rectal prolapse. Br J Surg 81: 302-304
Ding S-F, Delhanty JDA, Zografos G et al 1994 Chromosome allele loss in colorectal liver metastases and its association with clinical features. Br J Surg 81: 875-878
Donato N, Dario C, Giovanni S et al 1994 Retrospective study on adjuvant chemotherapy after surgical resection of colorectal cancer metastatic to the liver. Eur J Surg Oncol 20: 454-460

Dunn D, Nair R, Fowler S et al 1994 Laparoscopic cholecystectomy in England and Wales: results of an audit by the Royal College of Surgeons of England. Ann R Coll Surg Engl 76: 269-275
Dunser M, Haussler B, Fuchs H et al 1994 Tumorectomy plus tamoxifen for the treatment of breast cancer in the elderly. Eur J Surg Oncol 19: 529-531
England DW, Chan SY, Stonelake PS et al 1994 Assessment of excision margins following wide local excision for breast carcinoma using specimen scrape cytology and tumour bed biopsy. Eur J Surg Oncol 20: 425-429
Eu K-W, Seow-Choen F, Goh HS 1994 Comparison of emergency and elective haemorrhoidectomy. Br J Surg 81: 308-310
Evans DGR, Fentiman IS, McPherson K et al 1994 Familial breast cancer. BMJ 308: 183-187
Farmakis N, Tudor RG, Keighley MRB 1994 The 5 year natural history of complicated diverticular disease. Br J Surg 81: 733-735
Fernando HC, Alle KM, Chen J et al 1994 Triage by laparoscopy in patients with penetrating abdominal trauma. Br J Surg 81: 384-385
Fong Y, Blumgart LH, Cohen A et al 1994 Repeat hepatic resections for metastatic colorectal cancer. Ann Surg 220: 657-662
Ford D, Easton DF, Bishop DT et al 1994 Risk of cancer in BRCA 1 mutation carriers. Lancet 343: 692-685
Forouhi P, Walsh JS, Anderson TJ et al 1994 Ultrasonography as a method of measuring breast tumour size and monitoring response primary systemic treatment. Br J Surg 81: 223-225
Frazee RC, Roberts JW, Symmonds RE et al 1994 A prospective randomised trial comparing open versus laparoscopic appendectomy. Ann Surg 219: 725-731
Fullarton GM, Darling K, Williams J et al 1994 Evaluation of the cost of laparoscopic and open cholecystectomy. Br J Surg 81: 124-126
Gazet J-C, Ford HT, Coombes RC et al 1994 Prospective randomised trial of tamoxifen vs surgery in elderly patients with breast cancer. Eur J Surg Oncol 20: 207-214
Gillen CD, Walmsley RS, Prior P et al 1994 Ulcerative colitis and Crohn's disease: a comparison of the colorectal cancer risk in extensive colitis. Gut 35: 1590-1592
Goh H-S, Chan C-S, Khine K et al 1994 p53 and behaviour of colorectal cancer. Lancet 344: 233-234
Gough DB, Donohue JH, Trastek VA et al 1994 Resection of hepatic and pulmonary metastases in patients with colorectal cancer. Br J Surg 81: 94-96
Green JA, Mudenda B, Jenkins J et al 1994 Serum p53 auto-antibodies: incidence in familial breast cancer. Eur J Cancer 30A: 581-584
Greig JD, John TG, Mahadaven M et al 1994 Laparoscopic ultrasonography in the evaluation of the biliary tree during laparoscopic cholecystectomy. Br J Surg 81: 1202-1206
Guiliano AE, Kirgan DM, Guenther JM et al 1994 Lymphatic mapping and sentinel lymphadenectomy for breast cancer. Ann Surg 220: 391-401
Guinee VF, Olsson H, Moller T et al 1994 Effect of pregnancy on prognosis for young women with breast cancer. Lancet 343: 1587-1589
Habib NA, Michail NE, Boyle T et al 1994b Resection of the inferior vena cava during hepatectomy for liver tumours. Br J Surg 81: 1023-1024
Habib N, Zografos G, Dalla Serra L et al 1994a Liver resection with total vascular exclusion for malignant tumours. Br J Surg 81: 1181-1184
Hadjiminas DJ, Burke M 1994 Intraoperative assessment of nodal status in the selection of patients with breast cancer for axillary clearance. Br J Surg 81: 1615-1616
Hainsworth PJ, Rhodes M, Gompertz RHK et al 1994 Imaging of the common bile duct in patients undergoing laparoscopic cholecystectomy. Gut 35: 991-995
Hallissey MT, Dunn JA, Ward LC et al 1994 The second British Stomach Cancer Group Trial of radiotherapy or chemotherapy in resectable gastric cancer: 5 year follow up. Lancet 343: 1309-1312
Hardwick RH, Shepherd NA, Moorghen et al 1994 Adenocarcinoma arising in Barrett's oesophagus: evidence for the participation of p53 dysfunction in the dysplasia/carcinoma sequence. Gut 35: 764-768
Harries SA, Amin Z, Smith MEF et al 1994 Interstitial laser photocoagulation as a treatment for breast cancer. Br J Surg 81: 1617-1619
Heesakkers JPF, Gouma FBJM, Thunnissen MHA et al 1994 Non-radical therapy for early gastric cancer. Br J Surg 81: 551-553
Hemming AW, Langer B 1994 Repeat resection of recurrent hepatic colorectal metastases. Br J Surg 81: 1553-1554

Hennigan TW, Allen-Mersh TG 1994 Duration of blood flow reduction to normal liver tissue induced by angiotensin, vasopressin and enothelin. Eur J Surg Oncol 20: 446-448
Heys SD, O'Hanrahan TJ, Brittenden J et al 1994 Colorectal cancer in young patients: a review of the literature. Eur J Surg Oncol 20: 225-231
Hill ADK, Walsh TN, Bolger CM et al 1994 Randomised controlled trial comparing Nissen fundoplication and the Angelchik prosthesis. Br J Surg 81: 72-74
Hinder RA, Filipi CJ, Wetscher et al 1994 Laparoscopic Nissen fundoplication is an effective treatment for gastro-oesophageal reflux disease. Ann Surg 220: 472-483
Hoffman GC, Baker JW, Claiborne W et al 1994 Laparoscopic assisted colectomy. Ann Surg 219: 732-743
Hohenberger P, Schlag PM, Gernth T et al 1994 Pre and post-operative carcinoembryonic antigen determinations in hepatic resection for colorectal metastases. Ann Surg 219: 135-143
Holm T, Cedermark B, Rutqvist L-E 1994 Local recurrence of rectal adenocarcinoma after 'curative' surgery with and without preoperative radiotherapy. Br J Surg 81: 452-455
Hsu PI, Lin XZ, Chan SH et al 1994 Bleeding peptic ulcer – risk factors for rebleeding and sequential changes in endoscopic findings. Gut 35: 746-749
Izbicki JR, Bloechle C, Knoefel WT et al 1994 Complications of adjacent organs in chronic pancreatitis managed by duodenum-preserving resection of the head of the pancreas. Br J Surg 81: 1351-1355
Jaakkola M, Silanaukee P, Lof K et al 1994 Blood tests for detection of alcoholic cause of acute pancreatitis. Lancet 343: 1328-1329
Jamieson GG, Watson DI, Britten-Jones R et al 1994 Laparoscopic Nissen fundoplication. Ann Surg 220: 137-145
Jones AL, Trott P, Cunningham D et al 1994 A pilot study of intraperitoneal cisplatin in the management of gastric cancer. Ann Oncol 5: 123-126
Jonsson B, Ashgren L, Andersson LO et al 1994 Colorectal cancer surveillance in patients with ulcerative colitis. Br J Surg 81: 689-691
Jordan PH, Thornby J 1994 Twenty years after parietal cell vagotomy or selective vagotomy antrectomy for treatment of duodenal ulcer. Ann Surg 220: 283-296
Kadar RP, Bourne TH, Powles T et al 1994 Effects of tamoxifen on uterus and ovaries of postmenopausal women in a randomised breast cancer prevention trial. Lancet 343: 1318-1321
Karanjia ND, Corder AP, Bearn P et al 1994 Leakage from stapled low anastomosis after total mesorectal excision for carcinoma of the rectum. Br J Surg 81: 1224-1226
Kawasaki S, Makuuchi M, Kakazu T et al 1994 Resection for multiple metastatic liver tumours after portal embolisation. Surgery 115: 674-677
Kennedy RH, AI-Mufti RAM, Brewster SF et al 1994 The acute surgical admission: is mortality predictable in the elderly? Ann R Coll Surg Engl 76: 342-345
Kerin MJ, Williams NN, Cronin KJ et al 1994 Stereotactic cytology in a regional breast-screening programme. Br J Surg 81: 221-222
Kinne DW 1994 Management of the contralateral breast. Ann Surg Oncol 1: 454-455
Kollmorgen CF, Meagher AP, Wolff BG et al 1994 The long-term effect of adjuvant post-operative chemotherapy for rectal carcinoma on bowel function. Ann Surg 220: 676-682
Kroll SS, Miller MJ, Schusterman MA et al 1994 Rationale for elective contralateral mastectomy with immediate bilateral reconstruction. Ann Surg Oncol 1: 457-461
Kroman N, Hojgaard A, Anderson KW et al 1994 Timing of surgery in relation to menstrual cycle does not predict the prognosis of primary breast cancer. Eur J Surg Oncol 20: 430-435
Lautenbach E, Forde KA, Neugut AI 1994 Benefits of colonoscopic surveillance after curative resection of colorectal cancer. Ann Surg 220: 206-211
Loder PB, Kamm MA, Nicholls RJ et al 1994 Haemorrhoids: pathology, pathophysiology and aetiology. Br J Surg 81: 946-954
Longo WE, Vemava AM, Wade TP et al 1994 Recurrent squamous cell carcinoma of the anal canal. Ann Surg 220: 40-49
Lundegardh G, Adami HO, Helmick Ch et al 1994a Risk of cancer following partial gastrectomy for benign ulcer disease. Br J Surg 81: 1164-1167
Lundegardh G, Ekbom A, McLaughlin JK et al 1994b Gastric cancer risk after vagotomy. Gut 35: 946-949
Macintyre IMC, O'Brien F 1994 Death from malignant disease after surgery for duodenal ulcer. Gut 35: 451-454

MacMillan RD, Purushotham AD, Mallon E et al 1994 Breast-conserving surgery and tumour bed positivity in patients with breast cancer. Br J Surg 81: 56-58

MacSweeney STR, Postlethwaite JC 1994 `Second look' laparoscopy in the management of acute mesenteric ischaemia. Br J Surg 81: 90

Mann DV, Hershman MJ, Hittinger R et al 1994 Multicentre audit of death from acute pancreatitis. Br J Surg 81: 890-893

McCormick PA, Dick R, Panagou EB et al 1994 Emergency transjugular intrahepatic portasystemic stent shunting as salvage treatment for uncontrolled variceal bleeding. Br J Surg 81: 1324-1327

McCahy P 1994 Continuing fall in the incidence of acute appendicitis. Ann R Coll Surg Engl 76: 282-283

McCulloch 1994 Description of the Japanese method of radical gastrectomy. Ann R Coll Surg Engl 76: 110-114

McGuire HH 1994 Bleeding colonic diverticula. A reappraisal of natural history and management. Ann Surg 220: 653-656

McMahon AJ, Russell IT, Baxter JN et al 1994b Laparoscopic versus minilaparotomy cholecystectomy: a randomised trial. Lancet 343: 135-138

McMahon AJ, Russell IT, Ramsay G et al 1994a Laparoscopic and minilaparotomy cholecstectomy: a randomised trial comparing post-operative pain and pulmonary function. Surgery 115: 533-539

Meisner S, Hoffmann J, Jensen H-E 1994 Parietal cell vagotomy. Ann Surg 220: 164-167

Melbye M, Cote TR, Kessler L et al 1994 High incidence of anal cancer among AIDS patients. Lancet 343: 636-639

Mendenhall WM, Sombeek MD, Speer TW et al 1994 Current management of squamous cell carcinoma of the anal canal. Surg Oncol 3: 135-146

Mittra I 1994 Breast screening: the case for physical examination without mammography. Lancet 343: 342-344

Mueller X, Rothenbuehler JM, Amery A et al 1994 Bleeding peptic ulcer: and audit of conservative management. J R Soc Med 87: 132-134

Mulcahy HE, Duffy MJ, Gibbons D et al 1994a Urokinase-type plasminogen activator and outcome in Dukes B colorectal cancer. Lancet 344: 583-584

Mulcahy HE, Patchett SE, Daly L et al 1994b Prognosis of elderly patients with large bowel cancer. Br J Surg 81: 736-738

Mulder J-WR, Kruyt PM, Sewnath M et al 1994 Colorectal cancer prognosis and expression of exon-v6-containing CD44 proteins. Lancet 344: 1470-1472

Nab HW, Hop WCJ, Crommelin MA et al 1994 Changes in long term prognosis for breast cancer in a Dutch cancer registry. BMJ 309: 83-86

Nakazato H, Koike A, Saji S et al 1994 Efficacy of immunochemotherapy as adjuvant treatment after curative resection of gastric cancer. Lancet 343: 1122-1126

Nduka CC, Monston JRT, Menzies-Gow N et al 1994 Abdominal wall metastases following laparoscopy. Br J Surg 81: 648-652

Nevin P, Muylder X, Belle YV et al 1994 Tomoxifen and the uterus. BMJ 309: 1313-1314

Nicholl JP, Ross B, Milner PC et al 1994 Cost effectiveness of adjuvant bile salt treatment in extracorporeal shock wave lithotripsy for the treatment of gall bladder stones. Gut 35: 1294-1300

Nordback IH, Pitt HA, Coleman J et al 1994 Unresectable hilar cholangiocarcinoma: percutaneous versus operative palliation. Surgery 115: 597-603

Nossal GJV 1994 Minimal residual disease as the target for immunotherapy of cancer. Lancet 343: 1172-1174

Novell JR, Osborne MJ, Winslet MC et al 1994 Prospective randomised trial of Ivalon sponge versus sutured rectopexy for full-thickness rectal prolapse. Br J Surg 81: 904-906

Ogiwara H, Nakamura T, Baba S 1994 Variables related to risk of recurrence in rectal cancer without lymph node metastasis. Ann Surg Oncol 2: 99-104

Palmer KR, Kerr M, Knowles G et al 1994 Chemotherapy prolongs survival in inoperable pancreatic carcinoma. Br J Surg 81: 882-885

Patel P, Mendall MA, Khulusi S et al 1994 Salivary antibodies to *Helicobacter pylori*: screening dyspeptic patients before endoscopy. Lancet 344: 511-514

Perissat J, Huibregtse K, Keane FBV et al 1994 Management of bile duct stones in the era of laparoscopic cholecystectomy. Br J Surg 81: 799-810

Peters JH, Hoeft SF, Heimbucher J et al 1994 Selection of patients for curative or palliative

resection of oesophageal cancer based on preoperative endoscopic ultrasonography. Arch Surg 129: 534-539
Porter DE, Cohen BB, Wallace MR et al 1994 Breast cancer incidence, penetrance and survival in probable carriers of BRCA1 gene mutation in families linked to BRCA1 on chromosome 17p12–21. Br J Surg 81: 1512-1515
Poston GJ 1994 Somatostatin and the treatment of gastric cancer. Ann R Coll Surg Engl 76: 172-174
Pytel J, Sigon R, Bidoli E et al 1994 Primary gastric non-Hodgkin's lymphoma – does surgery still play any role? Eur J Surg Oncol 20: 525-536
Que FG, Nagorney DM 1994 Resection of 'recurrent' colorectal metastases to the liver. Br J Surg 81: 255-258
Quine MA, Bell GD, McCloy RF 1994 Appropriate use of upper gastrointestinal endoscopy – a prospective audit. Gut 35: 1209-1214
Rieger NA, Jamieson GG, Britten-Jones R et al 1994 Reoperation after failed antireflux surgery. Br J Surg 81: 1159-1161
Robertson CS, Chung SCS, Woods SDS et al 1994 A prospective randomised trial comparing R_1 subtotal gastrectomy with R_3 total gastrectomy for antral cancer. Ann Surg 220: 176-182
Robinson MHE, Pye G, Thomas WM et al 1994a Haemoccult screening for colorectal cancer: the effect of dietary restriction on compliance. Eur J Surg Oncol 20: 545-548
Robinson MHE, Marks CG, Farrands PA et al 1994b Population screening for colorectal cancer: comparison between guaiac and immunological faecal occult blood tests. Br J Surg 81: 448-451
Robinson IA, McKee G, Nicholson A et al 1994c Prognostic value of cytological grading of fine-needle aspirates from breast carcinomas. Lancet 343: 947-949
Rotman N, Pezet D, Fagniez P-L et al 1994 Adenocarcinoma of the duodenum: factors influencing survival. Br J Surg 81: 83-85
Saad Z, Bramwell V, Duff J et al 1994 Timing of surgery in relation to the menstrual cycle in premenopausal women with operable breast cancer. Br J Surg 81: 217-220
Sagar PM, Gauperaa T, Sue-Ling H et al 1994 An audit of the treatment of cancer of the oesophagus. Gut 35: 941-945
Sarin S, Boulos PB 1994 Long-term outcome of patients presenting with acute complications of diverticular disease. Ann R Coll Surg Engl 76: 117-120
Sause WT, Pajak TF, Noyes D et al 1994 Evaluation of preoperative radiation therapy in operable colorectal cancer. Ann Surg 220: 668-675
Schein M, Assalia A, Bachus H 1994 Minimal antibiotic therapy after emergency abdominal surgery: a prospective study. Br J Surg 81: 989-991
Scholefield JH, Ogunbiyi OA, Smith JHF et al 1994 Treatment of anal intraepithelial neoplasia. Br J Surg 81: 1238-1240
Scholl SM, Fourquet A, Asselain B et al 1994 Neoadjuvant versus adjuvant chemotherapy in premenopausal patients with tumours considered too large for breast conserving surgery: preliminary results of a randomised trial: S6. Eur J Cancer 30A: 645-652
Scott-Coombes DM, Williamson RCN 1994 Surgical treatment of primary duodenal carcinoma: a personal series. Br J Surg 81: 1472-1474
Sitzman JV, Wu Y, Cameron JL 1994 Altered angiotensin-II receptors in human hepatocellular and hepatic metastatic colon cancers. Ann Surg 219: 500-507
Smith AC, Dowsett JF, Russell RGC et al 1994 Randomised trial of endoscopic stenting versus surgical bypass in malignant low bile duct obstruction. Lancet 343: 1655-1660
Sperti C, Pasquali C, Piccoli A et al 1994 Radical resection for ampullary carcinoma: long-term results. Br J Surg 81: 668-671
Stangl R, Altendorf-Hofmann A, Charnley RM et al 1994 Factors influencing the natural history of colorectal liver metastases. Lancet 343: 1405-1410
Stewart GJ, Lawson JA, Morris DL 1994 Octreotide inhibits development of hepatic metastases from a human colonic cancer cell line. Br J Surg 81: 1332
Svanes C, Lie RT, Svanes K et al 1994 Adverse effects of delayed treatment for perforated peptic ulcer. Ann Surg 220: 168-175
Tate JJT, Lau WY, Li AKC 1994 Laparoscopic cholecystectomy for biliary pancreatitis. Br J Surg 81: 720-722
Tjandra JJ, Fazio VW 1994 Stictureplasty without concomitant resection for small bowel obstruction in Crohn's disease. Br J Surg 81: 561-563
Tsao JI, Loftus JP, Nagorney DM et al 1994 Trends in morbidity and mortality of hepatic resection for malignancy. Ann Surg 220: 199-205

Tudor RG, Farmakis N, Keighley MRB 1994 National audit of complicated diverticular disease: analysis of index cases. Br J Surg 81: 730-732
van Eijck CHJ, Krenning EP, Bootsma A et al 1994b Somatostatin receptor scintigraphy in primary breast cancer. Lancet 343: 640-643
van Eijck CHJ, Slooter GD, Hofland LJ et al 1994a Somatostatin receptor dependant growth inhibition of liver metastases by octreotide. Br J Surg 81: 1333-1337
van Lanschot JJB, Tilanus HW, Voormolen et al 1994 Recurrence pattern of oesophageal carcinoma after limited resection does not support wide local excision with extensive lymph node dissection. Br J Surg 81: 1320-1322
van Leeuwen FE, Benraadt J, Coobergh JWW et al 1994 Risk of endometrial cancer after tamoxifen treatment of breast cancer. Lancet 343: 448-451
Varty PP, Delrio P, Boulos PB 1994a Survival in colorectal carcinoma associated with previous extracolonic cancer. Ann R Coll Surg Engl 76: 180-184
Varty PP, Linehan I, Boulos PB 1994b Intra-abdominal sepsis and survival after surgery for colorectal cancer. Br J Surg 81: 915-918
Veronesi U, Luini A, Mariani L et al 1994 Effect of menstrual phase on surgical treatment of breast cancer. Lancet 343: 1545-1547
Vogel SB, Drane WE, Ros PR et al 1994 Prediction of surgical resectabiltiy in patients with hepatic colorectal metastases. Ann Surg 219: 508-516
Watson DI, Reed MWR, Johnson AG et al 1994 Laparoscopic fundoplication for gastro-oesophageal reflux. Ann R Coll Surg 76: 264-268
Watkin DS, Haworth JM, Leaper DJ et al 1994 Assessment of the common bile duct before cholecystectomy using ultrasound and biochemical measurements: validation based on follow up. Ann R Coll Surg Engl 76: 317-319
Williams NS, Hughes SF, Stuchfield B 1994a Continent colonic conduit for rectal evacuation in severe constipation. Lancet 343: 1321-1324
Williams RJ, Windsor CJ, Rosin RD et al 1994b Ultrasound scanning of the acute abdomen by surgeons in training. Ann R Coll Surg Engl 76: 228-233
Williams RJL, Hittinger H, Glazer G 1994c Resource implications of head injuries on an acute surgical unit. J R Soc Med 87: 83-86
Williams SGJ, Peters RA, Westaby D 1994a Thrombin – an effective treatment for gastric variceal haemorrhage. Gut 35: 1287-1289
Willson PD, Kunkler R, Blair SD et al 1994 Emergency oesophageal transaction for uncontrolled variceal haemorrhage. Br J Surg 81: 992-995
Wils J, Bleiberg H, Rougier Ph 1994 Adjuvant treatment of colon cancer. A plea for a large scale European trial. Eur J Cancer 30A: 578-579
Wilson YG, Rhodes M, Ibrahim NBN et al 1994 Immunocytochemical staining of pS2 protein in fine needle aspirate from breast cancer is an accurate guide to response to tamoxifen in patients aged over 70 years. Br J Surg 81: 1155-1158
Wyatt JP, Aitken RJ 1994 Evaluation of hospital and general practice follow up after surgery for colorectal cancer. Br J Surg 81: 145

Index

Abdomen, acute
  triage by laparoscopy, 253
  ultrasonography, 253
Abdominal aortic aneurysms, 19-41
  imaging, 31-32, 142-143
  inflammatory, 21
  infra-renal
    pathogenesis, 22-23
    treatment and outcome, 19-21
  pathogenesis, 21-24
    atherosclerosis and, 24
    immune response and, 23-24
    proteolysis and changes in extracellular matrix, 23
  repair
    cardiac risk assessment and revascularisation, 20-21
    conventional technique, 20
    endovascular, 28-36
    indications for, 19-20
    inflammatory aneurysms, 21
    infra-renal aneurysms, 19-21
    retroperitoneal/transperitoneal approach, 21
    spinal cord damage, 28
    thoracoabdominal aneurysms, 27-28
  screening, 24-26
  thoracoabdominal, 26-28
    complications of surgery, 28
    surgical management, 27-28
Abdominal vascular pathology
  computed tomography, 142-144
  magnetic resonance imaging, 142, 144
Acid phosphatase, as marker for bone metastases, 118, 119
Adenocarcinoma
  gastric, role of *Helicobacter pylori*, 70-71
  pancreatic, imaging, 138, 139-140
Adriamycin *see* Doxorubicin
Alginate dressing, skin graft donor sites, 176
Ambulance services, 105
Amoxycillin, 69, 71
Anaesthesia, cardiopulmonary bypass, 49
Angiotensin converting enzyme (ACE) inhibitors, cardiac support, 52
Anorectal surgery, 242-243
Antithrombin III in cardiopulmonary bypass, 48
Anus
  cancer, 243
  fistula, imaging, 145
  intraepithelial neoplasia, 243
Aortomyoplasty, 55
Appendicectomy, 253
Appendicitis, 253
Aprotonin, 20
  cardiopulmonary bypass, 50
Arginine, enteric nutrition, 155
Atherosclerosis
  and aortic aneurysms 24
  effects in cardiopulmonary bypass, 48

Balloon, intragastric, 210-211
BCG immunotherapy, superficial bladder cancer, 80-85
Beta blockers, cardiac support, 52-53
Bile duct
  imaging, 244
  malignant obstruction, 245
  stones, 244
Biliary disease
  gallstones, 243-245
  malignant, 245
Biliary tract
  computed tomography, 139
  magnetic resonance imaging, 140, 141
Biliopancreatic bypass, 206-207
Biphosphonates
  malignant hypercalcaemia, 121, 122
  osteolysis inhibition, 119-120
Bismuth compounds, 71
Bladder, orthotopic reconstruction, 85-86
Bladder cancer, superficial
  classification, 77
  follow up regime, 79-80
  investigation, haematuria clinics, 77-78
  management
    carcinoma *in situ*, 83-84
    intravesical agents, 80-84
    prevention of recurrence, 82-83
    PT1G3 tumours, 84-85
    urinary tract reconstruction after cystectomy, 85-87
  metachronous, monoclonal origin versus field change, 87
  non-random chromosomal deletions, 86-87
  prognostic factors, 78-79, 87-88
Blind loop syndrome, 206
Body Mass Index (BMI), 199-201

Bombesin, 191-192
Bone
  metabolism, markers, 116-117
  remodelling, 109-110
Bone metastases
  breast cancer, 109, 116
    diagnosis, 114
    hypercalcaemia, 121
    mechanism of metastasis, 110-111
    treatment, 118, 120
    tumour markers, 117
  diagnosis, 111-115
  hypercalcaemia, 120-122
  incidence, 109
  lung cancer, 109
    treatment, 119
  markers, 116-118
  mechanism of metastasis, 110-111
  myeloma, 116, 118
    treatment, 120
  osteolytic, 113, 114
  prostate cancer, 109, 117
    mechanism of metastasis, 110-111
    treatment, 118-119, 120
    tumour markers, 117
  sclerotic, 113
  treatment
    assessment of response, 115-118
    endocrine, 118-119
    orthopaedic management, 123-125
    radiotherapy, 122-123
    systemic, 118-120
Bowel, large *see* Large bowel
Bowel disease, CT and MRI imaging, 144-145
Bradykinin, 188
Breast
  benign disease, 253
  cancer
    diagnosis, 250-251
    preventive surgery, 252
    prognosis, 250
    role of menstrual phase in surgery outcome, 250
    screening, 249-250
    treatment, 251-252
Buckwalter operation, 203, 204

CA15-3 as tumour marker
  bone metastases, 117
  breast cancer, 251
Caecostomy, malignant large bowel obstruction, 5, 11
Calcitonin, malignant hypercalcaemia, 122
Calcium, urine excretion, metastatic bone disease, 117
Calcium alginate dressing, skin graft donor sites, 176
Cancer
  hormone treatment, 185-187
  see also sites and types of cancer
Carcinoembryonic antigen (CEA) measurement, 247
Cardiac support, 51-55
  devices for, 53-55
    pumps, 53
    total artificial heart, 54-55
    ventricular assist, 54
  myoplastic procedures, 55
  pharmacological, 51-53
Cardiomyoplasty, 55
Cardiopulmonary bypass (CPB), 43-50
  anaesthetic management, 49
  blood conservation, 49-50
  blood trauma, 47
  hormonal changes, 47
    modulation, 48
  indications for, 50
  neurological sequelae, 47-48
    minimising, 50
  oxygenation, 45-46
  pathophysiology, 46-48
  perfusion, 43-45
  risk minimisation, 48-50
  systemic inflammatory response, 46-47
    modulation, 48
Cardiotomy suckers and blood trauma in cardiopulmonary bypass, 47
CD44v6 and colorectal cancer prognosis, 240
Cholecystectomy, laparoscopic, 243
Cholecystojejunoileal bypass, 202
Cholecystokinin (CCK), 188, 190
Clarithromycin, 71
Clodronate, osteolysis inhibition, 119-120
Colectomy
  and ileorectal anastomosis, Crohn's disease, 239
  laparoscopic-assisted, 242
  subtotal, malignant large bowel obstruction, 11-13
Colitis
  computed tomography, 145
  ulcerative, malignancy and, 238-239
Colorectal cancer
  chemotherapy, 185
  Duke's stage, 240
  incidence, 183, 184
  inflammatory bowel disease and, 238-239
  outcome, 184
  prognostic factors, 240-241
  radiotherapy, 184-185
  screening, 240
  surgery, 184
Colorectal cancer, obstructing, 1
  gastrin and, 190
  prognosis, 14-15
  resection and delayed anastomosis, 7-8, 15
  resection and immediate anastomosis, 8-11

staged resection, 5-6
subtotal colectomy, 11-13
Colostomy, malignant large bowel obstruction
Hartmann's operation, 7-8
transverse colostomy, 5
Computed tomography (CT), 129
abdominal vascular pathology, 142-144
bone metastases, 114
bowel disease, 144-145
liver, 133-136
obstructive jaundice, 139
pancreatic neoplasia, 138-139
principles, 129-131
spiral, 130-131
abdominal vascular pathology, 142-144
biliary tract, 139
liver, 135-136
pancreas, 138-139
Confidential Enquiry into Peri-operative Deaths (CEPOD), 98
Contraction, wound healing, 171
Crohn's disease
imaging, 145
malignancy and, 238-239
surgical procedures, 239
Cystectomy, urinary tract reconstruction following, 85-87
Cytokines, wound healing, 172-173
chronic wounds, 174

Deoxypyridinoline, as marker in metastatic bone disease, 117
Digoxin, 51
Diverticular disease, 239-240
Doxorubicin (adriamycin), superficial bladder cancer, 80, 81, 83
Duodenal ulcers
laparoscopic highly selective vagotomy, 236-237
parietal cell vagotomy, long-term effects, 236
role of *Helicobacter pylori*, 66-67, 68
Duodenum, adenocarcinoma, 238
Dyspepsia, non-ulcer, role of *Helicobacter pylori*, 65

Embolism, gas, cardiopulmonary bypass, 48, 50
Emergency surgery, 253-254
Enteral nutrition
access routes, 156-160
feeds, 153-154
categories, 153
disease specific, 154-155
elemental, 154
glutamine in, 155
polymeric, 154
Enzyme linked immunosorbent assay (ELISA), *Helicobacter pylori*
diagnosis, 64
Epidermal growth factor, 176
Epidermal growth factor receptor, 187
bladder cancer, 87
Epirubicin, superficial bladder cancer, 80, 81, 82, 83
Epithelial growth factor (EGF), wound healing and, 172, 173
chronic wounds, 174
skin graft donor site, 175
Epithelialisation, wound healing, 170-171, 173
Epodyl, 81
Euthyroid sick syndrome, 47
treatment, 48
Extracorpoeal membrane oxygenation (ECMO), 56
Extracorporeal CO_2 removal ($ECCO_2R$), 56
Extracorporeal shock wave lithotripsy (ESWL), 244-245

Feeding tubes, naso-enteral, 157, 158
Feeds *see* Nutrients
Fibroblast growth factor, basic (bFGF), 173
Fibronectin, wound healing, 171
Fibroplasia, wound healing, 171
fetus, 180
Fluorescence in situ hybridisation (FISH), chromosome aberrations in bladder cancer, 86
5-Fluorouracil (5FU)
gastrointestinal cancer treatment, 185
liver cancer, 248
Flutamide, 119
Folinic acid, gastrointestinal cancer treatment, 185
Fractures, metastatic bone disease, 123-124

G proteins, 187, 189
Gall bladder, carcinoma, 245
Gallstones, 243-245
Gastrectomy, gastric cancer, 237-238
Gastric adenocarcinoma, role of *Helicobacter pylori*, 70-71
Gastric bypass, 202-203, 205-206
Gastric cancer
risk, after surgery for benign ulceration, 237
treatment
adjuvant therapy, 238
surgical, 237
Gastric lymphoma
non-Hodgkin's, 238
role of *Helicobacter pylori*, 69-70
Gastric ulcers, role of *Helicobacter pylori*, 67-68
Gastric wrap (band, clip), 211
Gastrin, 188, 190
Gastrin releasing peptide (GRP), 188, 191-192

Gastritis, role of *Helicobacter pylori*, 65-66
Gastro-oesophageal reflux, Nissen's fundoduplication, 235
Gastrointestinal cancer, 183
 incidence, 183, 184
 outcome, 184
 treatment
  chemotherapy, 185
  hormonal, 185-195
  radiotherapy, 184-185
  surgical, 184
Gastrointestinal endoscopy, use of, 236
Gastrointestinal surgery, review of new developments, 235-260
Gastrojejunostomy, loop, 202, 205
Gastroplasty, 203, 212
 vertical band, 208-209
Gastrostomy, percutaneous endoscopic, 158, 159-160
Glucocorticoids, malignant hypercalcaemia, 122
Glutamine
 enteric nutrition, 155
 parenteral nutrition, 155
Glycosaminoglycans, wound healing, 171
Gomez operation, 203, 204, 211-212
Gourlay and Cleator operation, 206
Growth factors
 peptide, 185, 187, 189-190
 wound healing, 172-173
  chronic wounds, 174
  fetal wounds, 180
  skin graft donor sites, 176

Haematuria clinics, 77-78
Haemocyanin, keyhole-limpet, superficial bladder cancer, 82
Haemopump, 53
Haemorrhoids, 243
Hartmann's operation, 7-8
 reversal, 8
Head injuries, 253-254
Heart, total artificial, 54-55
Heart failure, support in *see* Cardiac support
Helicobacter pylori, 61-62
 diagnosis, 63-65, 236
 epidemiology, 62
 eradication treatment, 71
 and gastric cancer, 191
 reinfection, 71
 role in gastroduodenal disease, 65-71
  gastritis, 65-66
  malignancy, 69-71
  non-ulcer dyspepsia, 65
  peptic ulcer, 66-69
 transmission, 62
Helicopter Emergency Medical Service (HEMS), 104
Heparin, intra-operative use in aortic aneurysm repair, 20
Histamine, 188
Hormone treatment of tumours, principles, 185-187
Hydroyproline, 171
 as marker in metastatic bone disease, 117
Hypercalcaemia, malignant disease and, 120-121
 management, 121-122
Hypergastrinaemia, 190-191
Hypothermia, cardiopulmonary bypass, 44
 pH management, 49

Immune response, aortic aneurysms and, 23-24
Indiana pouch, 86
Inflammation, wound healing, 169-170
Inflammatory bowel disease, 238-239
 hepatic metastases, 246-248
 malignancy and, 238-239
 outcome, 241
 surgery, 240-241
  outcome, 240-241
  recurrence after, 241
Injury Severity Score (ISS), 95
Inotropic drugs, cardiac support, 51-52
Insulin-like growth factor-1 (IGF-1) in wound healing, 172, 173
Interferons, intravesical, superficial bladder cancer, 82
Intestinal failure, nutritional support, 149
Intraortic balloon pump, 53
IVOX, 56

Jaundice, obstructive, computed tomography, 139
Jejunoileal bypass, 202, 203-205, 213
 complications, 204, 205
 with ileogastrostomy, 206
 reversal, 204, 205
Jejunostomy
 needle catheter, 157-158
 percutaneous endoscopic, 158-159

Keloid, 178
Kock pouch, 86

Lansoprazole, 71
Laparoscopy
 cholecystectomy, 243
 colectomy, 242
 emergency surgery, 253
 highly selective vagotomy, 236-237
 Nissen's fundoduplication, 235
Large bowel obstruction
 causes, 1
 diagnosis, 1-3
 malignant, 1
  decompression and delayed resection, 5-7
  diagnosis, 1-3
  management, 3-18
  perforation, 13

prognosis, 14-15
resection and delayed anastomosis, 7-8
resection and immediate anastomosis, 8-11, 15
subtotal colectomy, 11-13
surgical options, 4-13
Lasers
canalization of large bowel tumour, 7, 13
interstitial photocoagulation, breast cancer, 252
malignant melanoma palliation, 230
Lithotripsy, extracorporeal shock wave, 244-245
Liver
cancer
metastatic, 246-248
primary, 248
computed tomography, 133, 134-136
with arterial portography (CTAP), 133-135
varices, 248-249
Luteinising hormone regulating hormone (LHRH) agonists, metastatic bone disease, 119
Lymphoma, gastric
non-Hodgkin's, 238
role of *Helicobacter pylori*, 69-70

Magnetic resonance imaging (MRI), 129
abdominal vascular pathology, 142-143, 144
biliary tract, 140, 141
bone metastases, 114-115
bowel disease, 144-145
liver, 136-138
pancreas, 139-142
principles, 131-133
Major Trauma Outcome Study (MTOS), 99
Malignant melanoma
biopsy, 219-220
education about, 231
local recurrence, 217, 226
excision margins and, 220-224, 226-227
surgical management, 227
metastases
distant, 215, 216, 219, 222, 227, 229
intransit (satellites), 215, 216, 218, 222, 227, 228
lymph node, 215, 216, 218, 222, 224-226, 227
natural history, 215-219
palliative treatment, 230
prevention, 231
prognostic factors, 219-220, 223-224
distant metastases, 219
lymph node involvement, 218, 224
tumour thickness, 215-216, 220-221
resource management, 230-231
staging, 216-217
intransit metastases, 217, 218
surgical management, 219-230
adjuvant treatments, 229-230
distant metastases, 229
isolated limb perfusion, 228-229
recurrent melanoma, 226-229
regional lymph nodes, 224-226
resection margins for primary melanoma, 220-224
Mammography, 249
Mastectomy, 251
prophylactic, 252
Melanoma, malignant *see* Malignant melanoma
Mesenteric ischaemia, acute, laparoscopy, 253
Metronidazole, 71
Milrinone, 51
Mitomycin
liver cancer, 248
superficial bladder cancer, 80, 81, 82-83
Mitrofanoff principle, 86

Nasogastric feeding, 157
Nasojejunal feeding, 157
Neuromedin B (NMB), 191-192
Neurotensin, 188
Nipple discharge, 252
Nissen's fundoduplication, laparoscopic, 235
Nitric oxide, inhaled, cardiac support, 52
'Nutraceuticals', 156
Nutrients
disease-specific, 153, 154-155, 156
enteral, 153-155
parenteral, 155-156
Nutritional status, assessment, 150-151
Nutritional support, 149
access techniques, 156-165
current status, 156
metabolic manipulation, 156
patient selection, 149-151
perioperative, 151-153
enteral supplementation, 152-153
postoperative enteral nutrition, 152
total parenteral nutrition, 151-152
substrate selection, 153-156
see also Enteral nutrition; Total parenteral nutrition

Obesity, 199
disorders associated with, 199, 200
measurement, 199-201
surgical treatment, 201-214
assessment of results, 212
biliopancreatic bypass, 206-207
follow-up routines, 213
gastric bypass, 202-203, 205-206
jejunoileal bypass, 202, 203-205
patient selection, 201
pre-operative investigations, 213

problems, 212-213
removal of excess skin after, 213
vertical band gastroplasty, 208-209
Octreotide, 193-194
Oesophageal cancer
incidence, 183, 184
outcome, 184
progression from dysplasia, 236
treatment, 184-185, 236
Omeprazole, 68, 69, 71
Osteoblasts, 109-110
Osteoclasts, 109-110
bone pathology, 111, 112
Osteolysis, systemic inhibition, 119-120
Oxygen, tissue, and wound healing, 174-175
Oxygenation, extracorpoeal membrane, 56
Oxygenators
bubble, 45, 48
cardiopulmonary bypass, 45-46, 48, 50
chemical, 46
membrane, 45-46, 50, 56
pulmonary support, 56

p53 gene
breast cancer, 250
as prognostic marker
bladder cancer, 87-88
colorectal cancer, 40
Pace operation, 203, 204, 211-212
Pamidronate
malignant hypercalcaemia, 122
osteolysis inhibition, 119-120
Pancreas
cancer
cholecystokinin and, 191
gastrin and, 190
incidence, 183, 184
outcome, 184
treatment, 184-185, 245-6
computed tomography, 138-139
magnetic resonance imaging, 139-142
Pancreatitis
acute
alcoholic, 246
outcome, 246
chronic, treatment, 246
Parathyroid hormone related protein (PTHrP), malignant hypercalcaemia, 120-121
Parenteral nutrition, access routes, 160-164
Pentagastrin, 190
Peptic ulcers
bleeding, 69
management, 237
perforation, 69
management, 237
role of *Helicobacter pylori*, 66-68
in ulcer complications, 68-69
in ulcer relapse, 68
surgery, 236-237
malignancy risk following, 237
surgical practice changes, 71-72
vagotomy, 236-237
Peptide hormones, 185
gastrointestinal, 187, 188
receptors, 187, 189
treatment of malignancy, 186
Peptide YY, 188
Perfluorocarbons (PFCs) as oxygenators, 46
PICP/PINP, as marker in metastatic bone disease, 117
Pimobendan, 51
Plastic surgery, wound healing *see* Wound healing
Platelet-derived growth factor (PDGF)
receptor, 187
wound healing, 172, 173
chronic wounds, 174
fetal wounds, 180
Positron emission tomography, breast cancer diagnosis, 251
Procollagen, 171
Prostate-specific antigen (PSA), as marker for bone metastases, 118, 119
Proton pump inhibitor, *Helicobacter pylori* eradication, 71
Pulmonary support, 55-56
Pumps
cardiac support
Haemopump, 53
intraortic balloon pump, 53
cardiopulmonary bypass, 43
and blood trauma, 47
centrifugal pump, 43, 47
roller pump, 43, 44, 47
Pyridinoline, as marker in metastatic bone disease, 117

Rapid urease tests, *Helicobacter pylori* diagnosis, 64
Rectal cancer
adjuvant therapy, 241-242
local recurrence, 241-242
obstructive, 13
radiotherapy, 184-185, 242
surgery, 184
see also Colorectal cancer
Rectal evacuatory disorders, 242
Rectal prolapse, 242-243
Rectopexy, 242-243
Renal artery stenosis, imaging, 142, 143
Respiratory failure, pulmonary support, 55-56
Retinoblastoma expression, prognostic marker in bladder cancer, 88
Revised Trauma Score (RTS), 95
Royal College of Surgeons, Working Party on Management of Patients with Major Injuries, 98, 99

Scars, 176-179
  proliferative, 178-179
  stretched, 177-178
Scopinaro operation, 206-207
Screening
  aortic aneurysms, 24-26
  breast cancer, 249-250
Secretin, 188
Serotonin, 188
Silicone gel sheeting, 179
Silicone oil cream, hydrated, 179
Skin graft donor site
  dressings, 176
  healing, 175-176
  pain control, 175-176
Smoking and wound healing, 175
Sodium nitroprusside, 52
Somatostatin, 185, 193
  cancer treatment, 193-195
    pancreas, 246
  receptor inhibition, liver metastases, 247
Somatostatin-receptor scintigraphy, breast cancer, 251
Spinal cord compression, stabilisation, 124-125
Spinal cord damage, surgery for repair of thoracoabdominal aneurysms, 28
Spine, stabilisation, metastatic bone disease, 124
Stents
  endovascular stented grafts, aortic aneurysm repair, 28-36
  relief of malignant large bowel obstruction, 7, 13
Steroids
  treatment of hypertrophic and keloid scars, 178
  in treatment of malignancy, 187
Stomach
  cancer
    conventional treatment, 184-185
    gastrin and, 190
    incidence, 183, 184
    outcome, 184
  horizontal partition, 203, 204, 211-212
Strictureplasty, small bowel, 239
Stroke, cardiopulmonary bypass patients, 48
Sutures, scar stretching, 177-178

Tamoxifen, 118
  breast cancer treatment, 251
  long-term effects, 252
  resistance, 251
Teeth wiring, 210
Tetracycline, 71
Thiotepa, superficial bladder cancer, 80, 81
Thyroxine, thyroid cancer treatment, 186
Tinidazole, 71
Total parenteral nutrition (TPN), 149
  access
    central venous, 161-162
    home-based TNP, 164-165
    peripheral venous, 160-161
  catheters
    central TPN, 162-163
    Hickman-Broviac, 162, 165
    multilumen, 163-164
    peripheral TPN, 160
  home-based, 164-165
  perioperative, 151-152
  vasodilators, 160
Transforming growth factor ß (TGFß) in wound healing, 172, 173
  scarless, 180
Transjugular intrahepatic portasystemic shunt (TIPSS), 248-249
Trauma, 93
  deaths from, trimodal distribution, 94
  general categories of, 94
  measuring severity, 95-96
Trauma centres, 93, 95, 97-98
  Department of Health project, Stoke on Trent, 99-104
    protocol for admission, 102
    results of study, 103-104
  RCS Working Party recommendations, 99, 100
Trauma Score (TS), 95
Trauma services
  Europe, 98
  history, 96-98
  UK, 98-105
    Department of Health project, 99-104
    future, 104-105
    history, 96-97
    pre-hospital care, 105
    quality control, 105
    reports/studies, 98-99
  USA, 97-98
Triamcinolone, treatment of hypertrophic and keloid scars, 178
Triglycerides, medium chain, parenteral nutrition, 156
TRISS, 95-96
Tumour markers, metastatic bone disease, 117-118

Ulcers
  chronic, healing, 173-174
  see also Duodenal ulcers, Peptic ulcers; Colitis, ulcerative
Ultrasound, acute abdomen, 253
Urea breath tests, *Helicobacter pylori* diagnosis, 64
Urinary tract
Urinary tract (contd)
  continent diversion, 86
  reconstruction following cystectomy, 85-86
Urokinase-type plasminogen activator and

colorectal cancer prognosis, 240

Vagotomy
laparoscopic highly selective, 236-237
obesity treatment, 211
parietal cell, long-term effects, 236
Vasodilators, cardiac support, 52
Vasopressin, 188
Ventricular assist devices, 54
Vesarinone, 51, 52
VIP, 188

Wound healing
chronic wounds, 173-174
fetal, 179-180
growth factors in, 172-173
hypoxic wounds, 174-175
inflammation, 169-170
phases, 169-172
proliferation, 170-171
remodelling, 171-172
scarless, 179-180
skin graft donor site, 175-176
smoking and, 175
see also Scars